TOTAL WELLBEING

Also by Dr Hilary Jones

Before You Call the Doctor
Your Child's Health
I'm Too Busy to be Stressed
Doctor, What's the Alternative?

Also by Dr Brenda Davies

The Rainbow Journey

We wish to dedicate this book to all of our patients, past, present and future.

Acknowledgements

We wish to acknowledge all those who have been instrumental in helping with the birth of this book. Both of us have had considerable support from our families who have coped with us while we have been putting down our thoughts and pulling the text together. Thanks particularly to Sarah Jones. She not only transcribed Hilary's part of the text and helped with communication and correspondence between us since we were often separated by the Atlantic Ocean, but also provided loving emotional support. Brenda's mother, Hilda Todd, was as always a constant source of inspiration, and her son and daughter Keith and Lesda lent their unending support also.

To the circle of friends who have supported each of us, listened to us, tolerated us and encouraged us while helping us keep our feet on the ground, we send love and gratitude. Brenda wishes also to thank the members of the International Healing and Psychotherapy Group who are simultaneously colleagues, friends and mentors. Loving thanks to Dr Ewa Walker who has always offered wise and loving counsel.

Our long-suffering editor, Laura Brockbank, has shown us endless patience and her encouragement, comments and guidance have been invaluable. The book could not have come into being without the whole team at Hodder & Stoughton, and we thank them also. Thanks also to all those patients who have taught us much and whose lives we have had the privilege to share.

Contents

Introduction 

Over the last few years we have witnessed a revolution. The practice of medicine, once so securely in the hands of doctors, is now returning to where it began, to the people themselves, their relatives and carers. Although much of this movement is to be desired, it would be sad if the best of modern medicine was lost in the process, as indeed much of ancient medicine was abandoned in the past and is only now becoming available again to those who want it. There has been ill feeling from modern doctors towards complementary therapists and vice versa, and we feel that the only healthy way forward is to integrate the best of both worlds, opening up a world of choice to help ourselves stay well and treat ourselves when sick. There is no reason why, with respect on both sides, doctors and therapists should not work hand in hand for the total good of the patient. We have much to learn from each other and from the long history of medicine. What was in the forefront of medical practice years ago, and was superseded by more modern methods, did not necessarily lose its efficacy and can be useful today. But similarly those who are in favour of the ancient might like to remember that every technique was at the forefront in its day and we need to respect the modern as well.

The so-called complementary therapies, while seen by some as new and untried, are in fact based in ancient wisdom which for one reason or another became lost in the medical revolution. Over the last century this swift development removed the care of the sick from the loving hands of family and friends to the more sterile environment of the doctor's surgery and hospital. Much of the essence of care became lost in routine and process, and the true basics of caring for the sick, or indeed the healthy, were abandoned. Indeed the term 'tender loving care', often abbreviated to TLC in patients' notes, is often the term reserved for those who are dying and for whom nothing else appears appropriate any longer; while the loving which could be a natural healing component of every transaction between carer and 'patient' tends to be either ridiculed or discouraged as over-involvement. The essence of many of the complementary therapies and particularly of healing is to love the patient and hold them in high regard and positive esteem as a whole person, not as a collection of symptoms, a 'case' or an interesting phenomenon.

Although complementary therapies are now preferred by many patients, many people are afraid of taking the plunge to try more in the field of alternative care. This is often due to the fear of then losing the support of their doctor to whom they may need to turn in the future should they need antibiotics or surgery, for instance. If we could remove the mutual suspicion and mistrust between professionals, and work together as a team, then we could have a system of truly holistic care which embraces the whole person, body, mind and spirit, with the best of ancient and modern, east and west. Many complementary therapies remain beyond the means of most people since they are not available on the National Health Service and even in the private sector, the insurance companies are taking time to catch up with their clients' desires to be treated with complementary medicine. This is in stark contrast to countries such as Cuba where doctors and therapists have blended modern and traditional forms of therapy into their primary healthcare system. There is no reason why we cannot do the same.

Over the last few years we have seen a surge of interest in spiritual matters not only in the general public but in the medical fraternity. But many doctors are still reluctant to discuss their spiritual experience with others, sometimes seeing it as too personal and sacred for discussion, but often fearing ridicule and abuse because of it. However, it is time to acknowledge that a great number of people in the UK, along with the rest of the world, now hold a new set of values, with a greater concern for themselves, their health and the health of the environment. There is serious searching for a new truth by many who are now reaching the age of spiritual maturity. As the 'baby boomers' reach middle age and get closer to becoming the senior citizens of the world, they demand a different way of living with a voice that must be heard. They are demanding, among other things, a new way of taking care of our good health and of achieving total wellbeing as well as the freedom to choose. They are demanding to take back their power previously relinquished to doctors, politicians and others and to reinvest it in themselves, listening to their own wisdom.

It is our hope that we can support and further this quest for wellbeing and choice by offering an integrated approach to health, encouraging you to use your own discernment in coming to the right decision about what is good for you. Underlying every principle is the fact that we need to love ourselves enough to give ourselves the best we can, and know that in doing so, we shall be carrying out an act of love and care to those around us.

As has been seen through the centuries, the wishes and desires of the people can eventually sway the establishment. We hope that in making your choices about your own health you can help steer the medical establishment towards total care, holistic in every sense of the word, but mostly that you can learn to keep yourself in a state not only of absence of disease, but of total wellbeing.

How to Use This Book

Our aim in writing this book is that if you're well, it will help you stay well and get even more healthy, and that if you're not, you can learn how better to take care of yourself using the best of both orthodox and complementary medicine, integrating both and learning how to use them hand in hand. We have begun with a chapter on the basics for good living. Although accidents may befall us, and events beyond our control will destabilise us from time to time, if you can live by those basics, you will generally be fit and well and able to deal with what life sends, recovering quickly from anything which gets through your defence system. Please read the chapter on the basics before you move on to the rest of the book, since this will be referred to throughout the text.

We have chosen 50 common health concerns. For each one, we have looked at it initially from the point of view of symptoms and diagnosis together with the orthodox approach to treatment. We have then taken the complementary approach, looking at nutrition, supplements, exercise and lifestyle, complementary therapies and emotional and spiritual aspects of healing. There is finally an integrated checklist summarising the best of both worlds. Our hope is that, in taking responsibility for your health choices and being open-minded enough to look beyond either what orthodox medicine offers or the alternative route, you will be able to feel more in control of your wellbeing.

Appendix 1 will give you a more in-depth look at your immune system, while Appendix 2 will introduce very briefly the spiritual energy system which will be referred to from time to time. If you want to learn about that in more detail, then we would refer you to Brenda's book, *The Rainbow Journey* (Hodder & Stoughton, 1998). There is also a list introducing briefly each of the complementary medical techniques mentioned and suggestions to help you find a good therapist. Because of the space available, this cannot be an exhaustive list nor do justice to the benefits that each can offer, but should you wish to read more about the various complementary therapies, Hilary's book, *Doctor, What's the Alternative?*, also by Hodder & Stoughton, is a good starting point.

Appendix 3 will give you a table of natural sources of vitamins and minerals, to which you can refer whenever the text suggests that you need more of a particular nutrient. Although we hope that you will use food wherever possible to give you what you need, there are some cases where this is simply not practical. It is sometimes difficult, when you have an infection and are feeling awful, to eat all the food required to get all the vitamins and other nutrients that you need. Where we feel that doses need to be particularly high, we will say so in the text, but otherwise, please follow the instructions on the container of supplements you buy. Also make sure that you buy from a reputable source. There have been studies which have shown that old stock contains little of what is stated as active ingredients. Your health-food shop or high-street chemist may be a good place to begin, but there are more specialised sources and catalogues available if you look around.

We hope that you can use the book as a source of reference to help you prevent as well as treat illness. At no time do we suggest that you should stop taking medication that you've already been prescribed. Often starting to take care of yourself in different ways will make you feel so much better that both you and your doctor will see that you need less medication. We would like you to feel empowered enough, however, to ask questions, look for a second opinion if necessary and become an active partner in your own health with those who from time to time you may need to care for you. We have both heard horror stories where someone has opted for some complementary care after which their doctor has refused to treat them. The solution is simple. If you doctor feels that way, then you really are better off finding yourself someone new anyway.

If you do have to take orthodox medication, then you can reduce the risks of interactions etc. by following some simple rules:

* Talk to your doctor and your pharmacist and ask as many questions as you want to. Don't be put off. Always ask your pharmacist about the possibility of interactions.
* Keep a list of all the medicines you're taking and show it to every health professional you see.
* Ask to have your medication reviewed regularly. It's all too easy to stay on medication too long. Conversely, however, some medication (e.g. antibiotics) needs to be taken long after you feel you're better. Take advice.
* Ask the pharmacist for the manufacturer's leaflet of any medication you're prescribed.
* Check if there's a black box warning that will list any particular problems with the medication, e.g. not to be taken during pregnancy.
* Check the dosage and administration.

You are a powerful human being and most of the time your body knows how to heal itself as long as it has the necessary components to help it do so. We hope that you can combine the best of both worlds, keep yourself healthy and enjoy life.

The Basics for Good Living

Although *Total Wellbeing* is intended to be a directory of common disorders and the traditional, complementary and more integrated ways to treat or manage them, we believe that generally the accent needs to be on wellness rather than illness. Therefore we would like to recommend a basic life plan upon which you can rely for good health and to which you can add or substitute according to your needs.

The basics are:

* nutrition, which includes water and air as well as food
* exercise
* some form of regular detoxification, whether that be a massage therapy, steam, sauna, or fast
* some form or relaxation
* meditation or other spiritual practice
* regular well-person screening according to your age, risk factors, etc.
* some intimate relationship even if that is with some kind of group or a pet
* some form of service to others
* supporting and enhancing your immune system

Nutrition

It's interesting to see how styles have changed over the years from the meat and two vegetables of 30 years ago to today's recommendations that we eat less protein (especially as red meat), a greater intake of fruit and vegetables, much less fat and refined sugars. This reflects not only our change in lifestyle (Brenda's grandmother looked after a husband and 14 children without the aid of a washing machine or store-bought bread!) but also changes in the levels of pollution and the stress of a different nature that we now have to contend with on a daily basis.

Although Edgar Cayce, the famous healer and psychic, talked of air as a nutrient many years ago, and the Indian healers have always done so, we seem to have forgotten that this most fundamental of substances is the basic nutrient of life. When you start to take note of the air that you breathe and the way that you breathe it, not only will you have immediate benefits in terms of stress and anxiety reduction, but you will become more eager to ensure that the air you breathe is clean rather than polluted by cigarette smoke, exhaust fumes, etc. The basis of yoga, one of the most ancient of the healing arts, is conscious breathing and we would recommend it to you as a practice that can start you on the road to better health, physically, emotionally and spiritually.

Water is the next most important nutrient and we would recommend that you check that your water is pure, invest in some sort of filtration unit and drink at least 8 glasses a day, simply as clear water, either hot or cold. All of the chemical reactions taking place in your body this very minute need water to help them proceed at the pace your body requires them to do. You might like to cultivate the habit of always having some water with you to sip throughout the day.

Food is what your body is made of so eat the best you can afford, organic if possible, and using fresh ingredients whenever you can. Although a low-fat diet is recommended, you need enough fat to ensure adequate absorption of the fat-soluble vitamins, A, D, E and K. Olive oil confers great benefits in terms of protection from some illnesses such as cancer and therefore do use it whenever you need fat if possible. You need at least a tablespoonful daily.

If you eat 7 or more portions of fresh fruit and vegetables a day, some whole grains such as rice (brown or wild) and cereals, then you should get enough fibre to protect you from colonic and some other cancers, but if not, then do add some wheat bran, sesame seeds or flax seed (linseed) to your salads or cereals. Carotenoids (in brightly coloured vegetables) are essential and effective antioxidants to protect your DNA from free radical damage and to prevent cancer and signs of ageing. Vegetables highest in antioxidants include beetroot, red peppers, kale, broccoli, spinach, tomatoes and sweetcorn as well as potatoes. The cruciferous vegetables, such as cauliflower, broccoli, Brussels sprouts and cabbage, have natural anti-cancer agents and should be a regular addition to your diet. Watercress acts in much the same way. See the chart on p. 543 for natural sources of vitamins and minerals.

Fruits highest in antioxidants include bilberries and strawberries as well as plums, oranges, red grapes, kiwi, pink grapefruit, apples, bananas, melons and pears. Soya milk or protein is great for reducing menopausal symptoms, especially hot flushes, and symptoms of premenstrual syndrome. However, it also appears to have a protective effect on the breast and prostate, reducing the risk of cancer and it can help reduce your cholesterol (LDL cholesterol) by about 10 per cent in about 9 weeks due to its isoflavone content. So if you can add soya to your basic diet, you'll be doing yourself a favour.

Salmon, herrings, sardines and mackerel all contain omega-3 fatty acids which are powerful anti-cancer agents, and should be included in your menu about 3 times a week, but if you're strictly vegetarian, you can get the same effect from flax seed (linseed) ground up on salads or cereals. In fact linseed contains both omega-3 and omega-6 fatty acids which are even more beneficial. Red meat is best avoided, especially if you have a family history of breast cancer (see p. 170), although wild game or organic meat is less harmful. Try to remove all fat including chicken skin and not to char it by cooking at very high temperatures. Those extra tasty burned bits from the barbecue are potentially lethal, we're afraid, since they contain carcinogens (cancer-promoting substances).

We shall recommend additions in the form of extra or substitute foodstuffs, or supplements, as we go along. But if you're well now, we want you to stay well, so please make whatever adjustments you need to over the next few weeks (not all at once) to ensure your continued good health. If you're under par, adjusting to a healthier lifestyle will have almost immediate benefits in terms of improved energy and mood.

EXERCISE

No matter what your age, from 8 to 80, exercise will improve your life. But if you're not used to exercise, then do add it to your regime gently, taking precautions to protcct your muscles by keeping them warm, and your heart by building up slowly and having a cool-down period when you're ending.

Walking is still probably the best exercise there is and ideally you need to start with about 10 minutes a day, building up over about 2 months to 45 minutes 4 or 5 times a week at a fairly brisk pace. If you want to lose weight, you may need a slightly more vigorous regime, and if you have painful joints, exercising in water would be good for you. Whatever you choose, make sure it's something you like and will enjoy. Brenda had difficulties with exercise for years until she found line dancing! Adding weights can also be fun, but again do it gently. Whether you begin by lifting a can of peas in each hand or go to a fancy gym, take it easy and always have an assessment from your GP before you begin on any new regime.

DETOXIFICATION

We are constantly surrounded by pollutants and we therefore need to detoxify ourselves regularly. There are several ways you can choose to do this, from adding dry skin brushing to your daily cleansing routine, to having a day a week when you take only fruit, fruit juices, water and herbal teas. It's a good idea to start and end the day with a cup of hot water which both detoxifies and stimulates your liver and kidneys and you might like to have a regular steam or sauna. Massage helps move toxins out of your tissues and is also a lovely way of getting some of your quota of touching! Essential for total wellbeing. We would highly recommend Jane Scrivner's wonderful book, *Detox Yourself* (Piatkus, 1998) which will leave you feeling squeaky clean, to say nothing of more flexible and several pounds lighter!

Have a look at the toxins checklist below. So many of us are living in polluted atmospheres, with cigarette smoke, fumes, geopathic stress (natural radiation arising from the earth, see p. 9), radon gas and electromagnetic fields playing havoc with our minds and bodies. There's always something you can do. Remember that a tree can deal with an amazing amount of pollution from car fumes, as can some plants, so if you have a garden you could plant a tree (or at least a large plant!) If not, you could plant one somewhere else to help the earth deal with all the mess she's trying to clear up. Peace lilies can neutralise some of the force field from computers, microwaves and televisions, so have some of them in your home and office. Spider plants are also good at reducing pollution in your home.

Toxins checklist

Self: Are you inadvertently eating or drinking pesticides, contaminated water or detergents? Check that your water is pure. It might be worth investing in a purification system (see p. 5) or buying bottled water. Try to buy organic fruit and vegetables where possible. Do you rinse your crockery and cutlery well to rid them of all traces of detergents? Do you check labels for additives? Cooking from fresh ingredients is always better and then you know exactly what you're eating. Do you drink a lot of canned drinks? Their sugar content can later cause blood sugar to fall with quite marked effect on mood, concentration and attention. Are you absorbing mercury from old fillings in your teeth? It might be an idea to get your dentist to check you out. Are you missing some health problem? Candidiasis (see p. 330) must be one of the most missed diagnoses. How about doing a detox with a regular fruit and water/herbal tea fast and a weekly steam and/or sauna?

Environment: Are you being bombarded by electromagnetic fields? From computer, electric alarm clock, electric blanket, television or other electric or electronic equipment? You could buy a screen to protect you from your computer and put plenty of plants around your office, especially peace lilies to neutralise electromagnetic stress. Switch off completely or remove equipment you don't really need. How about a Zen alarm instead of your radio alarm clock? Lovely to be awoken by gentle chimes. Do you have a geopathic stress problem in your home or workplace? Geopathic stress is caused by energy that arises out of the earth especially from geological faults. You can have your home checked or you could buy a neutraliser (available from Dulwich Health, tel. 0181670 5883). Is the air you breathe clean? Would it be worth having an ioniser and an air filter system? Do you have synthetic carpets? They can release toxic fumes unless you treat them with a carpet guard spray.

RELAXATION

We live such stressful lives that most of us actually have to learn how to relax these days. Are you one of those people who needs to fill every moment with something 'useful', can't stand to be kept waiting, or gets furious at how long it takes for the lift to arrive? If so, you need to learn to relax and rest a little. Your stress and your blood pressure will come down, you'll stop being in 'alarm mode' with your muscles and mind alert and ready for action, and your whole self will be able to rest and refresh itself. If you have any doubts whatsoever about the effects on your body of being tense, then just clench your fist for 20 seconds and observe carefully what happens to the circulation in it. Notice those white patches? And the red bits? That happened in 20 seconds. Think what happens to your neck, spine, shoulders, etc. by having your shoulders constantly raised, your muscles tensed – often for years. Time to do it differently if you don't want to end up with a stiff, aching body and a similarly rigid mind.

And what about your mind? Well, the same holds true. If you don't relax and allow yourself time to just be, to think, to ponder and smell the roses, then you're not only missing a great deal of the pleasure of life, but you're also missing out on a good deal of the natural function of your brain, the really creative stuff, which usually only comes to the fore when you're not actively doing anything.

Whether you choose to learn a specific relaxation technique, to shut your eyes and listen to a favourite piece of music or to use a relaxation or meditation tape or CD such as Hilary's *Classical Relaxation* CD (Polygram) or Brenda's *Just Be* (available from Nigel Shakespeare, tel. 0171 535 7907), please do take at least 20 minutes a day and *relax*.

Meditation or Spiritual Practice

Some people may feel that relaxation and meditation go together. That can be the case, but not necessarily. There are so many benefits from meditating regularly that it really deserves a separate place of its own. Some would say, if you can add only one more thing to your routine (you *are* a busy person after all!) then the thing to choose would be meditation.

There are numerous ways to meditate, from the very simple to the elaborate. If you want to learn transcendental meditation, you will usually need to go to a Meditation Centre to do so. However, there are many books on the market to teach you or you could use a meditation tape as a guide to begin with.

From lowering your blood pressure, to improving your circulation, from helping your memory to relieving stress-related illness, meditation has a better track record than any medication. It has been well researched over the years and we would highly recommend that you try it. Always start with some conscious breathing if only for a minute or two and then allow yourself to suspend the day and all that it contains. Soon you will be able to find a place of absolute peace and silence that already exists inside you. Wonderful!

If you belong to some church, synagogue or other religious community, then you're probably familiar with religious practice, if not necessarily spiritual. You could have a spiritual moment watching a sunset, singing your baby to sleep or walking in a forest. Sitting on the beach, listening to music or silently holding someone's hand may lift you to that place of bliss, that peak experience. Whatever is good for you, try to treat yourself to it regularly and enjoy. It will enhance your life.

Regular Screening with your Health Practitioner

Although this needs to begin as a good practice from childhood, it becomes even more essential as we get older. So many of the illnesses that can otherwise ravage our lives, can be prevented or halted if detected early enough. If you have risk factors such as a family member who has had heart disease or breast cancer, if you're post-menopausal or live a particularly stressful life, please add a regular appointment with your GP to your diary. There are well-persons' clinics where you can have your blood pressure checked along with other non-invasive investigations. However, having a regular blood sample taken to test liver, kidney and thyroid function is wise, as is having stools examined for occult blood (microscopic amounts of blood invisible to the eye) as you get older. Breast examinations, easily carried out at home on a monthly basis, need to be augmented by a professional examination and mammogram from time to time. Talk with your doctor to see what they recommend. Dental check-ups and eye exams are also part of your responsibility in taking care of the extraordinary machine you've been given. It never ceases to amaze us how much more care many of us take of our cars than our bodies! Go and have an MOT for yourself!

Intimate Committed Relationships

We know that for some people this seems impossible, especially if you live alone, are less mobile than you'd like, are grieving or confined in some way. But it just is a fact that without some meaningful contact with others, our spirit becomes weak and we become ill. There is incontrovertible evidence that those who have good relationships live longer, recover more easily from illness or surgery and stay healthier. In one study it was found that people suffering from malignant melanoma (a virulent form of skin cancer) who attended a support group for only 6 weeks, survived years longer than others who did not, simply because they developed a feeling of belonging, being useful to others and being committed to someone else's wellbeing apart from their own.

If you are not in a relationship or live alone, could you have a pet? (There are programmes in some hospitals that allow pets to visit those who have had heart attacks or who are having painful procedures or chemotherapy, with quite dramatic results.) Could you look after someone else's pet? Could you join some club or organisation that allows you to meet others regularly? Could you go to a day centre? Could you do some voluntary work? The essential is to develop a sense of belonging and commitment.

Service

We who work in the caring professions are very lucky, for we're fulfilling this very necessary human need all day long. Mothers with children at home, those who have someone to care for, who work at the local hospice or rattle a tin for a charity on flag day, are all living out this basic human need. Look at what happens to many women when the children leave home and suddenly they aren't there to cook for. So many of the mid-life difficulties for both sexes are exacerbated by no longer feeling useful.

Whatever your age, you can find some way of being of service, not in a codependent way, but to render some useful function in the world. Brenda's father at the age of 80 still used to do odd shopping for 'the old people' in the village. An elderly friend of her mother's picks up the evening newspaper for her mum and takes it to her room. Her 3-year-old grandson carries flowers in his wheelbarrow for her daughter-in-law to plant. Someone walks along the road, smiles and says 'Good morning' and brightens someone's day. The cashier hands us our change and smiles. Someone on the telephone takes time to open with a pleasantry and end with 'Have a nice day'. Service. It's so easy, benefits the whole world and not just ourselves. What a gift to give and receive, to be able to improve our own lives while improving those of others.

SUPPORTING AND ENHANCING YOUR IMMUNE SYSTEM

Your immune system helps protect you from illness and infection and also ensures that your whole self stays in a state of good maintenance and repair. When for some reason our immune system is low, we're more vulnerable to illness. However, sometimes our immune system is too sensitive and we're then at risk of allergic reactions, asthma, ulcerative colitis or autoimmune illness, where our bodies start to attack parts of themselves as though they were foreign.

The immune system (see Appendix 1) consists of a complex network of organs (thymus, spleen, tonsils and lymph nodes), specialised white blood cells and substances found in serum (the fluid part of the blood in which blood cells and platelets are carried) such as complement, interleukin and interferon.

We are becoming more aware through the study of psychoneuroimmunology that our thoughts and emotions also have a great impact on our immune system and our ability to stay free from illness. In short, happy people with a positive attitude and who laugh a lot have a better chance of staying free from illness or recovering quickly should illness strike. If you're able to live by the basic tenets already described, then the likelihood is that your immune system will be strong. However, all of us from time to time forget to take care of ourselves, work too hard, are hit by a series of stressful events, are grieving or shocked. At such times becoming ill may almost be a kind of safety valve which makes us stop and listen to our bodies and take stock of our lives. In most cases, your immune system will be able to take care of things and get you well if you let it, but that means you need to stop, rest, drink lots of water and take care of yourself – or better still let someone take care of you for a few days while you conserve your energy to fight whatever ails you.

Smoking and alcohol threaten your immune system, as does refined sugar, so these need to be cut out. Free radicals, formed as by-products of fighting infections, of breaking down food to release energy, by ultraviolet light and pollutants such as exhaust fumes and smoke left to their own devices, can cause damage to cells and also to the very stuff of life, DNA. So dealing with them by the use of antioxidants is essential, especially if you're stressed or ill. Fruit and vegetable juices and, when you're ready, nutritious food, will help you right yourself, although the addition of echinacea, astragalus and vitamin and mineral supplements will help. Adding Vitamins A (1000 IU twice daily), B complex (one tablet of strong Vitamin B Compound), C (2000–3000 mg daily), E (800–1200 IU) daily, with 50–100 mg CoEnzyme Q10 (CoQ10), carotenes (naturally occurring pigments in fruit and vegetables which are powerful antioxidants), selenium (200 mcg daily) and zinc (30 mg), plus some thymus extract if you have a viral illness, or spleen extract if you have a bacterial illness, will top up your armoury and give you the best chance of getting well quickly. If you're pregnant or a sexually active woman of child-bearing age and not using contraception, don't take Vitamin A since at high doses it can be associated with birth defects.

There are times, however, when our immune system fails to deal with the situation, when we're overwhelmed by infection, when our bodies are under attack, for instance by cancer, when we're grieving and needing our energy to deal with that; at these times we need extra help in the form of antibiotics or other medication. If that is where you are, then taking care of yourself includes using the best that modern medicine has to offer and incorporating it into an active plan of self-healing. It is that integration of the two that is the basis of this book.

We wish you a happier, more healthy life.

Complementary Therapies

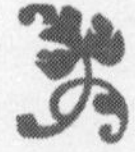

The following is by no means a comprehensive list of complementary therapies, although it includes all those mentioned in the text and is intended to give you a brief introduction to each. There is literature available about them all should you wish more detail than is within the scope of this book. We recommend that you find a therapist who is well trained and qualified and who belongs to a professional body with a system of registration, code of ethics and conduct, and internal regulation. Sadly, it is all too easy for those who have a little knowledge to call themselves therapists but be unequipped to deal with problems which may arise during the course of treatment. Any good therapist should be willing to discuss their qualification with you and to furnish you with proof of their registration with their professional body upon request. It's perfectly reasonable for you to ask how long someone trained and how long they have been in practice and indeed to check that there is a register you could see. It is only by insisting upon such validation that we can ensure that the complementary therapy movement continues to gain strength and acceptance as a sound and safe addition to orthodox medicine. In general terms it would be wise to avoid anyone who professes a cure, who tells you to stop other medication, who makes adverse comments about your orthodox practitioner or who refuses to answer any of your queries to your satisfaction. If you have any doubt as to the professionalism of your practitioner, whether orthodox or complementary, then you may be wise to look elsewhere.

Many of the complementary therapies are ancient and have been used on an ad hoc basis for years, their nuances steeped in regional folklore. Thus many of them are available on a do-it-yourself basis. Aromatherapy oils and crystals, for instance, are widely available, and are sometimes undervalued for their quite potent effects. If you wish to use any of the techniques below as a therapy, we recommend that you consult a therapist who will not only prescribe for you, but who will be aware of the cautions you need to adopt and of conditions where certain remedies are contraindicated.

Although some therapies stand alone as an alternative to orthodox medical care, we feel that an integrated approach using the best of both worlds is much wiser and the only sensible way forward. Sadly, there has been antagonism from both the medical camp and from the alternative and complementary field. Hopefully we're moving to a point where each can celebrate the wisdom of the other and can learn to practise in harmony for the ultimate good of the patient.

If you require further information about any of these therapies, please turn to the list of useful addresses on p. 549.

ACUPRESSURE

This is an ancient method of healing, using the meridians which are stimulated by pressure from the hands of the practitioner to promote a healthy flow of chi, the life force mentioned by various names in all the ancient civilisations and healing schools. When this flow is blocked, there is also a block to good healthy energy which keeps us alive and well. You can learn the pressure points yourself and do much to relieve headaches, menstrual cramps, anxiety, nausea, etc.

ACUPUNCTURE

This is an ancient oriental practice using the same meridians mentioned above and around 2000 points along them which are stimulated by the use of fine stainless steel needles that are inserted through the skin in order to right the flow of chi.

There is usually little if any pain and no bleeding. Occasionally a tiny electrical current may be used to aid the stimulation and sometimes the process of moxibustion, where herbs are burned at the site of points, will facilitate more healing.

Alexander Technique

The practitioners of Alexander Technique call themselves teachers who through a series of lessons help their pupils to improve their posture and thereby remove much of the stress and tension that exists in all our bodies, and which over time can be the cause of illness and disease. Pupils learn to be aware of their bodies and how they use them, often in maladaptive ways and with a good deal more effort than is necessary. Renewed flexibility and grace have a marked effect on the emotional as well as the physical state.

Aromatherapy

The use of the essential oils of various parts of a wide variety of plants, either in massage, diffused into the atmosphere or in baths, compresses, etc., allows for quick access to the circulation and the limbic system, a part of the brain which deals with emotions. High-quality pure oils are used and can be very potent. They should not be seen as perfumes but as powerful substances to be used with care in tiny quantities. If you're pregnant, have epilepsy or are taking other medication, especially for high blood pressure, then see a qualified aromatherapist rather than trying to do it yourself.

Art Therapy

Wonderful to help unlock emotions by the use of colour and form where they may be otherwise inaccessible. Don't worry if you have never been able to draw or paint – the therapy is more about your emotions than your creative ability, although you may find that you are much more talented in that area than you ever knew.

Autogenic Training

A system of exercises aimed at giving you more control over the internal systems of your body by inducing profound relaxation. It combines a meditative technique with affirmation to bring about an internal state which can be very healing.

Ayurvedic Medicine

An ancient Indian medicine which is based upon balancing the energies of the body by the use of diet, exercise, meditation and massage. Its philosophy touches every aspect of life, from what we eat to how we move to our body build. The examination of the pulse alone gives the practitioner an amazing amount of information about the patient and along with a detailed history can lead to recommendations to help rebalance all aspects of living.

Bach Flower Remedies and Australian Bush Essences

Flower remedies are made from flowers and spring water and possess the ability to affect mood and alter our emotional state. Dr Bach's Rescue Remedy contains 5 such essences and is useful to carry for emergencies.

The Bates Method

A series of exercises designed to improve eyesight when used with relaxation and dietary advice. The use of vitamins and supplements which act upon the visual pathway are part of the treatment.

Biofeedback

This powerful method of learning to change our inner state at will can have a profound effect upon our physiological and psychological wellbeing and the need for medication in certain illnesses. The effects of our mental efforts are made visible on a screen which monitors progress. Biofeedback relies upon the connection between mind and body and needs to be practised regularly, rather like meditation.

Chiropractic

This method of manipulation of the skeletal system releases joints and muscles that are stiff or painful to restore normal functioning, occasionally years after the original injury. In many cases the symptoms would appear to be unrelated to the problem that the chiropractor uncovers. Manipulation is quick and usually painless although the sound of the release may be quite alarming. Advice will usually be given about various aspects of your life which may have perpetuated the problem and which, if uncorrected, may cause it to recur.

Clinical Ecology

This comprehensive treatment examines the environment in which we live and the effect it has upon our physical and emotional state. Examination of hair, blood and skin responses to various substances helps the practitioner give advice about diet, pollution, stress, etc.

Colour Therapy

This underestimated therapy can have a profound effect upon our mood and feelings of wellbeing as well as our performance and self-esteem. From the use of colour in our homes and choice of clothes to the skilled assessment of the electromagnetic vibrations emitted in our aura (see p. 539), the colour therapist can help rebalance our energy system by the use of colour.

Cranial Osteopathy

Gentle and precise manipulation of the bones of the skull help restore its natural movement and balance allowing subtle rhythms to be re-established, the absence of which may have caused symptoms throughout the entire body. You may feel as though nothing is happening since the manipulation is so fine and delicate. It can be effective for conditions and symptoms that seem to be totally unrelated to the head.

Crystal Healing

Different crystals resonate with varying frequencies of light and hence emit vibrations that can help augment our own healing energy and help us regain a healthy balance. Although there are therapists who are highly skilled with gems and crystals, this is one of the therapies that you can learn to use to good effect yourself.

Dance or Movement Therapy

Apart from being an enjoyable hobby that will keep you supple and fit, dance and instinctive movement can have deeply therapeutic benefits, enabling you to touch emotions which are otherwise inaccessible, to heal your chakras (see p. 539) and generally to balance your energy. Try anything from moving to music to stamping to a drum beat to humming and moving your body while in the shower.

Healing

Healing is an active partnership between the healer and the person receiving healing, during which energy is transmitted from a higher source through the healer who is used simply as a conduit. The aim is to bring mind, body and spirit into harmony and balance, and to prompt the innate healing power of the individual to restore healthy functioning where possible. The person receiving healing may feel nothing, or have a sensation of heat, cold or vibration. Benefits may vary from a sense of peace to a remission of symptoms. The healer may choose to touch the patient (laying on of hands) or to work a few inches away from the body in the aura.

Herbalism

Another holistic therapy which aims to restore balance to the whole being, in this case using plants or parts thereof, for their medicinal properties. A herbalist may mix several herbs to help you although there are many available for your own use in their more simple forms. Sadly, we have lost our animal instinct to use whatever nature provides for whatever ails us. This ancient art helps us do just that again.

Homeopathy

The theory of treating like with like is the basis of homeopathy. To alleviate symptoms, minuscule amounts of substances are chosen that would cause the same symptoms in a healthy person if taken in larger quantities. There is no intention to suppress or mask symptoms, but rather to help the body deal with the underlying cause and move back to a state of balance. Thus there may be a temporary exacerbation of symptoms before they disappear. The greater the dilution of the remedy, the greater its potency. Not only the symptoms, but your personality type, your build, etc. are all taken into account by the homeopathic practitioner in choosing a remedy that is tailor-made for you.

Hydrotherapy

Literally therapy with water, this can include anything from baths to steam rooms, underwater massage to sitz baths (see p. 345) and Jacuzzi. Often other agents are added to intensify the benefit of the water, such as oils, Epsom salts or seaweed. The aim is to detoxify and relax or in some cases stimulate.

Hypnotherapy

The theory is that if the conscious mind can be distracted, the subconscious can be accessed. A state of trance results which may vary from a sense of relaxation to a trance so deep that surgical operations can be carried out without pain. Also suggestions that are beneficial to the subject can be made, which will remain in the mind after the person returns to normal consciousness. Nothing can be done against your will and you remain in control throughout the process. The more the subject is willing to cooperate and relinquish control, however, the more effective the therapy can be.

Light Therapy

Many people deprived of bright daylight will develop disorders ranging from depression to sleep problems. Light therapy, which uses a full-spectrum light akin to sunlight, usually dispensed by a lamp, can help. Some skin disorders such as psoriasis have also shown improvement by exposure to light.

Magnetic Therapy

This covers a wide range of therapies using magnets to balance the body's natural energies and restore health. Magnets can be placed in mattresses and pillows on which to sleep, in various pads and applications to be used locally, for example for backache and also as massage tools to heal pain. They have been found useful in the treatment of sleep disorders, low energy, arthritis, MS, ME, irritable bowel syndrome and stress. Other possibilities are still being researched.

Massage

Relaxing or stimulating, human touch in the form of massage has markedly beneficial effects on the recovery from a variety of illnesses. It forms part of several other therapies and is now used for all age groups from premature babies, who gain weight better than those who are not massaged, to the elderly, who sleep better, have improved self-esteem and better circulation. It can also aid detoxification, reduce stress and help lymphatic drainage, as well as having a high feel-good factor.

Meditation

Whether guided, accompanied by a mantra, practised alone or in a group, meditation may be one of the most healing practices you can add to your daily routine. It can be as simple as withdrawing for a few minutes from the daily grind and being very still in mind and body, or as ritualistic a spiritual practice as you wish to make it. The beauty of it is that it can be practised anywhere, anytime, and profound states can be reached where there is absolute peace while in a state of complete awareness. A teach-yourself therapy, it can be even more profound if you treat yourself to learning with a master.

Music Therapy

Music is one of the most mind-altering substances known to man and whether your choice is classical, rock or pan pipes, your internal environment cannot fail to be changed by it. As a therapy it has great benefits, but do not underestimate the value of simply spending some time alone immersing yourself in melodious sound. It will open your creativity, soothe or stimulate your mind and allow those who are otherwise inaccessible, such as those with severe Alzheimer's and autistic children, to be contacted.

Naturopathy

This therapy relies on the fact that the body can probably heal itself of most ills if it is supported in its attempts to so do. Therefore using diet, exercise, natural products and rest, the naturopath will help you restore a state in which you are in balance again internally and health is restored. Some of the edicts appear to be in direct opposition to orthodox medicine, as the philosophy suggests that we leave the symptoms to the body to sort out while it is given all the tools to help it do so.

Nutritional Therapy

Before there were medicines, in a time when our ancestors grew their own food and ate what was available and in season, most illnesses were treated using food itself as medicine. By adjusting the diet, our forebears were able to deal with a multitude of problems for which we now look either to a pill or to a doctor. Nutritional therapy encourages us to return to basics and give our bodies what they need in terms of good, wholesome, nutritious, clean, simple food and copious amounts of clean, fresh water. There are so-called super-foods which have amazing healing properties dealing with illnesses as diverse as cancer and colitis, and which are preventative for much more. (See Basics for Good Living on p. 4).

Osteopathy

The art of osteopathy is intended to diagnose and correct problems in the musculoskeletal system and to give help with posture etc. to prevent the recurrence of such difficulties in future. Pain, stiffness, immobility and deformity can result from bad postural habits, old injuries, recent trauma or stress and your osteopath will skillfully pinpoint these and help you correct them. Sometimes massage or even acupuncture is used as an adjunct to manipulation.

Qi (Chi) Gong and T'ai Chi

Related to each other, these therapies focus mind, body and spirit to move the life force (chi) and to strengthen our inner selves. T'ai chi uses a series of prescribed, ritualistic movements, whereas Chi gong relies more upon flowing, instinctive movements which bring the mind as well as the body to a state of peace. Both have the effect of increasing flexibility and stamina, balance and grace.

REIKI (REIKE)

This therapy uses the flow of energy in the natural paths of meridians within the body. Closely allied with therapeutic touch, it releases blockages both emotional and physical, and promotes relaxation and healing.

REFLEXOLOGY

Vertical energy lines starting and ending in your hands and feet connect all the organs that lie in their path. Hence stimulation of the ends of these zones, by massage, has a direct effect on internal organs which are otherwise often inaccessible. Everything from your lymphatic system to your pineal gland is represented on the sole of your feet and hands and your therapist will be able to diagnose and try to correct problems by sensitively isolating and massaging the correct area. As with acupressure, you can learn many of the points yourself, but for a full diagnosis as well as treatment, see a good therapist.

RELAXATION

Most of us spend our time in a state of tension of which we're often unaware. Only when symptoms develop or someone suggests that we relax do we focus on the lack of relaxation we exhibit. Relaxing both body and mind allows us to benefit from better blood circulation with the healing properties that brings, better oxygenation of our tissues, the complete absorption of the nutrients from our food and the effective elimination of waste products. Better sleep, digestion and motility are but a few of the gains which can be achieved with only a few minutes of input daily.

SHIATSU

This comprehensive therapy combines massage, acupressure and some manipulation, both to diagnose and to treat, improving circulation, promoting relaxation, stimulating one's own innate healing energy and generally improving balance in all areas. A profound detoxification can occur, so drink plenty of fluids to carry toxins away and have as much rest as your body indicates it needs.

THERAPEUTIC TOUCH

This is somewhat akin to spiritual healing although the language used by the proponents of the two techniques varies greatly. What the spiritual healer will talk of in spiritual terms, the therapeutic touch practitioner will explain in terms of quantum physics. However, the techniques are very similar, involving either the laying on of hands or healing into the aura.

TRADITIONAL CHINESE MEDICINE (TCM)

This term includes not only acupuncture, herbal medicine and diet, but also a specific philosophy that all of nature is represented by yin and yang which need to be harmony and balance if there is to be good health and peace of mind. The concept of the life force, chi, being in constant movement in good health and of illnesses being a result of blockages to its flow, is also fundamental to other forms of healing such as spiritual healing, Chi gong and T'ai chi. Traditional Chinese Medicine practitioners may use a host of related techniques in an aim to restore the delicate balance of yin and yang and thereby restore health.

VISUALISATION

This underestimated healing therapy can be practised very simply by anyone. The idea is to harness your imagination and creativity to project a world which is more desirable. By the use of vision and affirmation, messages are given to the subconscious about what to create, giving the subject a sense of control and power to make life happen. Just as every physical object is manifested following a visual image, our lives can similarly take shape in the way in which we wish, by using the power of visualisation to mould them.

YOGA

Another ancient practice involving mind, body and spirit using exercises which integrate the whole of you. Breathing slowly and deliberately while performing slow movements and postures gives you control over your body and mind. It is impossible to remain stressed while consciously breathing, and stretching your muscles helps stimulate the release of endorphins, which elevate mood and give a sense of wellbeing. Increased flexibility, strength and stamina, balance and poise add to good posture and grace of movement. It is useful in a host of ailments and no matter how young or old you are, you can benefit.

Surgery

Surgery is understood by most people to be a form of treatment of disease, injury or other disorder by direct physical intervention. It may also involve the investigation, diagnosis and management of injuries or other disorders carried out with surgical instruments as opposed to those using drugs, diet or changes in lifestyle.

In days gone by a surgeon's adage might have been 'if in doubt cut it out' and many patients were apparently willing to subject themselves without question to whatever procedure a surgeon suggested. These days, however, patients are better informed or are likely to be aware of non-invasive alternatives. No surgical intervention is entirely risk free and merely being considered for surgery can provoke anxiety and apprehension in many people.

To begin with, somebody facing surgery is already obliged to deal with the emotional impact of nursing a symptom or a disease and may have already been through the harrowing period of time during which diagnosis was made. Some of the investigations themselves may have been invasive, conferring some risk. And sadly, thanks to massive publicity of those rare cases where things go wrong, anybody facing surgery is all too aware of the attendant risks and unforeseen consequences of surgery. For children, admission to hospital, especially when surgery has been suggested, can be especially traumatic and it needs to be handled well so that any damage to the child's psychological development can be avoided.

In all cases patients and doctors need to work together to allay fears, eradicate uncertainties, improve information and include patients in taking decisions about the type of treatment. Making the hospital stay as comfortable as possible goes a long way towards making the surgical experience as emotionally satisfactory as it may be physically life-saving.

Admissions to Hospital

There are three main types of hospital admissions: those where the person is admitted urgently through accident and emergency; those which are organised by the GP, and those which are arranged by a specialist in an outpatient department for further urgent investigation. Prior to admission, it is helpful if you address any uncertainties and are sure in your own mind about what is going to be done, how it's going to be done and why. It is also important to know what the likely outcome of the treatment is going to be. An Admissions Pack should detail where and when to report and what items you need to bring into hospital.

Cancellations

The last-minute cancellation of a surgical procedure is always psychologically difficult to accept and doctors should try to avoid this happening at all cost. However, with reduced resources, the cancellation of a non-urgent operation in favour of an emergency is clearly unavoidable. Regrettably patients scheduled for non-urgent procedures can find that their operations are cancelled not just once but several times. If this should happen to you, try to obtain some kind of firm commitment from the specialist as to when you are likely to be recalled for your operation. Make them aware of the degree of pain you are suffering, how it is affecting your employment and how many dependants you have relying on you. If while waiting for your next appointment your condition changes significantly, make sure that priority is given to your operation and do not be afraid to pester your family doctor for support and help.

Informed Consent

At some point before the operation you will be expected to sign a consent form. Legally you must understand what procedure is being planned, why it is being planned and who is going to carry it out. You should be aware of all alternatives to the treatment suggested and what the anticipated outcome is. Sometimes the next of kin is asked to sign the consent form if the person facing surgery is either too young or too ill (e.g. unconscious) to sign the consent form themselves. In this situation you should understand the full implications of the consent form and make sure that all possible information is available. Always ask about the risks of the procedure. There is always a balance of risk and benefit and it is important that whoever signs the consent form can put the risk and benefit into proper perspective. By law a doctor has to give sufficient information and a reasonable portrayal of the facts so that the person facing a surgical procedure can make an informed choice.

Before the Operation

It's perfectly reasonable for you to ask as many questions as you need in order to make a choice about the surgery you're to have and whom you want to perform it, although of course within the NHS your choice may be limited to whoever covers your area. Nevertheless it's still acceptable for you to ask for a second opinion if you wish. Spend some time talking to the professionals (you could visit the ward and talk to the nursing staff, for instance) and gather as much information as you can about your condition and the procedure. However, if you're one of those who would rather not know what's going to happen, that's also OK. As a psychiatrist, Brenda often sees people who are afraid of what's going to happen or who feel lost and anxious afterwards about what was removed etc. A simple diagram of the anatomy and an outline of the operation usually allays their fears. Ask your surgeon if that can be done for you if you wish so that you know what's going on.

Before the operation the consent form needs to be signed, the operation site marked out, the notes reviewed, any allergies noted and the results of all pre-operative tests checked to make sure that you are fit for surgery and anaesthesia. The anaesthetist will visit you and talk to you about anaesthesia and about what you are likely to experience and pre-medication may be prescribed which will help you feel more relaxed. You will have no food or drink usually from at least 6 hours before the procedure and will be taken to theatre wearing a gown, and perhaps a special paper hat and pants, and sometimes stockings depending upon the operation you are having. You will have a wrist label which will be checked along with your notes on several different occasions to ensure that you are the right patient having the right operation.

The following recommendations for nutritional healing, exercise and lifestyle, complementary therapies and emotional and spiritual healing are appropriate for the whole period surrounding surgery, both before and after the actual operation.

Nutritional Healing

Although your doctor will check that you are not anaemic and that you're generally fit for surgery, there is much you can do to ensure that you are at optimum nutritional status as far as your condition will allow. For as long as possible pre-surgery, have as good a diet as you can, full of all the natural foods we mentioned on p. 5. However, add extra sources of Vitamins B, C and E, all of which help wound healing. Zinc and magnesium are also essential to the natural healing process, so to help both your surgeon and yourself, top up these too. Add anything you need to ensure that your immune system is on top form and set to deal with the added stress that surgery is bound to put upon you. Look at the section on wound healing on p. 333 and add whatever supplements you need. The vitamins and minerals mentioned above can also be taken as supplements of course, especially if your appetite is poor because of your condition. Check with your doctor what you're doing if you have any doubts. Since gingko biloba may have an effect on blood clotting, mention this if you're taking it. If you're anxious about your surgery, then try to ensure that you take your Vitamin B, calcium and magnesium at night to help you sleep for the few nights prior to going into hospital. You may also like to try some of the other methods mentioned on p. 468 if you are not sleeping well.

Exercise and Lifestyle

Try to keep your body and mind as fit as possible in the pre-operative period. If you're able to exercise, great. If not, then even some simple gentle stretching will help you keep toned and will also help your body recover after surgery. Keep your mind alert too, which will not only allay your anxiety but will help you feel in control of the situation rather than a victim on whom surgery is being performed. Once you have made your choices and the decision to go ahead with the surgery, try to let go and trust the surgical team to do its best for you.

Mike was due to have surgery to remove a kidney. Being a sole proprietor in his business, he had been working till 10 p.m. every night to try to clear all work and prepare for any eventuality before going into hospital. He arrived at hospital feeling stressed and exhausted and had difficulty in winding down and relaxing before his operation.

Irene has 3 young children. She was due to have some gynaecological surgery and her mother was coming to stay while she was in hospital to look after the children. Her husband had arranged to work shorter hours to spend more time with the children and also to visit. Nevertheless, Irene spent the last week or so before going into hospital baking and cooking in order to leave the freezer full of ready meals. She also intended to try to clean the whole house to leave things spic and span for her mother.

Do take time to rest, relax and destress yourself prior to the surgery. We have seen patients like Mike and Irene who feel that dealing with home and work is more important than resting before going into hospital. That may be tempting, but is really unwise. Try to make the few days before surgery a time of preparing yourself.

Complementary Therapies

Have a massage, perhaps, vaporise some lavender oil and take it easy. In fact look at the anti-stress strategies on p. 482 and incorporate what you can into your timetable without making it even more stressful. Some Arnica will help prepare for the shock of surgery and is also a good measure for a week or so afterwards. If you're very anxious, have some hypnosis or listen to a meditation tape to help relax you. A good hypnotherapist will teach you self-hypnosis to use when you are preparing yourself for the surgery. Add to your night-time routine an Epsom salt or Moor bath which will help you sleep soundly. A moor bath is prepared using a healing mud which you dissolve in the water.

Emotional and Spiritual Healing

Do avoid the guilt which sometimes seems to surround those on a spiritual path who then have to go down the orthodox route and have surgical intervention. It's perfectly fine for you to have the treatment you need whether orthodox or otherwise. Having some healing up to the surgical procedure can often shrink tumours, help reduce or minimise other disease and make for easier, less extensive surgery than would have been otherwise necessary. You may find yourself needing to grieve for the part of you that is being operated on, especially if the surgery involves losing part of yourself. If you know that's going to happen, you might want to have a little ceremony, either alone or with your chosen supporter or healer, to prepare for the loss and begin the process to separate from it.

Hannah has had diabetes for much of her life and at 72 she is facing amputation of her left foot due to gangrene. Naturally she is very distressed at the prospect of the surgery, but spending 6 sessions with a healer who encourages her to grieve for the loss and come to terms with it before the surgery actually takes place, helps her to relax prior to the operation and also helps her recovery afterwards. She is also seen by a counsellor who answers her queries and allays her fears about how she will manage afterwards by informing her of the support services she can expect to have.

For some people there are no negative emotional consequences of surgery, but instead a feeling of almost being reborn, of being so glad to be alive and of having a new beginning. Healing can be quick and uneventful. So, do as much healing as you can pre-operatively and the whole process will be easier for everyone. There is some interesting research on the post-operative progress of those patients who were prayed with or for, before and during surgery, compared with the progress of those who were not. Not only was there more rapid healing, but complication rates were down, infection rates lower and hospital stays shorter. The choice is yours.

Why not ask someone who cares for you to be with you at the hospital and be waiting for your return from theatre. Although the nursing and medical staff will do all they can to help you feel at ease, there's nothing like a loving smiling face you know to wake up to. Perhaps that could be extended to your return home. Having someone either to stay or pop in and bring you nice treats to eat for a few days will work wonders. If that person could be on a similar spiritual level to yourself, that would be even better.

AFTER THE OPERATION

The speed of recovery varies from person to person and clearly depends on the type of operation or procedure carried out. Pain control is vital and many studies have shown that less post-operative pain relief is required when the patient is fully informed of the events in which they are playing a central role.

Unfortunately in today's National Health Service circumstances are not always ideal. Medical and nursing staff are extremely stretched and lack adequate resources. There is always a shortage of beds and hospital managers are under pressure to discharge patients as early as possible. However, hospitals are not allowed by law to discharge patients until satisfactory discharge arrangements have been made within the community and nowhere is this fact of more importance than in the discharge of elderly frail patients who still manage to lead independent lives.

When it comes to the time for discharge from hospital, some kind of management plan is very helpful. This will be drawn up by the surgeon and nursing and medical staff, and will be discussed with you before you leave hospital. You need to know when you should next attend the outpatients' department for follow-up and what symptoms or difficulty you are likely to encounter over the next few days. There should be a discharge letter for your family doctor and at least a few days' medication to tide you over that period until your GP has the information with which to prescribe for you.

Wound care should be carried out either by the district nurse or yourself. If you are to do it yourself make sure you know exactly what you have to do, whether you are permitted to shower etc., so that you will feel comfortable about what is happening. Ask your surgeon if you may apply some aloe vera juice or Vitamin E oil to promote healing and reduce scarring.

Before you finally leave hospital ask as many questions as you need, make sure you understand the answers and check that there is someone you can telephone if you need more information. Usually the ward will be quite happy for you to phone if you have queries.

SOME SPECIAL NOTES ABOUT CHILDREN

Children faced with a stay in hospital will always be apprehensive and frightened as they are not only coping with the illness itself but with a separation from their parents, the people on whom they most rely, and with the daunting environment of the hospital ward. We know that happy children always make quicker recoveries from surgery and much has changed in recent years to make a stay in hospital, even with a surgical operation, as much fun as possible. Most children's wards now are gaily decked out with colourful murals and are full of toys, books, games and computer electronics to keep them happy for days.

Zac was 6 when, because of very frequent and severe tonsillitis he was booked to go into hospital for a tonsillectomy. He had recurrent nightmares when he discovered this, regressed to wetting himself and exhibited frequent temper tantrums at school. A pre-operative visit to the children's ward, however, dramatically changed his preconceptions of hospital. He was given toys and books to read about going into hospital and, much to his mother's surprise (her own anxiety had inadvertently been fuelling his own), he actually actively began to look forward to going to hospital and thrived on the attention this attracted from his friends. His operation went smoothly and he has been fit ever since.

Ali is 8 and is having chemotherapy for a relapse of his leukaemia and has spent the last 8 months more in hospital than out. Although his parents and relatives remain anxious, Ali himself has made great friends on the hospital ward, he is much loved by the nursing staff and has almost established a room of his own in the leukaemia unit. He has no fear of needles or injections and faces his current medical ordeal with interest and courage.

Specialist paediatric nurses no longer wear impersonal identity badges. Instead, their name tags give their first names or their nicknames. They have a range of psychological and play techniques to overcome the fear of needles and injections.

These nurses are skilled in using distraction and relaxation to combat pre- and post-operative pain and they have at their disposal booklets in many different languages, including Bengali, Cantonese, Somali and Urdu, with which to meet the needs of black children and other ethnic minorities. Many children's wards use drawings and pictures to familiarise children with the hospital environment and to give them an idea of what they face. Many paediatric wards arrange special visiting days for children a week or so before the day of their admission, which enables them to have a good look around, to meet their specialist nurse and to be given cuddly toys who just happen to have illnesses or ailments identical to those of the child and which they can take home and nurse prior to their admission a week later when they will be similarly nursed themselves. In many paediatric wards, parents are often allowed to stay over night to be close to their children. The National Association for the Welfare of Children in Hospital (NAWCH) and Action for Sick Children do sterling work in making a sick child's health care as smooth, satisfactory and untraumatic as possible.

Integrated approach

1. Prepare as well as time will allow by having good nutrition, supporting your immune system and familiarising yourself with the hospital and the procedure you are about to have.
2. Don't be afraid to ask questions and make sure you understand the answers.
3. Only sign the consent form when you feel you have enough information to make an informed choice about what is going to happen to you.
4. Ask for pain relief when you need it since lowering the pain can reduce the stress upon you and enhance your healing process.
5. Post-operatively, rest adequately and take advice on exercise etc.
6. Both before and after the operation, do some relaxation and meditation as well as using other complementary therapies.
7. Always check with your surgeon or the ward staff about what you intend to do and make sure that there are no contraindications to your plan.
8. If you have a child needing surgery, take care of your own anxiety since it may well adversely affect your child.

Abortion

To many people the word 'abortion' refers to a medically induced termination of an unwanted pregnancy. But in fact the term refers to both induced abortion as well as spontaneously occurring abortion or 'miscarriage'. Induced terminations of pregnancy are brought about artificially, either at the mother's own request because her pregnancy is unwanted and unplanned, or because doctors have advised it on medical grounds. These might be because of a genetic abnormality in the fetus, for instance, or because of physical illness in the mother from active breast cancer, heart disease or kidney failure.

There are many reasons why the developing embryo is aborted, and although the circumstances may be very different in each case, the physical effects and emotional impact on the woman, in the short and long term, may have close similarities.

Miscarriage

Miscarriage is the spontaneous expulsion of the developing embryo before the 24th week of pregnancy. This used to be thought a critical cut-off time as fetuses delivered before then were not thought to be viable. However, with the incredible technical improvements and special intensive care premature baby units now available, some infants may survive from 22 weeks onwards.

It is estimated that overall something like 1 in 5 pregnant women miscarry, so no woman should think that she is alone or unique when she suffers this traumatic experience, or that she is in any way a failure. Most miscarriages occur before the 10th week of pregnancy, in the very earliest stages. Many women do not even realise they are pregnant because their miscarriage happens so early and it may simply be confused with a late period.

Often, chromosomal or other fetal abnormalities are the cause, but any kind of severe infection or illness in the mother may also be responsible. In the earliest stages of pregnancy a low progesterone level can prevent the fertilised egg from implanting in the lining of the womb. Autoimmune disorders, where the mother's own antibodies for some reason reject the implanted embryo, are another factor. In the later stages of pregnancy, between 12 and 22 weeks, miscarriage might be caused by genetic abnormalities in the fetus, weakness in the neck of the womb allowing the uterine contents to be lost (cervical incompetence), muscular lumps called fibroids in the wall of the uterus or an abnormal internal shape of the womb.

Symptoms

Many women notice a small amount of very light bloodstained discharge at some stage in early pregnancy and this is often due to normal cellular changes at the neck of the womb (an erosion), or to implantation of the embryo very low down in the uterine cavity. In the case of a miscarriage, however, the bleeding will be heavier. There is obvious bright red blood which is much more than just 'spotting', and more importantly the onset of cramp-like pains in the lower abdomen similar to those of a bad period. If these two symptoms occur together, medical advice should be sought immediately, especially if they occur after 12 weeks of pregnancy.

Elizabeth has been trying to have a baby for some time and was delighted when 5 weeks ago, she was found to be pregnant. About a week ago she noticed some spots of blood from her vagina, and her GP suggested she take a few days off work and rest. This morning she started to have a dragging backache and later quite strong lower abdominal pains rather like very bad period pains. Her husband took her to the emergency room at the hospital. On examination her cervix was found to be partially open. Elizabeth has an inevitable abortion.

Types of Miscarriage

We will describe different types of miscarriage so that it is clear which type of treatment is needed. In a 'threatened' abortion, the fetus remains alive within the womb and the bleeding is really a warning sign. The pregnancy often continues normally. In an 'inevitable abortion', the fetus has already died and is in the process of being expelled from the womb through the opened cervix. The doctor can see this when he looks directly at the cervix through a vaginal speculum when he examines the woman during a pelvic examination. Elizabeth, one of our case histories, was in exactly that situation. This type of abortion may be 'complete' when all the uterine contents have been lost, or 'incomplete' when part of the placenta and fetus remain behind. In a 'missed abortion', the fetus had died some time previously but has been retained along with the placenta within the uterus. This becomes clear when symptoms arise or ultrasound tests show that the baby has no heartbeat and is failing to grow.

Medical Care

If a miscarriage is suspected, the woman concerned is usually given bedrest. Although this may not determine the eventual outcome of the problem, it certainly helps to combat the stress involved in these circumstances and at least helps the pregnant woman to feel she is giving her growing baby every possible chance. Ultrasound scanning can show that the fetus is either present or is not within the womb and that there may be a heartbeat. It also shows whether the implantation has taken place within the fallopian tube, in which case the pain and bleeding will be due to an ectopic pregnancy in which the baby is developing in the wrong place and cannot possibly survive. Sometimes a pelvic examination is conducted by the doctor to determine the uterine size and whether the cervix is open or closed. Where a miscarriage is incomplete and the bleeding is heavy, a surgical procedure known as a dilatation and curettage (D&C or 'scrape') is performed to prevent further symptoms such as continued heavy bleeding and pain and also to avoid complications in the future such as intrauterine infection. The woman may be prescribed antibiotics to prevent infection and other medications may be administered if bleeding is a problem. Fifteen per cent of women, whose blood group is rhesus negative, are also given anti-D immunoglobulin to prevent problems occurring in any future pregnancies as a result of rhesus incompatibility. This condition arises only if the baby had inherited rhesus positive blood from the father and the baby's cells crossed over into the mother's circulation, resulting in the production of maternal antibodies that would in turn damage the baby when they crossed back again. The anti-D immunoglobulin would stop this happening at a future time.

When threatened abortion occurs after 12 weeks, immediate medical attention is important because many miscarriages of this type may be treatable. An incompetent cervix, for example (where the neck of the womb opens prematurely), can be stitched shut with a tough nylon stitch known as a Shirodkar suture, as in Amy's case (see below), and uterine relaxants and bedrest can maintain the pregnancy until the growing baby becomes viable, even if born prematurely.

Amy is 18 weeks pregnant. Her previous two pregnancies ended in spontaneous abortion at 16 and 17 weeks respectively. She was reassured by her clinician who, on this occasion, placed a Shirodkar suture into the neck of the womb to prevent a further occurrence. Although she has remained anxious about the outcome, she is starting to relax in the knowledge that another mid-term abortion is unlikely.

Some women seem to miscarry recurrently and after 3 miscarriages, they are medically referred to as 'habitual aborters'. Tests to discover why this happens may include genetic studies, investigations for hormonal problems and infections, as well as a special X-ray (called a hystero-salpingography) of the lining of the uterus and fallopian tubes. Once an underlying cause has been identified it can be treated appropriately. Even where no identifiable reason is found, a successful outcome of pregnancy occurs in a good proportion of cases and any antenatal care is especially thorough and frequent in this group of women.

The Outlook

So be reassured: most women who miscarry do go on in the future to have a normal pregnancy. Better diagnostic facilities and treatments have made this possible.

Induced Abortion (Termination of Pregnancy)

Under the terms of the Abortion Act, a medically induced termination of pregnancy can be carried out up to the 24th week of pregnancy. A minimum of 2 doctors are required to sign a certificate that specifies the reason for the operation; this can include social, emotional and physical reasons. A termination can only be carried out if the continuance of the pregnancy would constitute a risk to the mental or physical health of the woman or her existing children, or if there is a substantial risk of serious handicap to the baby. The latter would apply, for example, if amniocentesis (a test on the amniotic fluid which surrounds the baby within the womb) showed severe developmental defects or chromosomal abnormalities such as severe spina bifida and anencephaly where the top of the baby's head is not properly formed. Terminations may still be carried out for social reasons, but these would still have to fulfil the criteria referred to above.

How Is a Termination Performed?

The earlier a termination is performed, the fewer the physical and emotional consequences. The procedure is done either under general or local anaesthetic and usually takes less than 10 minutes. The neck of the womb is dilated with curved metal rods and the lining of the womb is then scraped with a curette, an instrument resembling a tiny sharp spoon, which removes the implanted embryo and the placental tissue.

In more advanced pregnancies, after the 16th week for example, the method described above is not suitable and a method calculated to expel the fetus by bringing about contractions of the uterus is preferred. A prostaglandin hormone is delivered into the uterus itself or applied in pessary form high up in the vagina, resulting in contractions usually sufficient to expel the fetus within 12–24 hours.

In most cases women recover quite quickly in the physical sense from an abortion, although they should expect some vaginal bleeding and mild cramp-like pain resembling a period for up to several days. Normal periods generally resume in 2–3 months provided there are no complications such as infection. Love-making can commence again within 2–3 weeks if desired.

Risks and Complications

Provided a termination is carried out in a properly equipped hospital by a qualified and experienced gynaecologist, the risks are small and complications are uncommon. However, any operation carries a small risk of infection, bleeding and even more serious complications, although the mortality rate for this operation is very much lower than that for full-term pregnancy itself. There used to be concern about a woman's future fertility, but evidence shows that single terminations alone rarely cause such problems.

Illegal Abortions

Mercifully, illegal 'backstreet' abortions are very much a thing of the past, at least in Britain, although they are still conducted routinely in other parts of the world. They are very high-risk procedures with infection, septicaemia, infertility and, not uncommonly, death being the ultimate penalty. Illegal abortions should be avoided at all costs.

Emotional Support

All the emotional support afforded to women who have had a miscarriage applies to women having terminations, especially as there is a much bigger element of self-determination involved with the procedure. Miscarriage, however devastating, may often come to be regarded as natural destiny over which the woman herself has no control, whereas a termination, for whatever reason, means that the woman herself has to make a difficult choice. For this reason lingering feelings of guilt and regret may emerge both in the short term and occasionally many years later.

Professional Psychological Help

All women benefit from advice or counselling when faced with miscarriage or termination. Whether she loses a baby that she desperately wants, or whether she decides to terminate the pregnancy herself because she is determined to put her career and personal life first, the woman will need help and support. Many factors play a part in decisions concerning abortion, including financial and social circumstances as well as physical ones. Often a woman is forced to make a choice about a termination as a direct consequence of failure of contraception and not a lack of family planning. The GP is logically the first port of call to turn to for help, but some family doctors have their own ethical and religious dilemmas, and will be unable to recommend an induced abortion themselves. Nevertheless they are legally obliged to refer any woman seeking a termination to another medical colleague who can help. Alternatively the woman can refer herself to organisations such as Marie Stopes, the British Pregnancy Advisory Service, the local family planning clinic or an NHS or private gynaecologist. The Brook Advisory centres are also a useful source of help and concentrate particularly on younger women under 25 (see Useful Addresses).

Tina has been referred for psychotherapy for depression. She has remained sad and depressed since a termination of a pregnancy 2 years ago. She admits that she had really wanted to have the baby, but that her boyfriend cooled off after the announcement of the pregnancy and she felt unable to have the child alone. On religious grounds she has always been anti-abortion, but at the time she could see no other way out. She said that she had known girlfriends who had had abortions and who had felt fine afterwards but she simply couldn't shake off the feelings of guilt and anger. She thinks of the child every day, wonders whether it would have been a boy or a girl, and visualises the child toddling now.

Emotional and Spiritual Healing

Abortion, whether planned or not, is a complex issue which involves physical, emotional and spiritual issues. If you have aborted spontaneously, it is a good idea to sit down with your partner and discuss how you both feel about the event and about other related issues such as becoming pregnant again. Try to confront your deepest fears and sorrows. If you have become a habitual aborter, addressing whether you both really want a child will often be rewarded by a change in the pattern.

Work on the second (sacral) chakra can help heal any previous spiritual wound that may be getting in the way of a successful pregnancy, and healing may also help you carry a pregnancy to term. Talking to the child in your womb and welcoming it can be a powerful and potent tool. Try to give priority to your pregnancy by reducing stress and work levels where possible. Maintaining a healthy weight, eating a balanced diet and stopping smoking and drinking will give your child the most healthy environment in which to grow. Obviously good nutrition is essential, and if you are vegetarian or vegan, this is a time to look very carefully at taking adequate vitamin and mineral supplements. Gentle exercise will help but douching should be avoided.

Should miscarriage still take place, always have some form of a ceremony for the child who has been aborted and give yourself time to grieve. No matter how painful, this is a normal phenomenon and it is best not to suppress it by medication. Take time to be gentle with yourself, have some counselling and let go of any misplaced guilt about not having been able to continue the pregnancy. It may seem fatalistic, but things often happen as they are meant to, so if the child is aborted, perhaps there were very good reasons why. Try to learn whatever you can from the experience.

Taking Your Time and Learning

It could be said that every pregnancy is planned at some level, even though we may be unaware of our intention. Also every pregnancy has a lesson for us, and whether it proceeds to full term or not, only when the lesson is learned can the incident be healed and closed. Though there are few physical consequences when abortion is performed well in proper hospital conditions, the memory of the interrupted pregnancy can live on in the tissues if not in the mind, not only while the physical body recovers from the trauma, but for a long time to come.

Termination may be sought for a variety of reasons and in approximately half of all cases there will be no emotional consequences other than relief. However, for the rest there often remains a mixture of guilt, remorse and sadness which, if neither recognised nor resolved, may continue for years unabated. For all, addressing the unfinished business with the child who would have been born can close the episode once and for all and allow the mother to resume her life fully. Such a ritual can take place alone, or better still in the company of witnesses who will honour both the woman and the child while feelings associated with the abortion are released. This can occur even before the termination takes place or at any time after it.

Do take some time deciding what you really want. Having a termination to satisfy family, partner or social demands may only end in resentment, bitterness and prolonged difficulties. Memory stored in our tissues can also cause difficulties, for instance unresolved emotional pain about an abortion could present as a fibroid or pelvic pain in later life. If you are truly unable to give a child what it needs and feel hostile towards it, then termination may be a courageous move. Have some counselling, let go of any guilt, learn to forgive yourself if necessary and share the experience with someone who is supportive to you. If, like Tina (see p. 45), having a termination goes against previously held beliefs, then do try to seek some counselling rather than hide the shame you may feel. There need be no effect on future pregnancies; however, if you continue to harbour guilt and shame, then you may see your inability to conceive as a just punishment. Don't underestimate the power of your mind!

Only you will know whether you are using abortion as an alternative to proper contraception. If you are, then perhaps you could look at better options for the future. Having unprotected intercourse carries with it enormous responsibilities, since each time the natural consequence could be a pregnancy. (And of course there is the possibility of contracting or spreading disease.)

If you have ever had either a miscarriage or an abortion, we would highly recommend that you read Isabel Kirton's wonderful book *Spirit Child* (Findhorn, 1998).

WARNING

Aromatherapy, so healing and gentle, can become a bit of a minefield during early pregnancy so do consult a well-qualified aromatherapist if you want to carry on using oils. The following list (by no means exhaustive) includes some of the oils which SHOULD NOT be used during pregnancy:

Basil	Calamus
Cedarwood	Clary sage
Hyssop	Jasmine
Juniper	Marjoram
Mugwort	Myrrh
Pennyroyal	Rosemary
Sage	Thyme
Wintergreen	

Rose should be used with caution and, as with all oils used in pregnancy, it should be well diluted and used in small quantities.

Integrated approach

1. Take time to consider your feelings about your pregnancy.
2. Consider the physical, emotional, spiritual and social circumstances.
3. Talk to partners, relatives, friends or counsellors.
4. Report any bleeding or pain as soon as possible.
5. Discuss any grief, anxiety, anger or regret to prevent it resurfacing later.
6. Arrange a ceremony for the child if this is appropriate, to help you move on.
7. If miscarriage has happened before, ask your doctor what tests may help in preventing recurrences in the future.

Addictions

John, aged 46, was a director of a computer firm and was accustomed to enjoying a 'liquid lunch' in the pub every lunchtime with some of his work colleagues. He also drank in the evening and found that the odd shot of whisky would calm his nerves. He visited the doctor for a screening examination and became angry and defensive when the doctor challenged him on the amount of alcohol he was drinking, and paid no attention when on examining it the doctor pointed out that his liver was enlarged. He need not have worried that the doctor's report might not go down well with his firm's medical department as he was prosecuted for drunk driving three days later and sacked anyway. This was also the straw that broke the camel's back in his private life as his wife and 3 children walked out on him. It was only then that John was finally forced to face the fact that he was an alcoholic and was able to accept that he had a problem and needed help to deal with it.

An addiction is usually regarded as a dependence on and a craving for some kind of drug. In recent times, however, the term has been adopted by the lay public and extended to include behavioural addictions such as sexual addiction and gambling. Abuse of any of these means that the addict is either persistently or occasionally using them to excess. The benefits to the addict of indulging in this kind of behaviour are fairly clear. The person feels happier and more confident when they are using the subject of their addiction excessively, they feel a sense of wellbeing and their ability to cope with the stresses and strains of modern life seems to be enhanced. However, many addicts are in fact running away from these tensions and unfortunately this very escapist behaviour tends to lead to short- and long-term consequences that merely increase the pressures upon the addict. There comes a time when an addict develops a tolerance to their addiction so that they have to take more of the drug or indulge in increasingly antisocial behaviour to achieve its original effect. Eventually they become dependent and experience unpleasant withdrawal symptoms when the drug or addictive substance is stopped.

Ray came for therapy in a last-ditch attempt to save his marriage. A few years ago he lost a great deal of money betting on horses and vowed to his wife that he would never fall into the same trap again. He did not place a bet for 5 years, although he was drinking rather heavily. A few months ago he started to gamble once again and lost most of their savings. Ray has a gambling addiction with a cross-addiction to alcohol.

Alcohol

One of the most commonly abused drugs in Britain is alcohol, with some 2 million people drinking excessively and up to half a million being physically and psychologically alcohol-dependent. For these people, when they stop drinking they experience confusion, agitation, sweating, nausea, itching, muscle cramps and feelings of panic. In the worst cases fits and delirium tremens can occur: frightening hallucinations terrify the victim and in the worst cases there is a mortality rate of up to 10 per cent. The psychological impairment associated with alcohol includes dementia, unsteadiness, altered sensation in the nervous system, loss of short-term memory, paranoia, depression and sexual dysfunction.

Excessive drinking also leads to physical complications such as cirrhosis of the liver, stomach ulcers, an inflamed pancreas gland, heart disease and infections. Many other drugs which are commonly abused bring about similar health consequences and also, like alcohol, lead to social difficulties within the family and at work, proneness to accidents, criminal behaviour and even vagrancy.

WHAT IS A UNIT OF ALCOHOL AND HOW MANY UNITS ARE SAFE?

One unit of alcohol = 1/2 pint of beer = 1 glass of wine = 1 measure of spirits = 1 schooner of fortified wine (e.g. sherry or port).

Up to 13 per week is relatively safe, but be careful driving and operating machinery when you've had any alcohol, no matter how little.

Between 14 to 24 spread over the week may still be OK, although the maximum if you're a woman is 21 per week (see women and alcohol, below).

At 25 to 35 you're risking liver damage and are possibly starting to hurt your brain. Stomach and digestive problems are also common.

If you're drinking 36 to 63, your liver, brain and digestive system are in trouble. Your concentration will be poor, your memory disturbed and you're probably having social and relationship problems, even though you may be the last to know! If you haven't got legal problems yet (e.g. drink driving etc.), they won't be long in occurring, and your employment is probably on the line too. You're performing much more poorly than you think.

If you're drinking more than 64 units per week, you're in danger. Your physical, mental, social and spiritual wellbeing are being damaged. Your liver, heart, brain and nervous system are all affected and you need help to stop now. Please don't try to stop by yourself. You could be at risk of severe withdrawal symptoms and delirium tremens and/or withdrawal fits. You need to either cut down slowly or better still go and talk to your GP who will suggest a reputable alcohol unit where you can detoxify.

Women and alcohol

In the 1960s problem drinkers were mainly older men; however, a third of those coming forward for help now are younger professional women. Official statistics are always low because many women are still afraid to ask for help.

Nevertheless in 1998 there are estimated to be over 3 million women with alcohol problems in UK.

Which women drink most?

1. Women in professional households (twice as likely to exceed the recommended limits than others).
2. Women working full time.
3. Those with higher incomes.
4. Those who have suffered some other form of psychological illness such as an eating disorder.
5. Those who have a relative who is or has been alcohol-dependent.
6. Ten per cent of women between the ages of 18 and 29 (compared with only 0.3 per cent of women over 65). These young women are far more likely than others to put themselves at risk from drunk driving, violence and sexual assault.

Why do women react differently to men with regards to alcohol?

1. They have more fatty tissue than men and less water available to dilute the effects of the alcohol.
2. They metabolise alcohol differently, since they have lower levels of the enzyme alcohol deydrogenase which breaks it down.
3. Because of the above they are more prone to alcohol-related liver disease such as hepatitis and cirrhosis.
4. They are more likely to suffer alcohol-related heart problems such as cardiomyopathy.
5. Alcohol raises oestrogen levels in women and therefore they are more susceptible to hormone-related cancers such as breast and ovarian cancer.
6. Fetal alcohol syndrome occurs in the babies of women who drink heavily during pregnancy although those who consume only one unit a day may produce children with behavioural anomalies.

Nicotine

Another very commonly abused drug is nicotine. Addiction to cigarettes is mainly psychological, but very heavy smokers can also become physically dependent on nicotine. People are these days aware that smoking is a major risk factor for heart disease as well as lung cancer and a host of other disorders, but people have great difficulty giving up as nicotine withdrawal may lead to intense cravings, feelings of restlessness, lack of concentration and anxiety and depression.

Maureen, 38, has been trying to stop smoking for 5 years. She's been smoking 40 cigarettes a day ever since she was a teenager, and no matter how hard she has tried to stop, she's smoking within a few days. With 4 children to look after, and a part-time job to hold down, she finds it is extremely difficult to deal with the stress and responsibility without the calming effect of a cigarette. Her smoker's cough and constant breathlessness, even when combined with exhortations from her family to stop, have apparently made no difference, and her husband is particularly concerned as Maureen has a family history of heart disease and lung cancer.

DRUG ADDICTIONS

There are many drugs other than alcohol that may be abused, including those that are illegally obtained from drug dealers, those that are initially prescribed by doctors for therapeutic reasons, and those that may be bought over the counter from chemists and pharmacies.

Elsie was prescribed Valium 12 years ago when she had a stillborn child. Over the years she tried repeatedly to withdraw from the medication, both on her own and in hospital, but in fact the dose steadily increased. Without it she felt anxious, agoraphobic and afraid. Elsie is addicted to prescribed medication in the form of benzodiazepines.

Heroin is one of the most commonly abused opioid drugs, producing a very fast dependence and severe withdrawal symptoms. Tranquillisers, which were without doubt overprescribed in the 1960s and 70s as a treatment for anxiety and insomnia, have proved extremely difficult for some people to stop because of persistent psychological dependence. Other commonly abused drugs include amphetamines (speed), cocaine, cannabis and LSD. Even common painkillers such as paracetamol and aspirin may be taken to excess by some. Teenagers particularly are still abusing solvents with a mortality rate, even now, of 200–300 deaths per year in Britain.

Kevin has recently 'dropped out' of college. What was originally a little flirtation with heroin has now become a major problem and he has been arrested and charged with possession of a Class A drug. He knows that his drug using is ruining his health, destroying his family relationships and damaging his friendships as well as jeopardising his studying, but nevertheless he continues to be a user. He has now admitted to himself that he is addicted to the drug and has come for help.

BEHAVIOURAL ADDICTIONS

Activities such as gambling, eating chocolate to excess or becoming sexually promiscuous are not drug addictions, but the consequences of the craving and the compulsion to continue the behaviour have many parallels in common.

Conventional Treatment

The sooner any kind of addiction is detected, the better. This maximises the chances of subsequent treatment being effective. Sometimes the addict will come voluntarily to the doctor because they have suddenly been confronted by the consequences of their addiction. However, often the doctor is brought in by another family member (usually the addict's partner), who can no longer cope with the effects of the abuse and is insisting that something be done.

The general approach by the doctor would be to ascertain the nature of the addiction, which would include the type of drug or substance or the sort of behaviour the addict is indulging in, how long it has been going on, how regular it is and whether there is any evidence of withdrawal symptoms. It is important to discover the extent of any psychological or social complications stemming from the addiction. Any kind of pre-existing problem such as depression, anxiety or more serious psychiatric disorder needs to be identified and taken into account as a possible causative factor. Sometimes, by the time the addict has sought help, their relationships have already suffered badly, with the victim slipping into a lonely and dangerous existence where they are rejected by family and friends only to have them replaced by heartless and shady characters of a notorious and dangerous drug subculture.

A full and thorough physical examination is essential to ascertain the overall condition of the addict, and sometimes urine and blood testing can be useful to measure the extent of any physical damage. An overriding factor is the motivation of the addict to change because clearly this will have a major bearing on the outcome of treatment. After the initial assessment decisions have to be made about whether the addict is going to stop their addiction completely or whether it would be better to tail it off gradually as treatment progresses. The treatment can continue on an outpatient basis if the addict is only a short-term drug taker, has a regular job and lives in a stable home environment. However, addictions with much more significant withdrawal symptoms, such as to opioids and barbiturates, will generally require in-patient supervision.

Treatment will obviously depend on the type of addiction, but medication can be used to counter frightening and unpleasant withdrawal symptoms, and psychological treatment in the form of individual and group psychotherapy over several months may be required. Long-term rehabilitation may mean that the addict resides with other recovering people in order to learn new social and living skills so that the risk of relapse is reduced. Behavioural counselling for pathological gamblers can be extremely helpful, and for those wishing to give up smoking, hypnosis, cognitive therapy and tobacco substitutes such as nicotine chewing gum are good and effective methods of treatments.

Furthermore, the partners and families of the addicts

themselves must not be neglected in all this as they have clearly suffered and will continue to suffer the consequences of what has happened to their relative. It is imperative that their needs are addressed as well, as the addict will continue to be in need of their help and support for some time to come.

Emotional and Spiritual Healing

The factors that make someone start to use an addictive substance or activity are often quite different from the factors that keep them using it. Involved in the development of addictive disorders are genetics, culture, peer pressure, the need to experiment and various personality traits as well as stress, boredom, conflict, etc. But other later factors become important including physical 'tolerance' to the addictive substance itself and also the drama of the addict's way of life. Some people will use a substance on a few occasions and be able to stop but others will become addicted and develop other difficulties in their lives.

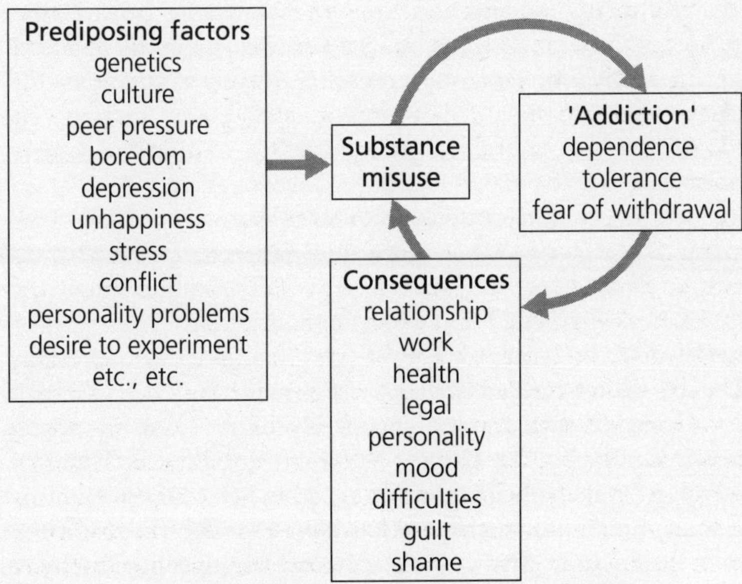

The Development of Addictive Disorders

At the heart of every addiction is a core of shame, with insecurity, poor self-esteem and a low level of self-confidence which can often be traced back to some problem in early childhood. In spiritual terms, addictions are usually the result of some damage at the time of the development of the root chakra, the first of the energy centres of the body to develop between birth and the age of 3 to 5 years. The block or damage to this chakra results in an ambivalence towards life, with poor stability and a sense of not belonging anywhere. Usually there is a desire to opt out of life in some way. Drinking, drug-taking, being addicted to food (or the lack of it), to sex, to love, to relationships is often the result. Once dependence is established, whatever the underlying cause, new and often more complex problems develop on several fronts – health, relationships, financial, employment, social, etc, although denial that there is a problem is a hallmark of addictive illnesses. Women who have addictive problems are sometimes denying not only their feminity but also their own personal needs, sabotaging themselves emotionally and steadily distancing themselves from what they truly desire. Although they may feel comforted temporarily by their addiction, the real problem, the yearning of their spirit, is rarely addressed at all.

If addicts can find a way to soothe the soul and reclaim a sense of power, the rest then follows. Most of all, forgive yourself and try to see this episode as having been something from which you were meant to learn, and when it's over, let it go with as much grace as you can. A word of caution, however. Those around you who have been hurt by your behaviour may not be able to let go as easily as you can. Bear with them as they try to struggle with their own pain. Just because you have stopped, they cannot necessarily close the door on the past. It may be time for them to have some professional help too.

Those living with or involved with addicts, however, must bear in mind that it may take a long time for the addict to grow into health. Any forcing of an end to the behaviour only results in relapse and a sense of failure and disappointment with an increasing belief that giving up and living differently is impossible. Usually family members and workers feel a great sense of urgency to get the person to stop. And because of the damage being done daily on all levels it is important that abstinence is achieved as soon as possible. However, love, compassion and patience are the hallmarks of good treatment, although love includes saying 'no', setting good boundaries and separating ourselves from anything which may endanger our own lives as the person we care for tries to move to a place of greater inner peace. Though putting down the addictive substance is usually seen as the first step, that usually isn't as easy as it sounds. The vulnerability and sensitivity that renders the addict terrified of life without their anaesthetic may return as the withdrawal stage is approached. Understanding this and having compassion can do a great deal to help the person try to move forward.

Nutritional Healing, Vitamins and Supplements

If you've been using any addictive substance, then the likelihood is that you've been neglecting other areas of your life including looking after your body and eating a healthy diet. The sooner you can get back to regular routine and a good eating plan the better. See p. 5 for a good basic eating plan. An assessment by a dietitian would be useful. The B vitamins are essential if you've been drinking a lot and antioxidants such as Vitamins C and E will help repair some of the damage caused on a cellular level. Vitamin K will help repair the clotting mechanism which may have suffered from liver damage. Take lots of fluids mainly in the form of pure water, although herb teas can be wonderful for helping you detox and soothing your anxiety while you're withdrawing. Try chamomile or kava. Milk thistle is useful to cleanse and support the liver, actually helping to regenerate cells in the case of cirrhosis and hepatitis. Dandelion and yellow dock will also help the liver and restore its ability to break down toxic compounds. Bupleurum root, popular in Japan, helps heal inflammation of the liver and reduce damage from toxins such as alcohol.

Exercise and Lifestyle

Starting to exercise again will help you detoxify and boost your confidence and overall feeling of wellbeing. It will also bring some discipline back into your life and help you feel back in control. Your circulation and breathing will be stimulated and this will make detoxification easier, improve your mood and move you much more quickly to a happier, healthier place. There's little more rewarding than seeing your body get in shape. Why not also look at other things you've neglected. A visit to the dentist, for instance, would be a good start.

Avenues of Help

Self-help groups such as Alcoholics Anonymous (AA), Cocaine Anonymous (CA), Gamblers Anonymous (GA), Codependents Anonymous (CODA) and Overeaters Anonymous (OA) are life-savers for those who are unable to get free of their addiction in any other way (see Useful Addresses). However, they are not the answer for everyone and it might be an idea to talk to a professional about what you really need. Until you acknowledge the severity of your problem it will be difficult if not impossible to deal with it. Counselling and support groups are useful and you may find that your family and friends will be very understanding once they see that you're determined to try to let go of your addiction.

It's important to address a whole range of life issues in treatment. Contributing factors such as abuse, abortion, violence, etc. need to be adequately dealt with. Relapse and cross-addiction as in Ray's case are common parts of the addictive process. It has been said that relapse is part of the treatment, and certainly every relapse offers new insights. Nevertheless, the accent should be on relapse prevention.

Complementary Therapies

Learning to meditate can completely change your life and now would be a good time to start. Get yourself a meditation tape or a book, or find a teacher. You could find your nearest centre for Transcendental Meditation at your local library or by phoning the centre in London (tel. 0990 143733). Reduction in anxiety can be achieved very quickly and a new sense of inner peace will reduce your need to return to addiction for solace. Relaxation, meditation and work on your root chakra (see Brenda's *The Rainbow Journey*, Hodder & Stoughton, 1998) will help ground you and build up your sense of self. Insecurities can be dealt with in psychotherapy where you can also learn to deal with peer pressure. The recovery from an addictive disorder can take a very long time and the fellowships (AA, NA, etc.) talk in terms of you never being cured but always being in recovery. Whether the latter is true or not is debatable, but don't expect the road to be shorter than 2 years, and it may be a good deal longer. Learning to have a whole new lifestyle based on peace rather than drama and chaos with healthy relationships and activities is important. You can expect better health physically, emotionally and spiritually, with more financial security and peace of mind.

Acupuncture can be very useful. A small pin inserted in your ear will help with cravings. Ayurvedic medicine could help rebalance your energy, detoxify, and reduce cravings while promoting healthy sleep and calming agitation. Homeopathy can be beneficial and sauna and massage are useful to help you detoxify. See p. 7 for a liver detoxification regime which is useful if alcohol is your problem. Vaporise some calming oils such as lavender or ylang-ylang in your home.

INTEGRATED APPROACH

1. Start by accepting you have a problem of addiction.
2. Identify the reasons why this may have come about.
3. Consider other methods of tackling these problems rather than running from them.
4. Reflect on how your addiction is harming your social and working life.
5. Reflect on how your addiction is damaging your health.
6. Think about how serious things could become if your addiction continues.
7. Resolve and promise yourself to act now before it is too late.

8. Seek advice and have a full physical check-up.
9. Include partners or relatives in your decision and determination.
10. Obtain help in dealing with underlying insecurities, poor self-esteem or lack of confidence.
11. Be realistic and remember that success takes time.
12. Stick to a healthy diet and exercise regularly.
13. Join a self-help group.
14. Strive to avoid relapses in 'using' but don't despair if this happens.
15. Try relaxation, meditation and other complementary therapies.
16. Obtain a suitable detoxification regime from your therapist.

AIDS

AIDS, otherwise known as acquired immune deficiency syndrome, appears to be a relatively new disorder among the human population and is caused by infection with HIV, the human immuno-deficiency virus. Damage to the immune system results in vulnerability to infections and cancers. Many people remain free of symptoms for many years after contact with the virus, although in the meantime they may act as carriers passing the virus on inadvertently to other people.

James is 27 and gay. He is currently in a committed and stable relationship with his partner although until two years ago he was fairly promiscuous and had had unprotected homosexual sex with a number of different partners mostly on a casual basis. When he felt a little out of sorts and lost some weight for no obvious reason he went to see his doctor for a check-up. The doctor, noticing some enlarged lymph glands in his armpits and groin, and knowing that James was in a high-risk group for AIDS, suggested a blood test. After fairly detailed counselling James accepted his disease and was later diagnosed as being HIV positive.

How Common Is It?

HIV infection is an international pandemic with 30 million people worldwide having been infected. The number is predicted to rise to 40 million by the year 2000 as nearly 10 000 new infections are estimated to occur every day. In Britain alone there are now about 30 000 individuals with HIV, with 2500 new infections every year.

The Effects of the Virus

The virus infects a special type of white blood cell known as a T-4 or T-helper lymphocyte which is essential for the body's immunity. In the early stages infected people show no sign of the disease and are asymptomatic carriers. Occasionally, however, they may have transient and rather vague symptoms such as weight loss, unexplained diarrhoea and a low-grade temperature, in which case they are sometimes said to have AIDS-related complex (ARC). Later on in the disease the immune system breaks down completely making the patient vulnerable to a variety of infections and cancers such as Kaposi's sarcoma and lymphomas. This syndrome is known as AIDS. The time it takes to develop from HIV infection to AIDS varies, the average time being 8–10 years. Once individuals develop full-blown AIDS the average survival time is 18–30 months.

How is AIDS Transmitted?

Although HIV has been isolated from many different body fluids, so far only semen and blood have been proved to transmit infection. In Britain HIV is mainly transmitted through having unprotected sex with an HIV infected person and by drug users sharing injecting equipment. Other less common routes of transmission include mother to infant infection and, rarely, accidental needle-stick injury. Before the risk of contaminated blood product transfusions was recognised, haemophiliacs were also exposed inadvertently to HIV transmission.

Many myths have sprung up regarding how AIDS may be caught and it is important to realise that HIV can only be transmitted through very close contact and not through simple social mixing. Activities for example which involve no risk whatsoever include touching and shaking hands, dry kissing without the exchange of saliva, embracing and cuddling, sharing glasses or cutlery or using public toilet seats.

Symptoms

Initially people infected with the virus will show no symptoms or, if they do, will only suffer a short-lived illness resembling glandular fever which then passes. Occasionally lymph gland enlargement is noticed. Minor symptoms include skin irritation on the face, weight loss, fever, diarrhoea and thrush infection in the mouth. More serious symptoms include shingles, herpes simplex infections, tuberculosis, salmonellosis and dysentery. The brain may also be affected leading to dementia. Full-blown AIDS which occurs much later features cancer of the skin such as Kaposi's sarcoma, opportunistic infections such as pneumonia and cytomegalovirus, fungal infections throughout the body and autoimmune diseases where the body's own immune system seems to attack its own cells such as blood cells and joints.

Rachel divorced her husband 4 years ago when she found out he was regularly sleeping with other women including prostitutes in Africa and the Far East, areas he regularly visited in the course of his business. In fact her husband is bisexual, something she only found out much later when a friend informed her in confidence. Rachel was mortified and had always had niggling doubts about whether her husband could have transmitted any sexually transmitted disease to her, including HIV. She has 2 children and did not really want to know the answer to her doubts, but when the anxiety and fear began to preoccupy her thoughts and make her depressed, she agreed to have counselling from her doctor and submitted to a blood test. Much to her relief it proved negative.

Diagnosis

A diagnosis of HIV infection can be suspected in anybody in a high-risk group who experiences unexplained weight loss or enlargement of lymph glands. Confirmation involves taking a blood sample to detect the presence of HIV antibodies, although a negative result does not necessarily rule out infection as it can take up to three months after exposure for the test to prove positive. Even positive results should be doubly checked in view of the implications, the main one being that most antibody-positive people are virus carriers and are very likely to develop AIDS and its numerous symptoms at some stage in the future. Counselling prior to a blood test for HIV is essential as far as advisability and implications are concerned and everyone should think carefully before embarking on a test. At the very least, anybody who even thinks they may have been exposed to HIV with or without a positive blood test result should be advised to practise safe sex in the future to protect others.

Preventing the spread of AIDS

* Never have unprotected sexual contact with anyone known or suspected to have AIDS or with people who have had many sexual partners in the past.
* Avoid having unprotected sex with people whom you do not know well or do not trust, and avoid promiscuity.
* Don't use intravenous drugs, but if you do, never share syringes or needles.
* Avoid sex with others who use intravenous drugs.
* No one who is HIV positive should donate blood, plasma, body organs, sperm or other tissues, nor should they ever exchange body fluids during sexual activity.
* Consider that oral–genital contact and wet kissing involving the exchange of saliva can theoretically transmit HIV and that consistent use of condoms may reduce HIV transmission.
* Hospital and other health-care workers should handle all blood products and needles and sharp instruments with great care at all times.

Conventional Treatment

There is no cure at the current time for AIDS, although there is a great deal of supportive treatment for the complications of this disorder such as antibiotics, anti-cancer drugs and radiotherapy. In the past HIV infection was usually treated using a single antiviral agent, although experience has shown that antiviral drugs are more effective when two or more are taken at the same time as combination therapy. Combination therapy provides more complete and sustained suppression of the virus than monotherapy and has resulted in a fall in death rate, fewer opportunistic infections and fewer admissions to hospital. Considerable progress is being made all the time in the development of new anti-HIV medicines and in Britain licensed therapies now include AZT, lamivudine, didanosine, zalcitabine, stavudine, ritonavir, indinavir, saquinavir and nevirapine. A number of other treatments are in late-phase development and are available now through open access programmes or on a named patient basis.

Medical Treatments and You

It is understandable that anyone with HIV will be anxious about the side effects and long-term safety of HIV treatment and will worry about emerging drug resistance in the virus itself. Tailoring the therapy to the individual coupled with thorough education remain key factors in looking after people who are HIV positive. Dementia, for example, is probably the most feared of all AIDS-related symptoms, raising the terrifying spectre of loss of control over everyday life, losing contact with partners, friends and family. Addressing those fears and keeping the patient informed, counselled and physically/emotionally supported at all times is vital.

The Outlook

Since the beginning of 1996, the use of combination therapy has seen a drop of 18 per cent in diagnosis of new AIDS cases at Britain's largest dedicated unit at the Chelsea and Westminster Hospital in London. At St Mary's Hospital in Paddington, mortality from AIDS has also fallen by 30–40 per cent and both hospitals have been able to treat fewer patients on an in-patient basis, using the more acceptable and user-friendly out-patient route. It is hoped that further improvements in preventive and therapeutic care will increasingly slow the progression of HIV infection to full-blown AIDS and that the intensity of treatment for sufferers will reduce to the extent that many people with the disease will be able to return to work and carry on a normal, active social life during treatment.

Supporting The Immune System

Although the conventional therapies must be the mainstay of treatment, there is much that can be done by the patients themselves to optimise health and minimise the damage done by the virus which, while not being the direct cause of death, cripples the immune system to the point that it can no longer sustain the body's defences against opportunistic infections and cancer. It is therefore in supporting the immune system and also in using natural antiviral agents that we can best help ourselves.

Nutritional Healing

Optimum nutrition is essential and since the body is fighting under extreme conditions, it needs to be supplied with nutrients in the most pure, easily available and unadulterated forms. So clean (i.e. pesticide-free) fruit, vegetables, water (eight large glasses per day), grains and other whole foods are essential. Juices provide easily assimilated, concentrated vitamins, minerals and enzymes and should form a part of the daily regime. These can be varied, of course, but should include green juices (such as wheat grass) in small quantities, diluted but drunk regularly throughout the day. Refined sugars have been shown to depress immune function for a few hours after their ingestion and should be avoided if possible. Flax seed (linseed) oil, organic olive oil and fatty fish such as salmon, tuna, mackerel and herring should provide enough fat for the absorption of the fat-soluble vitamins. Animal fats and other products should be kept to a minimum, especially since the antibiotics and oestrogen found in meat may be unhelpful. Soya products, seaweed, shiitake and mitake mushrooms add important nutrients which all help boost the immune system. The daily protein requirement is generally about 0.8 g/kg of body weight; however, this needs to be increased to about 2 g/kg of body weight where weight is falling. Whey protein is a useful and easily digestible addition to the diet at the level of about 1 g/kg of body weight. Avocados, peanut butter, almonds and sunflower seeds will help keep calories up and prevent weight loss. There's some interesting research on the benefits of turmeric (curcumin), and although it appears that it may have to be taken in fairly large quantities (it is available as capsules) it's worth adding a regular curry to your diet. Garlic has enormous benefits. Please use this amazing herb wherever you can. Not only is it packed full of minerals, but it has amino acids, is a natural antibiotic and antiviral agent and contains Vitamins A and C.

Vitamins and Supplements

Obviously a good multivitamin and multimineral is recommended (choose one with a long list of ingredients), but we advise adding Vitamin C (500–1000 mg 3 times daily), Vitamin E (400 iu) 3 times daily and a strong Vitamin B complex daily also. Selenium and zinc are essential as antioxidants and could be taken as extra supplements along with beta carotene (palm oil is the best natural source) and lipoic acid which appears to reduce the activity of the enzyme that allows the HIV virus to replicate its DNA. Vitamin E and selenium appear to slow down the progression from HIV infection to AIDS. Vitamin A and beta carotene appear to have a beneficial action on T-cell production. Carnitine, an amino acid, also protects the immune system. Bromelain, an enzyme found in pineapple, is a natural antiviral agent. Japanese studies show promising results when liquorice is given to HIV patients, but do monitor potassium levels or add bananas and orange juice if taking liquorice over a period of a couple of months or more.

Exercise and Lifestyle

Reduce stress as much as possible. A good way to do this is to meditate for 20 minutes or so twice daily. Creative visualisation, guided meditation or prayer would be beneficial, so do try to take time out of your daily schedule, whatever other demands there are upon you. A positive attitude is essential to reduce fear and tension which in themselves can depress immune function. Exercise such as yoga and T'ai chi or Chi gong help mind, body and spirit simultaneously and are strongly recommended. Breathing exercises, good rest and sleep are essential. Cigarettes, alcohol and high caffeine intake are unwise. Try to make sure that you see your friends regularly and have good social support.

Complementary Therapies

Spiritual healing can do a great deal here and achieving a peaceful state helps boost the immune system and optimises the body's own energetic resources. Touch is important and a regular massage with or without aromatherapy oils will help reduce tension and relax your body so that it can best utilise energy. Homeopathy may be useful especially if you are frightened or despairing. Use Ignatia where there is despair and grief about the illness or losses in your life or the fear of not getting well; Thuja where there is or has been a high sex drive followed by rapid exhaustion and emaciation. See a good homeopath for a full assessment. Various herbs are useful, the most important of which are astragalus and legustrum, ideally taken together. Ginseng will help energy, boost the immune system, detoxify the liver and is also a natural anti-cancer agent. Aloe vera with its amino acids, minerals and live enzymes is useful. Although one would imagine that echinacea would be good here because of its activity on the immune system, it appears that it is not useful where the immune system is so badly compromised already.

Emotional and Spiritual Healing

This is such an emotive illness which has been surrounded by considerable guilt and shame for many of those who suffer from it, and suspicion and judgement for many of those who do not. Rarely has an illness raised such emotional issues and caused so many people to look at themselves and assess their own lives. There needs to be much healing for the individuals who are afflicted with AIDS, for the families who have relatives who are sufferers, and for the community at large which needs to integrate the suffering into its ranks and care. Though great strides forward have been made in the treatment of AIDS, there has been some concern of late that the outlook is not as good as it may have appeared two or three years ago. Many AIDS sufferers have lost friends and partners to the disease and many families sadly await the demise of their loved ones. So not only are those involved struggling with their own physical problems, but they are often also dealing with grief and with impending death. There are counselling services set up in every community to deal with this modern disaster, and it would be wise for every sufferer and family or friend to avail themselves of this service. Healing can be of great benefit here in that it can help bring a sense of inner peace, reduce stress and bring comfort. In some cases, however, it can do more than this and actually reverse or arrest some of the changes taking place. Learning to talk openly about the feelings surrounding the possibility of death can ease grieving and sometimes open up a new understanding of the process of dying and what may follow. In whatever way you are associated with this illness, either as primary sufferer, friend or relative, or simply as a member of the human race, try to open your heart with love, empathy and compassion, and cease any judgement. There is much for us all to learn.

INTEGRATED APPROACH

1. Take all possible precautions to avoid contact with HIV.
2. Have regular check-ups and report any symptoms, especially if you are in a high-risk group.
3. Remember that as someone who is HIV positive you have a deep responsibility to other people.
4. Your love, understanding and support may be vital for someone diagnosed with AIDS.
5. Enjoy a healthy lifestyle, a well-balanced diet and nutritional supplements.
6. Experiment with all of the complementary therapies.
7. Do not forget that the outlook for patients who are HIV positive continues to improve and that combination therapy increasingly allows people to lead a normal and active social and working life.

Allergies

Allergies may result in a variety of symptoms affecting various different parts of the body. Most common among them are skin rashes, hayfever, asthma, sore red eyes and abdominal pain with nausea and vomiting. Severe symptoms, however, can lead to life-threatening swelling of the lips, tongue and throat, and even clinical shock with collapse and ultimately death. The underlying reason for an allergic response is an exaggerated reaction of the immune system to a number of different substances.

Molly dreads the summer months because every year, as soon as the warm weather begins, she develops red itchy eyes, a streaming or congested nose and an itchy feeling at the back of her throat with occasional wheezing when she rushes about. She found eyedrops, nasal sprays and non-sedating antihistamine tablets only moderately effective, and has to seriously curtail her outdoor activities at a time when all her friends and colleagues at work are able to enjoy life to the full. Molly's quality of life is suffering because of severe hay fever.

What Causes Allergy?

Our bodies are bombarded all the time by foreign proteins called antigens. Some antigens like the sting of an insect or the outer coat of a bacterium are harmful and potentially lethal, whereas others do us no damage whatsoever when we come into contact with them. Our immune system recognises antigens and assists us in forming antibodies to combat them. These antibodies, together with certain white blood cells called lymphocytes, become sensitised when first introduced to the allergen and when the immune system is next in contact with the same antigens there is an interaction which usually brings about the eradication of the allergens. In allergy, an exaggerated immune response is generated against even harmless substances which are effectively mistaken for potentially harmful substances.

Common Symptoms

Allergy brings about the release of chemicals such as histamine which causes blood vessels to open up and leak fluid, and muscles to go into spasm. Skin can erupt in a rash with white blotchy itchy areas called weals, the bronchial air passages can constrict and produce mucus, causing asthma, the eyes can become red and the nose can run as in hayfever, and the stomach and intestines can become inflamed leading to diarrhoea and vomiting. In the most severe cases complete closure of the respiratory passageways may lead to asphyxia, and flooding of the lungs with fluid can lead to respiratory failure. In less dramatic cases symptoms may be vague and non-specific so that allergy may not be identified as the cause of symptoms until after many months of patient investigation.

David, 24, is lucky to be alive. He went out for an Indian curry when halfway through his lips began to swell, his breathing to labour and he quickly became unconscious and had to be transferred to hospital. Here he was given intravenous adrenalin and positive pressure oxygen treatment which saved him in the nick of time. He had developed a severe anaphylactic reaction to peanuts which, along with peanut oil, are present in a vast number of food preparations, many of which remain unlabelled to this effect. He now carries emergency treatment wherever he goes.

Diagnosis

Often the diagnosis of an allergy is extremely obvious. The itchy, blotchy rash on the skin which occurs directly after handling certain plants and the similar signs developing beneath a necklace or a bracelet made from cheaper types of metal are unmistakable. Equally, foodstuffs such as shellfish or strawberries which always produce the same reaction in the same person are characteristic of true clinical dietary allergy. Often, however, allergic symptoms are difficult to pin down to any given substance. People often come into the doctor's surgery with an allergic reaction, and despite detailed scrutiny of their recent diet and environmental contacts there is no hard evidence as to the cause. Sometimes the responsible agents can only be discovered through exhaustive tests where the skin is challenged by exposure to various suspected antigens. These patch tests are widely used to diagnose contact dermatitis. Suspected antigens are applied to the skin via adhesive patches and after a period of time, the skin beneath the patch is observed. Tests can also be done for hayfever, pet allergy and hypersensitivity to house dust mite in the same way. In addition, blood tests known as RAST and CAP can be very useful in identifying true food allergies to ingredients such as milk, eggs, fish, shellfish, certain fruits, wheat, soya, peanuts (a member of the legume family) and nuts. Sometimes only blind-food challenges and strict elimination diets will throw further light on the causes of any given allergy.

Liz has noticed that after eating ice cream her eyes and face become puffy and she has to clear her throat of mucus. Her partner complains that after eating any dairy produce she snores quite loudly. Liz has an allergy to dairy produce.

Food allergies and intolerance

Food allergies are more common than most people think and usually some symptoms can be picked up within a couple of hours of eating the substance to which we are allergic. Symptoms of food intolerance, however, may be delayed by up to 72 hours and may be less easy to trace to a particular food. Therefore keeping a food and symptom diary is useful to detect any pattern. Food intolerance or allergy may prevent weight loss (see the section on obesity p. 242) because an inflammatory substance, prostaglandin E2, released during allergic reactions, inhibits the body's ability to burn stored fat. People who suffer food allergies may not produce sufficient pancreatic enzymes to break down protein molecules into the less harmful amino acids. Diagnosis is essential and although you can do it yourself to some extent (using Dr Coca's Pulse Test on p. 76), it is more accurate to have an immunoglobulin G test (IgG test) performed.

Conventional Treatment

Since allergens are responsible for allergy and its symptoms, the best preventative treatment involves avoidance of the allergen concerned. Someone who is allergic to eggs, for example, must avoid eating eggs and any food containing eggs as an ingredient. People allergic to peanuts, of whom there are a growing number and in whom the reaction can be especially severe, should scrutinise the nutritional labelling on foods extremely carefully, especially as peanut or arachis oil is widely used throughout the food chain.

People with hay fever, for whom grass pollen, tree pollen or moulds may be the cause, can try to avoid contact with these allergens by keeping bedroom and car windows closed, and wearing wraparound sunglasses and a mouth mask, but unfortunately the effect is limited as it only takes a few grains of pollen to trigger the reaction.

Antihistamine drugs remain the mainstay of preventative treatment because they neutralise the effect of histamine, one of the main chemicals responsible for the exaggerated immune response. The antihistamines stop the swelling so often seen in allergy, and many modern antihistamines are non-sedating and long acting. They are, however, of little value in more life-threatening reactions when more powerful drugs are needed urgently. Antihistamines are also of benefit to people with allergic eczema whose sleep is often disrupted by intense and persistent itching, as the older types of antihistamines are sedating and can allow a good night's sleep as well as soothing the irritation.

Other medications such as steroids and sodium cromoglycate can often prevent symptoms from occurring when taken on a regular basis. Steroids come in cream, tablet and injectable forms. Hyposensitisation or 'neutralising immunotherapy' may be effective in about two thirds of cases, but unfortunately this requires 2–3 years of treatment and a huge commitment on the part of patient and physician alike. This technique exposes the sufferer to tiny but increasing doses of the allergen over a period of time so that the immune response can come to terms with the allergen without producing the exaggerated response of allergy.

DR COCA'S PULSE TEST

Although it is essential to have a diagnosis made by a physician, you can check the possibility of food intolerance using the following method. Take your pulse before eating and then every 30 minutes thereafter. Your pulse rate will usually go up by 20 to 40 beats/minute after eating foodstuffs to which you are intolerant or allergic.

Once a specific allergen is isolated, try to eliminate it from your diet for at least 3 months. The fact that you are intolerant to it now doesn't necessarily mean that you can never eat it again, although for some substances like the peanut and arachis oils allergies mentioned earlier, reintroduction could be disastrous. Sadly, the foods to which you're intolerant are usually those you particularly crave, so giving them up may not be easy. A good place to start is to eliminate dairy produce, but expect mucus and headaches for a few days till your system clears. Spicy foods can worsen the food allergies by acting upon cells lining the small intestine, allowing allergens to enter the bloodstream.

Nutritional Healing

Your body's response to allergens may be reduced if you eat more fatty fish (salmon, tuna, herrings, mackerel) containing omega-3 fatty acids, although an even more potent source is flax seed (linseed) oil. Onions and garlic are anti-inflammatory and also build up the immune system, as do juices such as alfalfa and pineapple. Allergies of any kind demand a diet laden with antioxidants such as the riboflavinoids, naturally found in brightly coloured fruits and vegetables. It is useful to rotate foodstuffs, repeating them only every 4 to 7 days. Beware tartrazine (yellow food colouring) which can cause allergic reactions and asthma attacks in some people and which also interferes with the body's use of Vitamin B_6. Bromelain, found in pineapple, helps break down proteins to their constituent amino acids and reduces the likelihood of their causing allergic reactions.

Vitamins and Supplements

Vitamin C plays an important part in keeping our lungs healthy and able to fight off assault by allergens. It can also reduce the amount of histamine produced by white blood cells, with levels going down by up to 40 per cent after 9 months of regular intake of 1000 mg 3 times daily. Vitamin C also has anti-inflammatory and antioxidant properties. Cigarette smoke destroys the lungs' Vitamin C, and supplementing the diet of the children of smokers with Vitamin C can reduce their chest infection rate and their tendency to develop asthma and other allergic conditions.

The B vitamin group are important. Those with breathing problems often have low B_6 levels and this vitamin given as a supplement can reduce the frequency and severity of asthma attacks (see also the sections on asthma and chest problems). Vitamin B_5 is a precursor of cortisone and is essential to our ability to reduce the allergic response. Brewer's yeast, oats and barley contain beta glucan which links to receptor sites on macrophages (special cells which help clear harmful substances from the bloodstream) to boost immunity. Too much can be counter-productive so take the dose recommended on the package. It is most effective if taken with Vitamin C. Liquorice root is good for inflammation as it slows down the breakdown of natural cortisol thereby prolonging its healing action. It also slows down the body's manufacture of substances that exacerbate allergic inflammatory reactions. Ma Huang (*Ephedra sinica*) has been used for centuries to help breathing, rather like ephedrine which relaxes and opens the airways. Gingko biloba, which has been found to have amazing effects on circulation and brain function, also has anti-inflammatory properties which make it a useful addition to your regime.

Of the minerals, selenium, zinc and magnesium are of major importance for those with allergies and are not usually found in sufficient quantities in our diet. A multimineral supplement will usually take care of most of your needs. A visit to a registered naturopath would yield great rewards.

Complementary Therapies

A homeopath would probably prescribe a constitutional remedy for you. However, other remedies which may be useful are Allium cepa (when you have a burning raw feeling in your nose with a tingling sensation and a lot of sneezing and when you feel worse in warm rooms and better outdoors); Nux vomica (if you feel irritable and chilled, with a nasal discharge during the day and congestion at night, feel worse indoors and are sensitive to the cold and want to be wrapped up); Pulsatilla (best for women and children with a daytime nasal discharge and night-time congestion, who are gentle but emotional, who are congested in warm rooms, hot weather or when lying down); Arsenicum album (when eyes are hot and watery); and Apis (where there is redness, swelling and inflammation).

Chamomile and peppermint aromatherapy oils are beneficial, as is eucalyptus if there is a lot of congestion. Herbs which are useful include astragalus which builds up the immune system and can be taken daily, as opposed to echinacea which is highly effective but should be taken on a 4 days on, 4 days off regime. Nettles, either as capsules or as an infusion (tea), parsley which inhibits the production of histamine, and ginger are also useful. Wild cherry bark and mullen leaf soothe and heal the mucosal surfaces inside the body. Talk to someone knowledgeable at your healthfood shop to find what might suit you best or, better still, consult a herbalist.

Traditional Chinese Medicine sees allergies as an imbalance of the liver and may suggest a detoxification regime. Acupuncture may help and an Ayurvedic physician may suggest changes to balance your diet.

Exercise and Lifestyle

It would be worth investing in an air purifier, and humidifiers are useful especially at night. Air-conditioning your car will protect you from allergens while driving in the country or the polluted atmosphere of the city. Switching to natural products for personal, home and garden use (e.g. soaps, shampoos, moisturisers, insecticides) will be beneficial. We survived long before there were hi-tech pesticides and detergents. The use of boric acid or garlic powder as pesticides and soaps to wash clothes worked well for our grandmothers and would work for us too and prevent us destroying the environment as well as preserving our health. Bleach is a very effective antibacterial agent and fungicide useful for household surfaces, but do be sure to dilute it properly and do not use it in combination with detergents. Men with moustaches might like to consider shaving them off but if not, do shampoo them twice a day since they can harbour allergens literally right under your nose. If you would like an assessment of your home for allergens, then you might like to contact the British Society for Allergy and Environmental Medicine or Action Against Allergy (see Useful Addresses). As always, exercise is good for you, but always warm up slowly and wear a mask if outdoors.

Emotional and Spiritual Healing

Allergies can result in considerable limitation of freedom which can be both frustrating and annoying, especially for children who have difficulty in understanding why they are not allowed to have various foods, play in certain places, or have pets. Though understanding is increased in adulthood, the resentment can continue and sometimes requires counselling or psychotherapy. Sometimes those who suffer allergies are ridiculed and misunderstood by their peers, leading to isolation and ostracisation which only adds to the problem. Great care must be taken to improve the understanding of both the sufferer and friends, family and peers so that risks are not taken with this potentially life-threatening condition. However it is important to keep the balance right between concern and sensible care and rendering the sufferer an allergy invalid. Parents need to learn to trust their allergic child as soon as possible and not to fuss excessively otherwise normal development which includes exploration of the world and taking risks will be restricted, resulting in an adult who is anxious and lacking spontaneity.

Spiritual healing can benefit the sufferer in several ways. First of all the sense of inner peace will calm an irritable system, but also allergies may reduce in severity and in some cases remit altogether. In the acute phase, healing can help while more conventional treatment is on the way, calming the patient and helping keep the allergic reaction to a minimum.

Emergency treatment

The most effective treatment for severe allergies, including food allergies such as from peanuts, is adrenalin. This substance rapidly constricts swollen blood vessels, and can reverse the enlargement of the lips, face and tongue and the constriction of the respiratory airways which occur in severe anaphylactic shock. It can also reduce the drop in blood pressure which may occur. It can be given in either inhaler form or by injection, and the Epi-pen autoinjector is ideal for this purpose. The Epi-pen is easy to use, has no visible needle and has a shelf life of 2 years. Allergic sufferers can carry it with them at all times and children and adults alike can be taught how to administer it themselves. Children should take Epi-pens to school or keep one on standby there as well.

Finally, anyone with a life-threatening allergy would be well advised to carry some kind of identity bracelet to alert other people to the fact, should they become unconscious or need emergency treatment in public. The Medic-Alert Foundation can supply identity tags in bracelet or neck pendant form which can immediately bring the sufferer's diagnosis to the attention of others in an emergency situation (see Useful Addresses).

INTEGRATED APPROACH

1. Confirm allergic reactions with a symptom diary, patch tests, blood tests or the pulse test.
2. Avoid the offending allergen wherever practicable.
3. Adopt nutritional healing regimes to combat allergy the natural way.
4. Try vitamin, mineral and herbal supplements.
5. Consider complementary therapies such as naturopathy, homeopathy, aromatherapy and Chinese herbal medicine.
6. Make your home and working environment as low-allergen as possible.
7. Use antihistamines, sodium cromoglycate, decongestants and inhalers to relieve persistent symptoms.
8. Use steroids sparingly preferably in inhaler form or as dilute cream.
9. If severely allergic, carry an Epi-pen with you at all times and wear a MedicAlert Foundation identity tag.

Anxiety, Panic, Phobias and Obsessions

Richard had always felt uncomfortable in social gatherings, even those as small as dinner parties, or when eating out in restaurants. After a promotion at work he was invited to dinner by his boss but felt extremely nauseous and was actually sick several times, and spent much of the evening in the toilet. After that he always avoids any place or situation where other people might be 'observing him' as he put it, and has become increasingly isolated. Richard has a genuine social phobia.

ANXIETY

Anxiety is an emotion everyone feels at some time or another as it is a normal response to the various kinds of stress in life. It produces a sense of apprehension or fear and is useful to some extent in that it seems to make you more alert, more efficient in what you do and helps you focus and concentrate on the job in hand. Too much anxiety, on the other hand, becomes a distinct hindrance. It makes you feel dreadful, psychologically and physically, and ultimately it leads to you not performing as well as you should and suffering the social and occupational consequences. Often the anxiety you feel is out of all proportion to whatever it is that is causing it and sometimes you just feel extremely anxious and panic-stricken for no obvious reason. When you are made fretful about a specific problem or situation to the extent that you avoid it at all costs, you can be said to have a true phobia and are suffering from phobic anxiety.

You often experience these conditions for the first time in early adulthood although many others never have them until middle age. Women seem to be affected more than men with about 3 per cent of the population overall being touched by it.

Melanie is 27, the PA to an executive in the city. She has recently been offered a promotion which would involve her in a considerable amount of travel but she felt that she couldn't take it because of her fear of flying. She has never been able to go on holiday abroad and is filled with fear at the very thought of it. Melanie suffers from a phobia.

Jenny, 33, has 3 young children, and spends much of her time worrying about their welfare. Her concerns encompass everything from whether they are having the right kind of food to whether someone might molest them. She has a constant knot in her tummy and feels nervous and jumpy. Sometimes she feels almost paralysed by her fears as her pulse races and she becomes sweaty and has to sit down for a while. Her mother was an anxious person and Jenny herself was a nervous child. Jenny suffers from an anxiety state.

Symptoms

The psychological symptoms of anxiety include fear, apprehension and foreboding – that terrible feeling that something dreadful is about to happen. Patients often find that their ability to concentrate properly is affected and that they become irritable, snappy and intolerant to minor problems such as noise, queues and criticism. On the physical side headaches, migraine, indigestion and chest pain may arise, and overactivity of the nervous system leads to symptoms such as breathlessness, palpitations, dry mouth, shaking, nausea and sweating. Often people are unable to sleep well and feel the need to go to the toilet more frequently.

Rick is 16 and about to take his GCSEs. He studies hard and has good grades. He sets high standards for himself and intends to go on to study medicine. The elder of two children, he knows that his parents, while being very supportive, expect him to do well. The teachers have said that he is capable of straight As. Over the last couple of weeks he has felt nauseous in the mornings and has had to leave the classroom on one occasion to get some air when he thought he was going to faint. He is now having difficulty getting off to sleep at night. Rick suffers from anxiety.

All these symptoms can be felt by people with phobias, but the difference for them is that they are usually only experienced when confronted by a specific situation or object. Common simple phobias include fear of spiders, heights or darkness. Many people are uncomfortable with these things, but they are not truly phobic unless their fear is totally out of proportion to the provoking factor and they cannot be reasonably calmed or reassured. Truly phobic people also go to extreme lengths to avoid the object of their terror and can sometimes become quite distanced from the rest of society as a result. Common phobias include agoraphobia which is a fear experienced in large open spaces or public places, social phobias such as fear of being sick or fainting in public, and the simple phobias such as fear of flying or of hypodermic needles.

OBSESSIONS

Obsessions are recurrent thoughts and feelings which drift into your mind completely involuntarily. If you experience these obsessions you know that your thoughts are senseless, and often unpleasant, but you are seemingly incapable of ignoring them or resisting them.

Tod is frightened that he is going to be contaminated with dirt and compulsively washes his hands many times a day. He can't travel to work on the bus because someone else will have sat on the seat, nor can he use the public telephone since others will have breathed into it. His possessions have to be arranged in a particular way and he becomes distressed if anyone moves anything. On one level knows that his fears are silly but nevertheless they constantly come into his mind almost like the melody of a song or the lyric of a nursery rhyme and he can't get rid of them. He remembers that as a child he had to count the number of times he put out the light and would also touch his teeth on the side of his cup 3 times before he started to drink. Tod can't remember when these behaviours disappeared but he knows they did and that they then came back again about 6 years ago when he was 20. Tod has obsessive–compulsive disorder.

Among the most common obsessions are fears of being affected by dirt or germs, constant doubts that you have locked the front door when leaving home, or fear that you may commit some violent act or be subject to some similar personal threat. Many people seem to brood constantly over a word, a piece of music or an unanswerable problem. All sufferers are handicapped socially in some way by these unwanted thoughts.

Many people with these obsessions are driven to compulsive behaviour that involves repetitive yet apparently purposeful acts, which are carried out in a ritualistic fashion. These acts are carried out in order to eradicate fears or to relieve anxiety and are really the physical manifestation of an obsessional state. There is usually no peripheral pleasure derived from performing these repetitive activities, but the sufferer feels increasingly anxious and fearful if they try to resist carrying them out. Common examples of compulsive behaviour are frequent hand washing and checking or counting, and these may be performed so many times that they can seriously affect social and work life.

Doctors describe somebody in this state as suffering from an obsessive–compulsive disorder, a form of neurosis that often starts in adolescence, and tends to come and go in severity over many years. True obsessive–compulsive disorder is relatively rare, but up to a sixth of the population will experience minor obsessive symptoms at some time or another. Much depends on the person's underlying personality. Many people are very orderly and fastidious by nature and, when combined with underlying nervous traits such as poor self-esteem and sensitivity to other people's comments, this can result in ritualistic behaviour. The condition is probably partly inherited although environmental factors certainly contribute.

The Outlook

The conventional approach to treatment is the use of behaviour therapy, sometimes combined with antidepressant drugs such as clomipramine or paroxetene which seem to have a specifically beneficial effect on this condition. Behavioural therapy is a method of treatment that is aimed at improving a patient's function and wellbeing by a direct change in behaviour. This can be carried out by a clinical psychologist or psychiatrist or sometimes by a family doctor who has a special interest in the condition. Two thirds of all people who suffer from obsessive–compulsive disorder respond well to the above treatment, although symptoms can return under stress. Without treatment and in severe cases, however, the affected person can become completely housebound and severely handicapped by the condition.

Psychological Treatment

One of the most important but simplest ways to allay people's anxieties is to listen and talk to them. It is still true that a problem shared is a problem halved and if a doctor can make sense of someone's worries and fears while at the same time explaining the reasons why they actually feel physically unwell with their symptoms, any other more potent treatment or medication may prove unnecessary. This kind of simple psychological support can often reveal underlying conflicts and difficulties for the patient, such as financial or relationship problems, which have contributed to the current situation. They need to be sorted out in themselves before the anxiety can really be brought under control. It is also important to find out whether the patient has been trying to escape from their anxiety and its symptoms through drinking too much alcohol or taking other drugs (see p. 50). This will only have created additional problems rather than solving any of the underlying ones.

Behavioural treatment using relaxation techniques can enable an anxious patient to recognise and relieve signs of muscular tension and to prevent irregularities in pulse rate or breathing which are otherwise involuntary. With physical relaxation, an ability to mentally relax and become calmer and more psychologically comfortable often follows. Behavioural therapy is also the mainstay of treatment for people with phobias. Graded exposure is an approach whereby the patient is progressively exposed to the feared situation one step at a time under specialist supervision. Patients learn to control their feelings of panic in the stressful situation with the therapist's help and eventually they find they can cope with even the most alarming circumstances in apparent calm and control.

Terri complains that although she has travelled to work on the Underground for a long time, over the last few months she has become unable to do so. When she even approaches the train her heart pounds, she feels nauseous and faint, thinks that she is going to suffocate, has pains in her chest and feels dizzy and weak. On two occasions she actually ran out of the station and went home rather than to work. Terri suffers from panic disorder.

Physical Treatment

When anxiety or a phobic disorder is severe and leads to distressing and unpleasant physical and psychological symptoms in the patient, something more urgent needs to be done. This is especially true if any depression or other mental or physical illness forms part of the overall clinical picture. Beta blocker drugs are very good at eradicating the physical symptoms such as palpitations, nausea and sweating that accompany anxiety, without producing sedation, mental blunting or addiction in the long term. Prolonged anxiety with depression is best treated with antidepressants with a sedating quality, but always under close supervision and with adequate instructions and warnings. Tranquillisers still have a place in the treatment of anxiety but, because of their well-known ability to lead to addiction, should only be used in low dosage and in short courses. Preferably the tranquillisers should not be taken every day. When taken in this way, observing these conditions, tranquillisers can dramatically improve the quality of many people's lives.

Emotional and Spiritual Healing

Any inner conflict that we feel unable to resolve can result in anxiety, and that includes behaviour that leads us to be out of line with our integrity. Are you aware of what you are carrying around that's making you feel anxious? How about staying away from 'news' that can add to your anxiety? I (Brenda) decided long ago that reading, watching or hearing about tragedies and disasters etc. was doing nothing for me except filling my head and my heart with pain. I don't need that, thank you. So I decided that every day I will send out as much love and healing as I can to wherever it's needed, and in that way I'm doing what I can, but I no longer need to know the details. It doesn't help anyone (least of all me) if I get so upset by what's going on that I'm rendered ineffectual by the pain of it all. If you spend just a few minutes whenever you think about it focusing on your breathing (see breathing techniques, p. 114) your anxiety will start to settle.

Sometimes it's impossible to pinpoint the cause of anxiety and related illnesses. Whatever the cause, spiritual healing can usually help by giving you some inner calm and peace. You may like to try some self-healing techniques including visualising the situation that causes you anxiety and seeing yourself become an amazingly powerful being who can overcome the difficulty with ease.

Exercise and Lifestyle

Relaxation is the cornerstone of treatment for anxiety and whether you choose to use a relaxation tape or have a few sessions with a therapist, that time would be an investment for the rest of your life. Although tranquillisers (such as Valium) can reduce anxiety within a matter of 20 minutes and can be very useful in the short term or when a specific event is causing the problem, there are generally better ways to deal with it. Tranquillisers when used inappropriately can reduce your performance, make you sleepy and are also habit-forming. Yoga, which balances mind, body and spirit, will help you, as will breathing exercises.

Complementary Therapies

Massage and aromatherapy are extremely useful here. Chamomile oil calms, soothes and induces relaxation while reducing anger and stress. Geranium calms and creates a feeling of inner balance. Jasmine is emotionally soothing and lifts depression while sandalwood relieves nervous tension and is a gentle sedative promoting a sense of wellbeing. Ylang-Ylang helps soothe anger, is relaxing and sedative, calming nerves, relieving stress and promoting sleep. Lavender is not only soothing, but also potentiates the qualities of all the aforementioned oils when it is used in conjunction with them.

Hypnosis is often of great benefit to those suffering from anxiety, but do ask your therapist to teach you to do self-hypnosis so that you can carry on the treatment at home and use it as an aid to help you sleep as well as deal with difficult situations. During panic attacks, dizziness is caused by breathing out too much carbon dioxide. Rebreathing from a paper bag will settle the dizziness very quickly as you breathe in your own exhaled air and re-establish the level of carbon dioxide in your blood.

Phobias like Melanie's can often (but not always) be traced back to some traumatic event and the recovery of that memory can be very helpful in systematically desensitising the person. Your therapist may help you relive the frightening situation in your mind again and again until you can do so with little or no anxiety. Eventually you will be exposed to the real situation, but not until you are ready to do so.

Tod's obsessional thoughts, and the ritualistic, compulsive behaviour he had developed to protect him from the fear, need behavioural therapy and probably medication also.

Aromatherapy has an array of oils that could help. For phobias try lavender oil; sandalwood or marjoram will reduce the fear. Panic attacks may respond to lavender. Homeopathic remedies that you may like to try include Aconite for fear of dying and Ignatia where you find yourself with a changeable mood and gasping for breath. Bach Flower Remedies offer Aspen, Rock rose and Rescue Remedy for fear and panic. Red chestnut is good for fear, especially if it involves the possible loss of loved ones. However, for the best results, have a consultation with a therapist who will prescribe for you. Australian Bush Essences are similarly effective. Hypnotherapy, reflexology, acupressure, biofeedback and autogenic training are all useful.

Monica, 34, is highly regarded at work because she is so tidy and fastidious. However, she has recently been late for work on a number of occasions because she is unable to leave her flat without cleaning it from top to bottom at least 4 or 5 times. She is plagued by the idea that there is grease and dirt throughout the kitchen and that layers of dust lurk everywhere. It takes her several hours to complete her self-imposed task and she sets her alarm for 4 a.m. in order to try to leave by 8. As a result she is exhausted when she arrives for work, and is now threatened with the sack. Monica has obsessive–compulsive disorder.

Nutritional Healing

It's important to cut down on artificial stimulants including drinks and food containing caffeine (coffee, tea, canned fizzy drinks, chocolate) as well as refined sugars which cause a surge of blood glucose with a later slump. Drinks sweetened with aspartame can result in anxiety and even panic if you drink too much of them. Alcohol can also cause anxiety even though it may have an initial sedating action. Try keeping a food diary to see if there are any foodstuffs that result in an increase in anxiety (see food allergies and intolerance, p. 63). Adding 2–6 tablespoonfuls of flax seed (linseed) oil to your diet each day can have quite amazing effects upon anxiety including long-term panic and agoraphobia.

Herb teas, of which kava is perhaps the most useful, include chamomile, hops, passionflower and skullcap. Kava tea, either hot or iced, perhaps flavoured with some lemon or orange juice, has a calming action and can even promote sleep. Although it is nonaddictive, long-term use appears to cause dry skin and excessive amounts can cause a kind of intoxication. Valerian, also non-addictive, can help reduce anxiety and promote natural sleep; however, don't use it if you're pregnant or breastfeeding, or with prescribed anxiety medication. Unfortunately it smells awful!

Orthomolecular medicine

Two pioneering psychiatrists started to treat schizophrenia many years ago with Vitamin B_3. The method now offers hope of conquering phobias as well as other chronic mental and physical disorders and behavioural conditions. There are claims that it can help alleviate depression, obsessive–compulsive disorder, attention deficit hyperactivity disorder (ADHD) and autism. The process involves careful laboratory testing for nutrients and toxins, hormones, brain chemicals, etc., food allergies, candidiasis, metals, trace mineral deficiencies, amino acids and vitamins as well as hypoglycaemia and adrenal insufficiency. If you would like further information, contact the International Society for Orthomolecular Medicine, 16 Florence Avenue, Toronto, Ontario, Canada M2N 1E9; tel. (416) 733 2117; fax: (416) 733 2352; e-mail: centre@orthomed.org. Web address: www.orthomed.org.

The Outlook

Patients with anxieties and phobias may always remain natural worriers who are prone to being cautious and tense at certain times. But with ongoing support and a commitment to relaxation techniques they can all learn to live with their strong responses to stress.

Integrated approach

1. Remember anxiety can have beneficial as well as unpleasant effects.
2. Recognising the physical symptoms of anxiety is vital.
3. Practise coping strategies to limit the extent of your anxiety.
4. Avoid environmental or dietary stimulants.
5. Ensure adequate exercise and relaxation.
6. Use complementary therapies and nutritional supplements.
7. Consider behavioural (cognitive) therapy and graded exposure techniques.
8. Ask about beta blocker drugs and, as a very last resort, short-term tranquillisers.

Arthritis

Jean, in her late forties, came to the surgery complaining of pain and swelling in her right knee with pain also in her left hip joint. She explained that she had loved dancing as a young woman, and just recently had taken this up again as a hobby partly to help her lose some weight. Her knee had been a little sore after the first time, but she thought that it would improve with more exercise. Instead it had become increasingly worse and now she found it painful to walk or to negotiate stairs, and the pain would often wake her at night as she couldn't find a comfortable position. She had also noticed over the years crunching noises when she bent either knee, but until recently these hadn't been accompanied by pain. Jean has osteoarthritis.

Arthritis, or rheumatism as it is often called by the lay public, means many things to different people. Essentially, it is inflammation in a joint or many joints resulting in pain, stiffness and swelling. It can be the result of many causes and is not a single, straightforward condition. It may affect one joint or many joints simultaneously in the body. It may merely produce a temporary mild discomfort or a severe pain that gets worse over a period of time resulting in disability or deformity.

So common is arthritis that up to 25 per cent of all consultations with family doctors are made up of discussions revolving around a patient's rheumatological complaints. There has been a huge increase in the awareness of generalised conditions that can affect the onset and progression of rheumatic diseases, and at the same time there has been a huge rise in the number and complexity of diagnostic and therapeutic procedures that may be used to treat these conditions. Unfortunately, increasingly sophisticated and accurate technology has not always been matched by improvements in sympathetic attitudes or practical help from doctors.

Much research continues into finding stronger and more

powerful drugs to combat arthritis, all of which can produce serious side effects, but little thought has been given to the underlying causes. Even the commonest drugs that we use in treatment rectify the symptoms rather than the underlying problem. Yet rheumatoid arthritis, for example, is a relatively modern disease. As an ailment resulting in sometimes gross and very obvious joint deformity, it has never been found in the skeletons of Egyptian mummies and it has not been depicted in the paintings of the Great Masters during the Renaissance period. In fact, typical rheumatoid arthritis only began to emerge at the beginning of the twentieth century. This suggests that some new environmental factor may have arisen which stimulated its outbreak at that time. This may have been a micro-organism, but equally it could have been due to our changing diet or new substances around us in our immediate environment. Since so little is known about the underlying causes of the various forms of arthritis, orthodox doctors should be less dismissive of much of the useful work being carried out to explore some of the newer and more controversial treatments.

Paula, now 42, complains that her fingers are often stiff and swollen in the mornings, that she can no longer grip the lids of jars and that sometimes she needs aspirin or something equivalent to reduce the pain so that she can get on with her housework. She has noticed that the swellings at the joints of her fingers don't disappear even when the pain subsides, as it often does sometimes for weeks on end. She says that when she has a flare-up she feels weak and tired and sometimes has a fever. Paula has rheumatoid arthritis.

There are many different types of arthritis, but of all those seen in general and hospital practice the following are among the most common.

TRAUMATIC ARTHRITIS

This is the result of injury to a joint. It is therefore as common in the elderly who stumble and fall as it is in younger patients pursuing various sports as a leisure activity. A joint may be sprained resulting in damage to the ligaments around it, or the capsule which binds it; it may be dislocated, where the articular bone ends are disrupted from their normal position so that they cannot function properly; or there may even be a fracture through the joint resulting in bleeding into the joint space and the likelihood of secondary arthritis in later years.

OSTEOARTHRITIS

Generally known as degenerative or 'wear and tear' arthritis, this type of arthritis is extremely common in older people or in those who have had operations on, or severe injury to, their joints. Other factors such as metabolic diseases or infections may be responsible, and certainly there is a large genetic component which may make some families more vulnerable to it.

RHEUMATOID ARTHRITIS

This is the most severe kind of inflammatory arthritis and is the result of an autoimmune disorder. Here, the immune system for some reason recognises the joints as foreign in some way, and produces antibodies which work against the joints, damaging them and their surrounding soft tissue. Beginning in early middle age, mainly in women, the smaller joints of the wrists, ankles, hands and shoulders become extremely painful, swollen and stiff. The disorder may come and go in lapses and remissions, but more often than not, it is gradually progressive, resulting in some degree of disability and restriction of movement.

STILL'S DISEASE

This is a form of rheumatoid arthritis occurring in children mainly under the age of 4. It is otherwise known as juvenile rheumatoid arthritis. Although this generally settles down after a number of years (unlike adult rheumatoid arthritis), it can still leave a child with stunted growth and irreversible joint deformities which can threaten their quality of life.

Infective Arthritis

When bacteria find their way into the joint from an infected wound or the bloodstream, a septic or infective arthritis is produced. Generally the joints will be red and hot as well as swollen and painful. This type of arthritis may be the result of viral infections such as rubella and chickenpox, but can also be associated with rheumatic fever and some sexually transmitted diseases such as non-specific urethritis and gonorrhoea.

Gout

This disorder occurs due to a build-up of uric acid in the blood. This is one of the body's waste products and when it accumulates in the joints, it forms tiny crystals which mechanically irritate the sensitive lining of the joint producing intense pain, swelling and redness. Usually it only affects one joint at a time, in particular the large joint at the base of the big toe.

Sero-Negative Arthritis and SLE

This form of arthritis produces symptoms and signs similar to rheumatoid arthritis, although the classic blood test which is normally positive in the latter condition is negative. This type of rheumatism is often linked with skin disorders like psoriasis and inflammatory bowel diseases such as Crohn's disease.

Eva has a butterfly-shaped rash across her face and is obviously in pain with marked swellings of her hands and wrists. She says that she is stiff in most of her joints in the mornings, her knees, ankles and wrists being the worst. She feels constantly tired, has had a number of chronic infections and looks pale and anaemic. Eva has systemic lupus erythematosus (SLE or lupus).

ANKYLOSING SPONDYLITIS

In this condition the pelvic joints and the spine become inflamed resulting in fusion of the vertebrae and a very stiff ramrod spine known as 'Bamboo Spine'. Sometimes the hips and knees can be affected as well, and the disease is seen more commonly in men.

Critical Tests for Correct Diagnosis

Often the doctor may be able to make a diagnosis from what the patient says, and from the initial examination of the joints. The joints in the hand of a woman with typical rheumatoid arthritis, for example, are unmistakable and the distribution of joint inflammation is different in this condition than it is in osteoarthritis. Also, there may be other signs in distant parts of the body other than the joints which help the doctor to reach a conclusion. Rheumatoid arthritis is a generalised disease which may affect almost every organ of the body. Osteoarthritis on the other hand purely affects the joints.

Common tests include:

* X-rays, which may show degenerative changes, narrowing of the joint space suggestive of thinning of the articular cartilage, and reduced density as seen in osteoporosis (brittle bone disease) and rheumatoid arthritis.
* Blood tests can show the presence of proteins characteristic of rheumatoid arthritis, and high levels of uric acid which are diagnostic of gout. Another important blood test is the ESR (erythrocyte sedimentation rate) which, although not specific for any one disorder, indicates general inflammation and the degree of disease activity.
* Another commonly conducted test is an aspiration of fluid from the swollen joint which allows the fluid to be examined microscopically for the presence of germs, uric acid crystals or other abnormal constituents.
* Bone isotope scans, MRI scans and CT scans may also be used to look in more detail at bones and the soft tissue

around them and these are often used in sciatica to detect nerve entrapment around the spine or in patients whose symptoms are suggestive of more serious bone disorders such as cancers.

* Finally, surgical procedures such as arthroscopy are sometimes carried out diagnostically. Here, a narrow arthroscope is inserted into the joint space under illumination to look for particles of cartilage floating free within the fluid, or a torn cartilage which remains attached to the joint lining but which is preventing normal joint function.

Prevention

Despite our improved understanding of the various conditions leading to arthritis, we still pay scant attention to looking after our musculoskeletal system, and our joints in particular. And we are still no nearer to knowing the exact cause of autoimmune types of arthritis such as rheumatoid disease. Lower back pain and slipped discs are almost endemic in our society today, yet very few people bother to adjust their lifestyle to prevent these common problems occurring. The cost to the health service and to industry as a result of back pain is enormous, quite apart from the cost in terms of human misery and discomfort. If only people were able to keep their muscles stronger and to correct poor posture at an early stage, many patients who have been crippled by arthritis could have enjoyed an active and pain-free existence. Even young, fit athletes who should know better take short cuts and strain their joints often irretrievably.

There is a tendency for doctors to seize upon their potent pills and anti-inflammatory medications as soon as the patient walks through the door with a painful joint, but advice about whether to rest a joint or whether to exercise it is vital because if you have taken the wrong option, you can clearly make matters worse. A few general points of advice would be:

* The muscle should always be kept strong through active exercise or passive physiotherapy, as these maintain the integrity of the joints whose movement they control.

* An acutely inflamed joint should generally be rested whereas a cold stiff osteoarthritis joint should be exercised with non-weight-bearing activity to lubricate it.
* Splinting the joints is useful when they are acutely inflamed, and any patient with arthritis in weight-bearing joints should be helped to lose weight in order to reduce some of the pressure and strain in those areas.
* Finally, patients should be given a realistic idea of the outlook of their condition. It is better for a middle-aged footballer with osteoarthritis to know that excessive training could make things worse and it seems kinder to encourage a young woman with rheumatoid arthritis to be realistic about her future, and to come to terms with the fact that she may have to curtail her lifestyle to accommodate her arthritis. But in all forms of disability there is much that can be done to keep the patient thinking positively and constructively.

BLOOD TYPE AND ARTHRITIS

There is some interesting work being done on blood type and arthritis. Those with blood group A are more likely to have rheumatoid arthritis and to benefit from a strictly vegetarian diet. Those with blood group B are more prone to osteoarthritis and will do well with fish and a vegetarian diet. Blood groups O and AB need a more individual approach to diet.

Conventional Treatment

The orthodox treatment of arthritis is entirely dependent on the individual type of arthritis. In traumatic arthritis, for example, treatment is largely based on the mnemonic RICE, standing for Rest, Ice, Compression and Elevation. The joint is rested to prevent further inflammation, ice is applied, compression bandages are put in place, and the joint is elevated in order to discourage further swelling. All forms of arthritis respond to anti-inflammatory medications, but stronger drugs such as steroids and gold injections may be used for autoimmune rheumatoid arthritis. Antibiotics would be used for septic arthritis and allopurinol is the best treatment for gout. In cases where progressive arthritis has produced deformities in joints and disability, two surgical procedures are commonly performed which can relieve discomfort and improve function. These are arthroplasty where the joint is replaced with an artificial substitute, and arthrodesis where the bones in the joint are fused together. This obviously reduces function but it has the benefit of eradicating pain totally.

Nutritional Healing

Research at the National Rheumatism Hospital in Norway showed that grip strength improved and pain, swelling, morning stiffness and tenderness were reduced in patients with chronic arthritic symptoms within only a month of starting to eat a vegetarian diet. Some people appear to have an allergic form of arthritis where certain foods seem to be toxic and provoke attacks. Elimination of food substances one by one can often pinpoint such triggers. Beef, meat products such as bacon and sausage, and dairy products are often the culprits. Why not keep a food diary along with a separate entry when you have a flare-up. That way you can pinpoint a pattern if there is one and start to eliminate foods in a sensible fashion. The basic eating plan suggests plenty of fish and seafood, rich in omega-3 fatty acids which can reduce inflammation in rheumatoid arthritis and gout as well as in SLE. Three to five servings weekly would be good. The bonus is that this can also have a preventive effect for heart attack, stroke and cancer. However, you should avoid mackerel and herring (see below). You may well see results in terms of reduction in inflammation within a month and may be able to come off your anti-inflammatory medication eventually without risking exacerbation. As always, please discuss any changes in medication with your doctor.

Low-purine foods are helpful in gout. These include rice, millet, starchy and green vegetables, fruit (especially cherries), cheese, eggs, nuts and milk. Celery is particularly good since it helps mobilise toxic products from the joints (see p. 103). High-purine foods which are best avoided are meat and meat extracts, sausage and other meat products, alcohol, yeast and yeast extracts (Marmite) and some seafood including mackerel, herring, anchovies, mussles, roe, sardines and scallops. Moderate-purine foods which you should be wary of but can have occasionally if you really like them are fish other than those listed above, chicken, peas and beans, mushrooms, asparagus, cauliflower, lentils, spinach, whole wheat and oatmeal. Garlic and onions reduce inflammation and should be taken daily. Pineapple juice and star fruit juice will help the swelling, and cabbage and carrot juice can reduce joint pain. Soya and avocado have been cited as relieving pain and improving joint function. Avoiding tea, coffee, tobacco, salt, food additives and preservatives will benefit inflammation.

Vitamins and Supplements

Glucosamine sulphate, an amino acid and derivative of glucose, is one of the essential building blocks in the production of both cartilage and connective tissue and is the supplement to take, although unfortunately it's quite expensive. It's fundamental to the maintenance of both the strength and the shock-absorption of our joints and not only does it significantly reduce pain and stiffness, but unlike other pain-relieving drugs, it promotes actual healing and helps restore function. Chondroitin sulphate (also expensive) appears to be less effective but is nevertheless worth a try. Sometimes they're found in combination but we haven't seen any research that shows this offers great benefit over glucosamine alone.

Cetyl myristeolate is the new kid on the block and is a natural immunity factor produced by some animals including mice, sperm whales and beavers. It's still undergoing investigation but seems to hold promise. Enzymes are an effective adjunct to other therapy and in some cases can replace anti-inflammatories. Immune complexes circulating in the bloodstream are often the cause of inflammation in SLE and other autoimmune diseases. Enzymes help by dissolving these while also protecting the kidneys from complications associated with this debilitating illness.

The humble pineapple contains bromelain which is a potent anti-inflammatory equalling aspirin in its ability to reduce inflammation in rheumatoid arthritis. There are studies which show that bromelain has been able to reduce pain and swelling in cases where even steroids have failed! And all this without side effects! It's important that it's absorbed properly, so bromelain tablets need to be enteric-coated so that they're absorbed from lower down in the intestine and not from the stomach. Enzymes are available in combinations of bromelain, papain, trypsin, chymotrypsin and pancreatin. Turmeric (curcumin), used daily by many Asians as an ingredient of curry, is a potent anti-inflammatory which is not only useful in arthritis but has also been shown to be useful for post-operative pain and inflammation as well as for AIDS. It can be purchased as a supplement, but adding delicious curries to your diet will also help. Capsaicin (found in red peppers) causes a reduction in the serum levels of prostaglandins which can cause inflammation of joints and, over time, destroy them.

Methylsulphonylmethane (MSM), a supplement with a long history going back some 30 years, has great potential for healing joints and reducing pain. It was shunned originally because it left users smelling of sulphur (not very nice!) but in newer products that problem seems to have been overcome and it's just undergoing a revival. You can take it as a supplement or even buy a cream to apply locally. Ginger can be effective against rheumatoid arthritis by breaking down inflammatory proteins, easing pain, reducing swelling and stiffness and helping mobility.

The last weapon in the supplement armamentarium is the antioxidant which mops up free radicals, reduces inflammation and swelling but also prevents further damage. Vitamins C and E, flax seed (linseed) oil and beta carotene are the most important. (See p. 163 for more on antioxidants.) In gout, Vitamin C helps mobilise the uric acid from the tissues and encourage its excretion via the kidneys, thus limiting damage and pain. Sometimes if uric acid is mobilised quickly, there can be an exacerbation. You can limit this by building up the dose of Vitamin C slowly when you begin – starting say with 500 mg daily and increasing over about a week or 10 days to 3000 mg daily. Adding folic acid (folate) will also slow down the liberation of uric acid and help prevent a flare-up. Minerals are essential for healthy bone and cartilage and also for supporting the immune system, while grapeseed extract will strengthen collagen in ligaments.

Exercise and Lifestyle

If your already compromised joints are carrying around too much weight, then of course they're going to hurt more and suffer more damage. So losing some weight is often essential, especially if you're affected in the larger weight-bearing joints such as knees and hips. Also keeping joints flexible and supple is important. If you haven't exercised for a long time, take it easy and always do some stretching while your muscles get warmed up and again before you finish your routine. In fact for some people, stretching is even more important than the rest of the exercise programme.

Yoga and pilates are particularly good since the accent is on stretching the muscles and therefore helping your joints in a gentle but very effective way. Yoga also puts an accent on breathing and aligning mind, body and spirit. You may think yoga is impossible for you if you feel stiff and painful. Look for a good teacher who will lead you gently at your own pace and help you regain some flexibility. You'll be amazed at the improvement not only in your flexibility but in your general level of stress and reduction in pain (see p. 481).

Complementary Therapies

As long ago as the late 1970s there was a collaborative study in Glasgow involving the Homeopathic Hospital, the University Medical School, the Centre for Rheumatic Diseases and the Royal Infirmary, looking at the use of homeopathy in arthritis. The conventionalists had to agree that the results in favour of homeopathy were significant. The following remedies heal from the inside out and have a long-lasting benefit:

Apis mel – where there is red, shiny swelling as in gout.
Rhus tox – where there is physical pain and stiffness which are relieved a little when you do a bit of exercise and get moving.
Dulcamara – for rheumatism which is worse in cold damp weather.
Pulsatilla – when the pain is fleeting, affecting one joint after another.
Colchicum – also good for gout.

Other remedies specifically for gout include Belladonna and Arnica, Rhododendron where joints are worse in the mornings and Calc carb, where there is worsening in cold and damp. Do get some advice from a homeopath.

Celery seed extract can be great for all arthritic pain including gout. It gets rid of the toxins in the joints, has a soothing and mildly tranquillising effect. Take 4–6 ml of celery seed tincture 3 times a day. Gravelroot can also be helpful. Drink at least 8 glasses of water daily to flush the toxins out once they are released. Aloe vera will help detoxify your whole system including your joints and boswellia acts like a non-steroidal anti-inflammatory (NSAI) agent. Prickly ash gets rid of deposits in joints and yucca is good for rheumatoid arthritis.

Reflexology and aromatherapy also have a part to play. Rosemary oil will stimulate circulation, chamomile is soothing and lavender will ease pain and promote relaxation. Better still, treat yourself to a consultation with a good therapist who will blend oils especially for you. Acupuncture, acupressure, osteopathy and chiropractic could be helpful too, and Alexander Technique will improve your posture and reduce the possibility of deformity. Detoxification by chelation removes heavy metals and plaque from your gut and colonic irrigation can help reduce inflammation. Reconstructive therapy involves the injection of Vitamin C, glutathione, shark cartilage and other potent nutrients directly into the ligaments and cartilage of affected joints to help rebuild and strengthen the joint. Obviously this is a highly skilled procedure and only available in some centres.

Emotional and Spiritual Healing

Not only can emotional and spiritual healing help the pain and in some cases reverse radiological evidence of arthritis, but it will also reduce your stress levels. Stiffness, especially in the lower limbs, can be the result of a blocked second chakra and doing some work on this will usually help. See *The Rainbow Journey* for exercises and meditations to help here. Meditation should become part of your daily routine to help reduce stress. (See the Basics for Good Living, p. 4). There is of course a great deal of emotional difficulty surrounding chronic pain. Depression is a not uncommon companion of physical illness that involves pain and loss of function. You may wish to see a counsellor to help you with this.

INTEGRATED APPROACH

1. Protect your musculoskeletal system through careful regular exercise and good posture.
2. Moderate your weight.
3. Report symptoms early and pinpoint the exact diagnosis.
4. Experiment with nutritional changes and supplements.
5. Try appropriate complementary therapies.
6. Consider physiotherapy, osteopathy, chiropractic and yoga as essential but non-invasive physical treatments.
7. Use pharmaceutical medications with caution.
8. Embrace modern surgical techniques warmly when offered, as pain, immobility and swelling can often be eradicated in individual joints.

Asthma

Peter, aged 7, developed a persistent dry cough at night which continued for month after month. During the day he was fine except for when he played football in the playground at school. This proved particularly troublesome during the winter on especially cold days. The first two doctors he saw examined him but found nothing. The third doctor, who had a special interest in asthma, correctly diagnosed the condition, which of course only showed signs during the night and when Peter exercised but not at other times. His mild asthma is now well controlled with a preventative inhaler.

Asthma causes repeated attacks of wheezy breathlessness which come and go and which vary in severity from day to day and even hour to hour. It affects children and adults alike. Many factors are capable of triggering the symptoms, notably allergies, infections and vigorous exercise in cold air, but the underlying response is the same. The lining of the small air passages in the lungs becomes inflamed, resulting in constriction of the muscle in the walls of the air passages which then become progressively narrowed. In addition, mucus is produced by cells lining the tubes, restricting the airflow even further.

There are two main types of asthma: 'extrinsic' in which an allergy is usually to blame, and 'intrinsic' where there is no obvious external cause for the condition.

Common, and becoming more common

About 5 per cent of the total population suffers from asthma, but in children of primary school age, up to 15 per cent are affected. Although slowing somewhat now, the rate of increase in asthma has been alarming with a fivefold increase in sufferers seeking help from their doctors between the mid 1970s and the early 1990s.

Currently, more than 3 million people in England and Wales alone have asthma with boys apparently twice as affected as girls, although the ratio is reversed in adulthood.

Trigger Factors

Asthma often runs in families along with hay fever and eczema. Other than the genes that the sufferer inherits, maternal smoking during pregnancy, passive smoking in childhood and exposure to allergens at a young age may contribute to the onset of asthma. Viruses and other infectious agents and exposure to certain occupational hazards such as antibiotics in drug manufacturing or flour in bakeries may be to blame. Once the condition has developed, a number of trigger factors can start an acute attack. These include inhaled allergens such as pollen and moulds, fur and fluff from domestic pets, exercising in cold air, food additivies, strong emotion or stress, environmental pollution, dust and fumes, house dust and house dust mite.

Signs and Symptoms

In children the first signs of asthma may merely be a persistent nocturnal cough where no infection is present. In adults wheezing, breathlessness and tightness of the chest are the commonest symptoms although children can suffer from these as well. The severity of the attack varies greatly, with some people only developing mild symptoms when they exercise vigorously while others remain quite incapacitated most of the time. In severe episodes the amount of oxygen in the bloodstream may be seriously reduced resulting in blue cheeks and lips, a pale sweaty skin and obvious anxiety.

Clive, aged 82, has been having bouts of breathlessness for 6 months. Sometimes they come on by themselves, but at other times they only arise when he goes for a walk or climbs stairs. After heart disease was ruled out by the doctor, he was given anti-asthma medication which resulted in dramatic improvement in his symptoms. He is a typical example of late-onset asthma, and its appropriate treatment soon restored his quality of life.

Preventative Treatment

There is a lot the family of an asthmatic can do to help reduce the severity and the frequency of the attacks. One of the most important measures is to try to control levels of house dust mites which exist in all homes throughout the country, however tidy and clean they may be. Special covers for mattresses and pillows impenetrable to the house dust mites, are effective but costly, and special sprays to kill the mites rarely control asthma symptoms when used alone. Ideally all soft furnishings should be kept to a minimum. Carpets should be removed from bedrooms and replaced with wooden or linoleum flooring, curtains can be replaced by blinds, and cuddly toys, in which house dust mites thrive, can be 'treated' as it were by being deep-frozen in the freezer overnight once a week. Warm air from central heating tends to make matters worse, so humidification of bedroom air is important and those people with severe asthma who are always made worse by coming into contact with a pet may need to consider parting with it, however much of an emotional wrench that might be. Passive and active smoking should be strongly discouraged, and anyone whose symptoms only begin when they exercise will be helped by having a good warm-up period before embarking on the vigorous activity. Asthmatic children will find that, provided their teachers understand that the need for immediate access to treatment is sometimes necessary, severe bouts of asthma can be avoided.

Conventional Treatment

There are three main types of medication used in the treatment of asthma, namely preventers, relievers and emergency drugs.

PREVENTERS

These reduce inflammation in the air passages and stop them being so sensitive to airborne allergens and other trigger factors. They need to be taken on a regular basis and their effect is gradual and slow. They usually come as inhalers in small aerosols and include steroids, sodium cromoglycate and nedocromil. Despite various myths and scare stories associated with the inhaled steroids, they are generally extremely effective preventative drugs in all patients with asthma, and are probably the most effective preventative treatment of all in these patients. Cromoglycate is often used when exercise is the main trigger factor for asthma. One other type of preventer is theophylline, a group of drugs which can be given in liquid form to children, and in tablet or intravenous form in adults.

Relievers

Reliever drugs work by relaxing the muscle in the walls of the air passages allowing them to open up again so that air gets in and out more easily. These are called bronchodilators and again are usually given in inhaled form. They are often used only when symptoms occur rather than all the time, although some asthmatics need daily doses of both reliever and preventer medication.

Inhaler techniques

A critical factor in the effectiveness of inhaled drugs is the technique that is used by the patient. The medication has no effect unless the drug reaches the lower part of the bronchial tree, and in order for this to occur, activation of the inhaler device must coincide with inspiration. This technique can usually be quickly taught and learnt, although some children continue to have difficulty with it. For them, special delivery devices can make life a great deal easier. Spacers are made from see-through plastic and act as a reservoir for the drug when the inhaler is sprayed into one end and the patient breathes in and out normally from the other. Other sorts of breath-activated devices include turbo-halers, disc-halers and rota-halers (see picture).

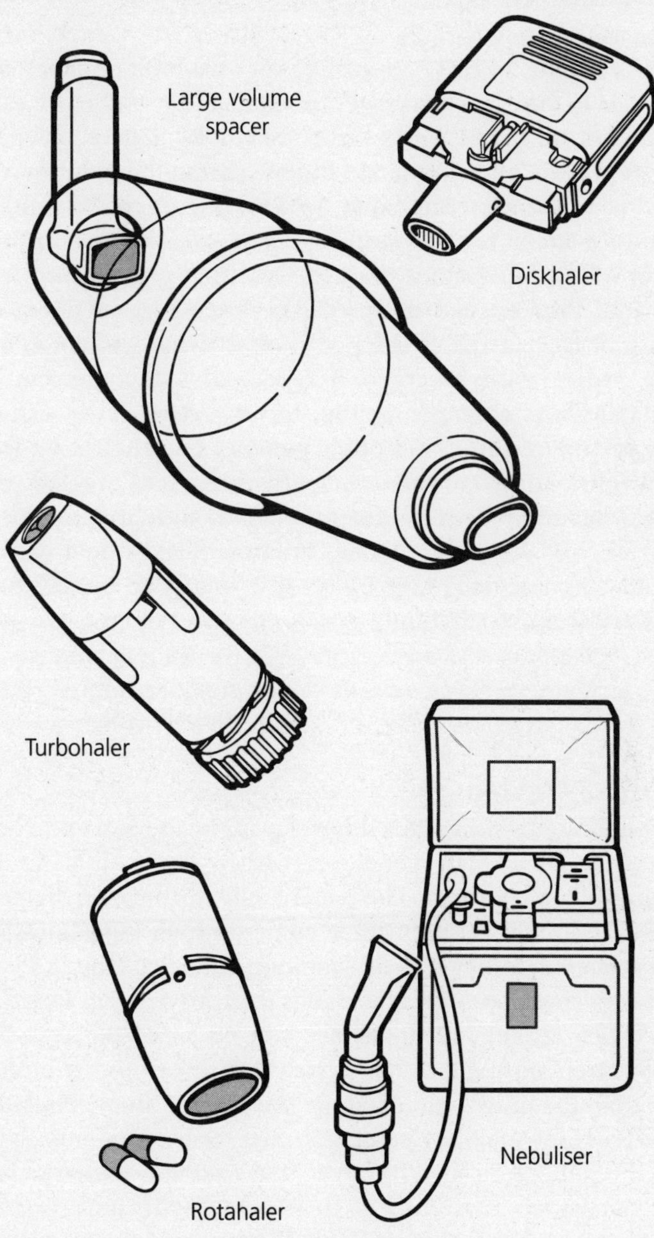

Asthma Delivery Devices

EMERGENCY DRUGS

In the emergency treatment of a severe acute attack, larger doses of a reliever drug as well as an anti-inflammatory preventer drug may be given together. For swifter and more effective action, a 'nebuliser' is sometimes used. This is a type of air compressor allowing air to bubble through a solution of a drug, producing a fine mist which can then be inhaled through a mask or a mouthpiece. The mist consists of very tiny droplets, much finer than those which are expelled from a normal inhaler, and it penetrates much further down the bronchial tree to reach the parts other drugs cannot reach. Some people with severe and recurrent symptoms borrow their nebuliser either from the doctor's surgery or asthma clinic at the hospital, and other patients buy their own from the chemist. In severe cases the patient may fail to respond to these usual methods of treatment and may need to be admitted to hospital as soon as possible. Treatment may then include oxygen therapy, oral steroids and possibly an intravenous injection of aminophylline, one of the theophylline group of drugs. The worst-case scenario is that the patient may be put on a ventilator to force oxygen under pressure into the lungs until the constriction in the airways can be reversed.

Positive Thinking

The whole aim of treating asthma is to allow the patient to be in control of their own condition rather than allowing the asthma to control them. The patient, the doctor and the practice nurse should between them come up with guidelines that the patient can follow if their condition changes. Many GP surgeries run specialised asthma clinics that provide constant help and advice. Treatment guidelines can be based on peak-flow measurements using a simple device that measures the outflow of air from the lungs on maximum forced respiratory exhalation (peak flow), or may be symptom-based, depending entirely on how the patient feels. Whichever way, asthma patients these days can become monitors of their own health and certainly remain the best judges of the level of severity of their condition at any one time. One critical factor is to recognise instantly when the asthma symptoms are out of control despite normal treatment, and are in need of professional reassessment. That mild to moderate asthma need not hold people back in their chosen lives and careers is amply borne out by the fact that many of our top athletes have won medals even in Olympic competitions despite being vulnerable to asthma. Positive attitude and an unwillingness to tolerate poor control of this preventable and treatable condition is essential.

TEN TOP TIPS FOR PREVENTING ASTHMA

1. Deprive house dust mites of moisture and humidity. Air all bedding and linen, open windows and ventilate the bathroom and kitchen when cooking, washing and bathing.
2. Keep dust to a minimum. Clean surfaces with a damp cloth and vacuum-clean all soft furnishings.
3. Wash bedlinen in a hot wash over 60°C to kill mites.
4. Enclose mattresses, pillows and duvets with special microporous membrane covers.
5. Remove bedroom carpets and have wooden, lino or cork tile flooring instead.
6. Use a high-efficiency filter-style vacuum cleaner.
7. Put children's soft toys in the deep freeze for 12 hours every week.
8. Use dehumidifiers and mechanical ventilation in the home.
9. Consider finding a new home for your domestic pet.
10. Avoid any contact with cigarette smoke anywhere in the home.

Nutritional Healing

Damage by free radicals – which can be produced from pollutants such as smoke, exhaust fumes, metabolism, ultraviolet light and the by-products of fighting infection – is a major factor in all illness, but none more so than in asthma where free radicals can cause restriction of the bronchial passages. Antioxidants can mop up these free radicals as they are formed and therefore prevent further damage. Fruit and vegetables are rich sources of antioxidants such as Vitamins C and E, beta carotene and lycopene. The basic eating plan (see p. 5) should give you most of what you need, although supplements would certainly enhance your diet. Eat plenty of onions and garlic. Dairy produce can cause a lot of mucus in some people. Try using goat's milk and products, sheep's yogurt or soya milk instead. Lowering your salt intake can decrease the frequency and severity of attacks. Food sensitivities may precipitate or exacerbate attacks and it might be worth considering a diet that is vegan with the addition of fatty fish such as salmon, herring, mackerel and tuna for 4 weeks and then reintroducing foodstuffs carefully, keeping a diary of any symptoms that occur. Taking a teaspoonful of honey every day can help too. Do check the label to make sure it is cold-extracted honey as it loses some of its benefit when heated and, according to Ayurvedic medicine, can also clog the system.

Vitamins and Supplements

There's some interesting research on the role of Vitamin B_6 in asthma. It's essential in the metabolic processes of serotonin and a dearth of it may allow serotonin to cause the airways to constrict. Supplements seem less effective in those who are constantly taking steroids but most helpful in children and others using theophylline. All the B vitamins are useful in reducing the stress that having such an illness inevitably causes. Other vitamins and minerals are important, especially magnesium, and a multivitamin/multimineral tablet daily would be wise. There is much exciting research about green tea and adding a couple of cups each day to your diet could have marked benefits.

Exercise and Lifestyle

Exercise strengthens the cardiovascular system and also promotes good respiratory function. Lifting weights can help strengthen chest muscles and not only will you look and feel better, but you will develop more power in your chest wall to help those breathing exercises when you need them. Yoga is a brilliant form of exercise for asthma sufferers. Not only does it teach you essential breathing techniques, but it also strengthens your body, keeps your muscles flexible (including those necessary for breathing) and promotes relaxation and natural healing.

Have a look at the stress in your life and how you can reduce it (see p. 481). Although some stress is a normal part of daily life, many of us live with unnecessary stress simply because we don't stop to challenge it. Just stop occasionally and see what you could offload to make your life more manageable.

Plants in your home, especially spider plants and peace lilies, can reduce pollution considerably rather in the way that trees help reduce the harmful effects of exhaust fumes. Just a word for menopausal women. There is a suggestion that women taking HRT are 50 per cent more likely than others to develop adult-onset asthma.

Complementary Therapies

The good news is that there are many complementary techniques that can help with this illness. It might be wise to choose something from each therapy and experiment with it rather than trying too many things and not knowing what it was that really helped.

The herbs that you could choose from include ginkgo biloba, garlic, liquorice, aloe and eucalyptus, all of which reduce mucus production and can therefore be useful as daily additions to your regime. Ginger and peppermint inhibit lung inflammation and, along with garlic, are natural antihistamines that help counteract allergic reactions and reduce both the frequency and severity of asthma attacks. Cayenne also makes the respiratory system less sensitive to infection and irritants. Ma Huang (Ephedra) is a natural bronchodilator.

Have a look at the section on allergies since some of the aromatherapy oils recommended there will help you. In particular, eucalyptus will help keep the airways open and is also antiviral and expectorant, while lavender will relax you and prevent panic from adding to the difficulties of breathing.

An aromatherapist may blend for you oils such as clove, cinnamon, melissa (lemon balm) and lavender which have been found to be very effective in respiratory conditions, especially where there is secondary infection. Acupuncture and Ayurvedic medicine could be useful too.

Emotional and Spiritual Healing

Spiritual healing can be effective both in the acute and the non-acute phases, and you may like to do some work on both your heart chakra and your throat since both of them can be linked with respiratory disorders and breathing difficulties. Clearing away any blocks that you have developed will help give you a free flow of your own healing energy. Learning to visualise light entering into your tissues, cleansing, healing and balancing them, will also help relax you when you do have an attack. When doing your breathing execises see the air entering your lungs as healing light opening the tubes and clearing passages. Learning to deal with an attack in fantasy while in a healing session or under hypnosis can have a marked effect when a real attack occurs. It's possible that in a session with either your healer or hypnotherapist you may become aware of the root cause of the problem and in some cases the disease can disappear completely. Be sure you choose a good therapist who is accredited (see p. 16) and don't give up after only a couple of sessions. Your therapist should be aware of your illness and be able to deal with you should you have an attack.

BREATHING TECHNIQUES

A bit like prenatal exercise which ensures that when you need it, you can do it, breathing exercises are essential for the asthma sufferer. Partners and close relatives or supporters can help you to be prepared in advance and to be able to slip directly into attack mode when necessary. Just quieting your breathing and counting it slowly will help not only with oxygen intake but with the anxiety that is precipitated by an attack. Breathe in slowly to a count of 8, have a short pause for a count of 2 and then out to a count of 8 while all the time visualising the air passages being open and free. If you can't manage a count of 8, don't worry and don't push it. Start with 4 or whatever you can cope with. Practise feeling your breath in various parts of your body. Look at what happens when you move your body. Notice that as you stretch you inhale and that you draw in more air than usual. See that moving your arms up one at a time increases the amount of air you inhale. Put your hands on your ribs and breathe in. What does it feel like? Can you make your ribs lift even further as you inhale? Then put your hands on your back at the bottom of your ribs. Does it feel different there? What about if you put your hands on your abdomen? Or stand on your toes? Or stand with your feet flat but with your whole weight sitting in your pelvis with your knees just slightly bent? Or lie back in your chair with your heels on the ground and your toes pointing up? All of these will make you more aware of your breathing and how the position of your body can quite dramatically affect the amount of oxygen available to you.

Then look at the rate of your breathing. What happens to your mood as you slow your breathing and make it more deep and regular? See how anxiety settles and you enter into a deep calm place within yourself. Your breathing becomes more efficient as your brain and all your tissues respond to the soothing rhythm and the extra oxygen. It is difficult to remain angry, anxious and upset while breathing slowly. Exhaling is usually automatic as your chest relaxes and your lungs are therefore squeezed gently by your chest wall. But you can learn to actively squeeze out a bit more air which will in turn result in increasing the capacity for more fresh air to come in.

Obviously clean pollutant-free air is essential for you, so if you live in the city or other polluted area you might like to invest in a face mask. Don't let anyone smoke anywhere near you and think about the possibility of investing in a clean air machine or an air filter.

INTEGRATED APPROACH

1. See your GP and, if necessary, someone with a special interest in asthma.
2. Observe triggers and avoid or reduce them as much as possible.
3. Eat a good healthy diet with lots of fruit and vegetables and take supplements as necessary.
4. Reduce salt in your diet.
5. Learn breathing exercises and practise them regularly.
6. Exercise regularly with a gentle warm-up.
7. Think positively.
8. Have good ventilation at home, at work and in your car.
9. Avoid smokey or other polluted atmospheres.
10. Reduce house dust mite levels in your home.
11. Use complementary techniques but always respect your illness and use medication as necessary.
12. Do not accept continual breathlessness or wheezing. These represent inadequate treatment.

Attention Deficit Hyperactivity Disorder (ADHD)

Chris, aged 2 and a half, was reported as being uncontrollable at the nursery. The staff simply could not cope with his tantrums, his bullying, his incredible restlessness and his inability to stay with any one task or game for more than a few moments. He was soon banned from the nursery, much to the displeasure of his parents who were made to feel irresponsible and inadequate. They also had to deal with his disruption at home. Chris's mental age remained at two thirds of the level it should have been while his educational standard suffered considerably, until he was diagnosed and treated as a normal child with attention deficit hyperactivity disorder.

Contrary to popular belief, ADHD is not a new diagnosis: it was first described nearly 100 years ago, although at that time it was referred to simply as hyperactivity. Many normal children who are just overactive and energetic have been falsely labelled hyperactive, and much confusion has arisen due to misleading media coverage suggesting that hyperactive children are difficult and naughty. Thankfully we now know an awful lot more about this condition and many of its associated myths can be dispelled. ADHD refers to a slight but demonstrable difference in brain function which causes a clever child to academically underachieve and to behave badly despite receiving caring and adequate parenting. While it is true to say that we hear more about this condition these days, it has not increased in frequency; rather, the medical profession has become more skilful at recognising it and diagnosing it correctly.

Between 2 and 5 per cent of all children are said to be affected by ADHD, which is thought to be due to a minor brain dysfunction resulting in differences in the fine tuning of the normal brain and which is referred to in the United States as 'minimal brain damage'. An imbalance in the brain's neurotransmitters noradrenalin and dopamine are likely to be responsible, and it is these substances which allow a normal brain to inhibit any tendency to hyperactive behaviour. In fact, areas of brain dysfunction can now be demonstrated using the latest brain-scanning techniques such as MRI and PET.

Symptoms

Children with ADHD exhibit two types of symptom, namely hyperactive impulsive behaviour and attention deficit learning weakness. The former results in fidgeting, restlessness, being excessively noisy and always on the go and talking incessantly. Affected children are impulsive, show impatience and intolerance and are easily frustrated. In the latter, their inattention causes difficulty in concentrating, they cannot give close attention to details, they fail to finish school work or simple chores, and they are forgetful and easily distracted. Physically they may be clumsy and accident prone. As they grow older the compulsive behaviour tends to improve although the learning and organisational problems may continue. ADHD is a strongly hereditary condition with most affected children having a close relative who has also suffered. It is mostly seen in boys who are 6 times more likely to be referred than girls.

The consequences for education

Max, aged 3, had always had a problem sleeping, refusing to go to bed much before 10 p.m. and remaining awake until the early hours and then frequently waking until rising full of energy just before 6. He exhausted his parents not only with this but also with his energetic and boisterous behaviour during the day. Some family therapy plus a behavioural therapy programme and a parent effectiveness course worked wonders for regaining control over Max's problem. His parents also found that eliminating food additives and colourings from his diet seemed to improve matters. Max settled after the age of 4 and did well at school.

If untreated, the condition can affect a child's learning right through their school years, although the problem first starts to come to the parents' attention somewhere between the ages of 2 and 3. Teachers often notice the disorder in children (provided they have been trained to recognise it), as characteristically the child will rush through their work, fidget and squirm in the class, call out inappropriately, take a long time to settle after a break and constantly fail to check work before it is handed in. Clearly this can affect their education in the future, especially as the condition is also associated with specific learning disabilities such as dyslexia.

It is vital to recognise ADHD since otherwise teachers who have not been trained to do so will label the child naughty and disruptive. Parents and teachers alike can find such children difficult or impossible to manage and may easily become excessively punitive. Excessive use of force and hostility then leads to resentment which unfortunately sows the seeds of irretrievable relationship problems. Because ADHD children overreact to taunting, they are often sought out by school bullies, and later blamed for the fracas that follows. A child's home life and environment should not be blamed for the condition, but it can certainly have an important bearing on the severity of the condition and its outcome. A devoted and talented teacher and a parent who is patient to the point of being saintly may be able to deal with the problem without need for treatment. Most ADHA sufferers, however, will need professional help and this involves behavioural advice, constant support at school and sometimes the use of stimulant medication.

Adequate information and advice to parents and teachers alike is vital. Generally speaking, society is encouraged to believe that children who behave badly have inadequate parents. In ADHD, however, it is the difficult child who is responsible for making competent, perfectly adequate parents seem at fault. Clearly there is much overlap between a normal energetic and fractious child and a child who has mild ADHD. Other causes of bad behaviour must be eliminated and care taken to ensure a correct diagnosis. Many ADHD children will need thorough educational assessment and many will require specialised help with reading and spelling. The stresses on parents and siblings must be addressed and many useful pointers can be given to achieve better behaviour through practical solutions. Dietary changes have often been suggested as part of the treatment although food intolerance rarely causes ADHD to develop per se. Some artificial colourings and preservatives can, however, make things worse, and clinical ecologists and allergists may be able to help in providing elimination diets to try in the hope of improving matters.

Stimulant Medication

This is central to the treatment of ADHD. The latest research suggests that without first priming the child with medication, other techniques such as educational and psychological treatments are relatively ineffective. Stimulants enable the child to focus, to listen and to be reached. Current medical thinking believes that before you can teach a child, you have to reach a child. The stimulants Ritalin and dexamphetamine have been used for some 40 years and over 150 controlled scientific trials have shown their benefit as well as their safety. When used correctly they are remarkably free of side effects and 85 per cent of ADHD children will be helped in the short term by one of these stimulants. Contrary to certain fears expressed in the media, there is no evidence to suggest that the use of amphetamine-type drugs leads in later years, to substance abuse or addiction in sufferers. Clearly this type of medication should only be given after a full explanation to the parents, and this will include pointing out that there is a major risk of failing to treat the child adequately in the first place. These drugs work by stimulating the mid-brain, which otherwise remains underactive and fails to damp down or control movements or sensations felt in the rest of the brain. When the mid-brain is stimulated, this extra activity is suppressed and the child becomes better able to concentrate, focus and learn.

Low-allergen diet

This should be followed for 4 weeks only, while keeping a journal of any changes in behaviour, attention, concentration, learning, etc. After 4 weeks, add one food at a time, give at least one portion a day and leave 5 to 7 days before adding another item. This way you will be able to see at a glance what causes the problem. In all cases when the diet is finally settled, rotate food items regularly, not repeating things more than every few days if possible.

2 meats.
2 carbohydrates (e.g. potatoes and rice).
2 fruits.
Vegetables (choose a good selection, e.g. cabbage, sprouts, cauliflower, broccoli, cucumber, celery, carrots).
Water.
Multivitamin/multimineral supplement.

Nutritional Healing, Vitamins and Supplements

The role of food dyes and additives in the development and exacerbation of ADHD has been hotly debated over the last 25 years. Several large food companies in the United States have funded research on the matter and have usually come up with results that tend to exonerate their products. However, some would say that their methodology is suspect and that closer examination of the results would lead one to a different conclusion. There is unequivocal evidence that at least one food colouring, tartrazine, does exacerbate the hyperactive behaviour in many children. In some children sucrose (sugar) also causes restlessness, agitation, irritability and disturbed behaviour when taken in large quantities, probably due to the sucrose precipitating an increase in adrenalin secretion. Glucose tolerance tests reveal that 74 per cent of hyperactive children have an abnormal result.

Food sensitivities have been generally dismissed in this country as a possible cause or exacerbating factor. However, there is evidence from Australian research that elimination diets in hyperactive children can have dramatic results on their behaviour. There is also some evidence that some children are simply undernourished and need a vitamin and mineral supplement which improves their attention, concentration and behaviour.

Docosahexaenoic acid (DHA), an omega-3 fatty acid found in breast milk, is found in lower levels in the brains of children with ADHD. This substance, necessary for the transmission of nerve impulses, makes up 25 per cent of the brain's fat content. Researchers in Scotland found that babies fed milk with no DHA generally had lower IQs than those taking either breast milk or baby food with DHA added. A Spanish study showed that dyslexics have less DHA in their brains than control groups. Since DHA is also found in fish oils it might be wise to supplement your child's diet with cod liver oil.

Complementary Therapies

Children with ADHD need plenty of individual supervision which can sometimes be combined with therapy for both the child and the harassed parent. There are therapists who work specifically with parents and children. Could you try to read to your child while he soaks in an aromatherapy bath? Some lavender or chamomile oil would be good and you will also gain the benefit of breathing the vapour. Having a vaporiser in the bedroom will help, but do set it long before bedtime and ensure that you extinguish the candle before you settle your child for bed. You could also combine cuddles with massage using the same oils well diluted. Amethyst crystals in the room may also help. You could always hang one in the window well out of reach but enabling it to catch the light and scatter it in the room.

Bach Flower Remedies and Australian Bush Essences may be useful, and a homeopath may have some remedies that will help. Although acupuncture is sometimes difficult in children, acupressure may be beneficial. Spiritual healing always works on some level and if your child would not be able to sit with you while you have healing together, then you could ask for his or her name to be put on an absent healing list. Don't forget that you would benefit too.

Another useful move would be to take an inventory of possible toxins in your child's environment and change what you can, noting the effect (see box on p. 7). In the real world it's impossible to rid ourselves of all toxins, but we can certainly try to pinpoint just what may be causing the problem and, if they can't be removed, use measures to neutralise them. A Feng Shui expert will help you provide a calm and healing atmosphere for both you and your child.

Although the diagnosis may have been made in childhood and you now have a difficult adolescent, or indeed as a young adult you are having problems, the suggestions above may still be of help. Self-esteem is usually low in the adult who was a hyperactive child and depression and impulsive behaviour may still plague you. There is healing to be done, so do get some help.

Emotional and Spiritual Healing

Toby is 33 and has never felt good about himself. He came along because he felt depressed when yet another relationship had failed and he found, when trying to assess his life, that he had achieved little despite considerable effort. Though he had had several quite good jobs which he felt he had managed to get because in the short-term he could be very charming, he could not deliver the level of dedication required after the honeymoon phase was over. In relationships his unpredictability and temper would usually lead to the breakup. On looking at his life history, it became apparent that Toby had been labelled an unruly, disruptive influence in class as a child since he could not sit still and concentrate on the content of lessons. He had received considerable punishment from both his father and his teachers because of this. His learning had suffered and his reading and writing skills were very poor. He had finally been left to his own devices and had virtually stopped attending school by the age of 14. Toby had undiagnosed ADHD.

The sadness which accompanies this illness cannot be underestimated as parents watch their children being 'naughty' and unruly and unable to fulfill their potential. Adolescents often find themselves in trouble and can be quite aggressive as their restlessness is exacerbated by the normal changes of adolescence. As young adults, or even older ones like Toby, their lives can be marred by the consequences of ADHD even if by then, the condition itself has abated somewhat.

Counselling and psychotherapy are useful for all concerned though it may be that the child will have difficulty in cooperating without the underlying causes being addressed and medication prescribed where appropriate. Parents also need support and counselling since their patience will be sorely tried and violence both verbal and physical towards children suffering ADHD is not uncommon as parents are constantly challenged and frustrated by impulsive and unacceptable behaviour and apparent refusal to obey the rules. Healing is useful for all and may have a very calming influence on the whole family. Dealing with problems of self-esteem and self-confidence are a priority.

The Outlook

In many cases ADHD completely disappears in puberty, although in others the hyperactivity decreases only to be replaced by moodiness, sluggishness and apathy in teenagers. Some perform badly academically and some resort to antisocial behaviour as a result. Very occasionally all the symptoms continue into adult life although this tends to be limited in most cases to an inattention and inability to sustain work output.

INTEGRATED APPROACH

1. Don't blame yourself or give up hope.
2. Talk the situation through with your doctor and know that if all else fails, stimulant drug therapy will make a difference.
3. Look to your child's diet and to possible toxins in the environment.
4. Keep a detailed journal of any changes you make so that you have a good record. Otherwise it can be difficult to pinpoint exactly what you did that made a difference.
5. Consult an aromatherapist and ask for a blend of oils for you to use for massage, for baths and to vaporise in your child's room.

6. Talk to your child's teacher and be sure that she/he understands the situation fully.
7. Take what help is available in terms of behavioural advice etc. That includes you if you are an adult who suffered from ADHD as a child.
8. Make sure that there is no other cause for the behaviour, for example a middle ear infection, constipation, vitamin or mineral deficiency, or heavy metal intoxication.

Backache

Andy works as a salesman for a computer company and used to like going to the gym and running 2 or 3 times a week to keep fit. Six months ago he was bedridden with severe back pain which hurt more when he coughed, sneezed or moved and was accompanied by pain going down the back of the left leg into the foot. Even now he is still plagued by stiffness and aching in the small of his back and he has not yet been able to resume his sporting acivities. Andy has a slipped disc.

Dave is a general practitioner who enjoys playing squash and rugby, but whose back pain has gradually been getting worse to the extent that he now finds visiting patients at home extremely difficult because of getting in and out of the car, and even sitting in the surgery for more than an hour is unbearable. Forced to become less physically active he put on weight which merely served to make the problem worse. Eventually after a series of negative investigations he had an epidural anaesthetic as an outpatient and walked away from the clinic pain free. A second similar procedure 6 months later resulted in complete freedom from back pain, and he has now resumed his sporting activities and can see his patients at home in half the time.

Back pain is a universal problem and the cause of significant suffering and disability. In the last month 30–40 per cent of the population will have experienced a certain degree of back pain, although thankfully the majority of attacks will settle more or less completely within a few weeks. Having said that, 70 per cent or more people will suffer at least 3 or more recurrences. Six per cent of all consultations with doctors are taken up with back pain, and millions of working days are lost at a cost of billions of pounds to industry. The cost to the NHS is consequently phenomenal. But the cost in human terms is what we are most concerned with here and this includes sleep problems, low mood, anxiety, lack of confidence, reliance on medication and poor self-esteem. Overall, the symptoms of back pain can lead not only to chronic discomfort, but to financial, emotional and interpersonal problems as well.

Mary is 61 and has severe pain running down her right arm into her hand and fingers. She also has discomfort in her neck which is worse when she looks upwards or looks over her shoulder. She has a slight dowager's hump and X-rays show a marked degree of osteoporosis with wedging of three of the vertebrae in this area which press on the nerves supplying sensation to her arm. She has brittle bone disease.

Symptoms

The symptoms of back pain are generally non-specific and poorly localised to any one area. No two people will report exactly the same symptoms, and the degree of disability caused by the back pain will vary immensely. However, there are patterns of pain which are helpful to the doctor in assessing the underlying disorder.

MECHANICAL PAIN

Over 90 per cent of cases are due to mechanical problems within the bones, joints, ligaments or muscles. Problems encountered in these parts of the body include prolapsed discs, inflammation within the facet joints which allow the vertebrae to move one on top of the other, inflamed cartilages and osteoporosis (brittle bone disease). Patients who suffer from mechanical low back pain are often aged between 20 and 60 with men and women affected equally. Patients often complain of long periods of mild pain interrupted by severe exacerbations. The pain that is felt is related to physical activity and tends to be made worse by prolonged standing or sitting and is relieved by movement. Lifting can often be difficult and sufferers find they cannot reach down and touch their toes without making the pain worse.

INFLAMMATORY PAIN

With inflammatory back pain where some inflammatory process is affecting the spine as well as other parts of the body, the back pain is characterised by morning stiffness with relief of the discomfort as the day progresses and the patient becomes more mobile. The back becomes straighter than usual with reduced movement in every direction, and often the dull ache can move downwards from the lumbar region into the buttocks and thighs.

NEUROLOGICAL PAIN

With neurological pain, the pain often starts in the spine but moves into the arm, into the chest wall or down into the leg, along whichever nerve route is being compressed mechanically by the disorder in the spine. A perfect example is sciatica which can cause pain going down the back of the thigh into the calves or even to the bottom of the foot.

Carol is PA to an ambitious and hard-working executive. She works long hours at her desk, mostly on a word processor, and notices more and more frequently a sense of tension in her neck with restriction of movement, pain in her shoulders and tingling in her fingers. She has developed some inflammation and minor displacement in the facet joints between two or three of her neck vertebrae; in other words, she has cervical spondylitis, resulting in referred pain in her arms, shoulders and fingers.

SINISTER PAIN

In 'sinister' back pain, the discomfort may be associated with weight loss and general malaise, and features pain which remains unrelieved by rest or movement, with progressive deterioration. Luckily this type of back pain accounts for less than 1 per cent of all types seen, and it always requires urgent investigation as it suggests a more serious condition such as infection of the vertebrae, osteoporosis or even malignancy.

REFERRED PAIN

Referred pain is pain felt in the back which actually comes from other organs of the body such as the kidneys, the pancreas, the aorta (the main artery taking blood from the heart to the lower part of the body) or the stomach. Again, the pain is not related to physical exertion, and is diffuse.

These patterns of pain are not in themselves diagnostic, but give the doctor a clue as to which systems in the body require the most urgent investigation. A great deal of information can be gained by talking to the patient and finding out how long they have had the pain, what makes it better or worse, what occupation they are in and what their general health is currently like.

Diagnosis

The diagnosis of back pain is one of the most difficult areas faced in modern medicine. Symptoms are often misleading and the pain is non-specific and diffuse. The physical examination can help to assess the patient's range of movement and the pattern of pain. It may also identify any complications such as nerve root pressure which may be affecting muscular power in the limbs, leading to abnormal sensation or even interfering with bowel and bladder function. Measurements of leg length can identify compensatory stresses and strains on the spine, and manipulation with the fingers can sometimes reveal specific trigger spots over the ligaments and muscles of the back.

Eventually, however, when pain persists more than the usual 6 weeks and the patient is still in constant pain, investigations are usually carried out to try to identify precisely where the trouble lies. Unfortunately the most convenient and the cheapest tests such as X-rays are rarely helpful, contrary to popular belief, as X-rays merely show the condition of the bones themselves rather than the soft tissues around them from which pain usually emanates. Ultrasound tests are sometimes carried out to determine whether the pain may be coming from other structures such as blood vessels, kidneys or the pancreas, and these tests are simple and non-invasive. When back pain is clinically significant and causing a lot of ongoing pain, magnetic resonance imaging scans (MRI) or computerised tomography scans (CAT) are carried out which show not only the bones and joints but the condition of the spinal cord and the nerves which arise from it as well. Blood tests are often done to show the presence of any general inflammation in the body, any blood disorder which can affect the bone marrow within the vertebrae, or any other chemical abnormality which may reveal problems in other organs that in turn are affecting the spine.

Because of the high cost of the scans, however, another modern approach is that of using an epidural anaesthetic as a partly diagnostic procedure. This anaesthetic bathes the spinal nerves with an anti-inflammatory steroid which is designed to take any mechanical pressure off the nerve and ease the symptoms. If the pain is relieved by such a procedure it successfully localises the problem to the nerves themselves rather than the facet joints which join the vertebrae together above and below. An epidural anaesthetic would not work if it were these joints that were inflamed but it does help where nerve compression is the problem.

The Mind/Body Link

Pain is pain, whatever the cause, but there are few areas in medicine other than back pain where the discomfort is quite so amplified by psychological factors. If you have chronic back pain you do not sleep well, you become anxious and depressed, you lack confidence, your job may be at risk, you often think poorly of yourself and it is easy to feel a failure. You can also become reliant on medication which can make you drowsy or affect your concentration, and all this takes its toll on even the most stoical of people. Your medical notes become thick files of referrals to various specialists and hospital departments and often you feel dismissed by conventional doctors who tell you that you must simply learn to live with your symptoms. Modern management schemes for the treatment of back pain attempt to overcome this narrow way of thinking, as you will see below.

Prevention

Bearing in mind that we spend approximately a third of our lives in bed, it would be wise for us to pay a little more attention to the kind of rest we get there and the strain that is often put upon our backs by sleeping on old mattresses that give little support. A study a few years ago found that many young people sleep on very poor mattresses and are set up for back problems for the rest of their lives. So how long is it since you changed your mattress? Does it give you the support you need? And what about your pillow? Does it amply support your neck to allow your spine to stay in a straight line while you sleep? It would be a good investment to purchase the best bed you can afford and couple it with a specially designed pillow. And if for any reason you have to lie on your back, make sure you have a pillow under your knees to take the strain off your lower back.

If you spend all day in an office, insist that you have a well-designed chair and that equipment such as computer screens are placed at eye level to avoid strain upon your neck. But good seating shouldn't stop in the office. Is your favourite chair really good for your back? And what about your car seat?

If you tend to have a weak back, go and talk to a physiotherapist about it and learn proper techniques for lifting, bending, sitting, etc. to minimise the difficulty. Although back exercises may seem like treatment, they are in fact a must for everyone. Remember that our spines were not originally designed to keep us upright, and the reason for so many people having back pain is that so few of us take as much care of our backs as we would of various pieces of household equipment. Now that the basics are out of the way, let's look at treatment.

Treatment

The first step in treatment is to obtain an accurate diagnosis so that appropriate treatment can be chosen for the underlying problem. Having established that, treatment may encompasses any or all of the following techniques.

REST

With acute back pain, rest is important to allow muscle spasm to settle. But the consensus of opinion is that since 15 per cent of muscle bulk around the spine can be lost after a full week of bedrest, it is better if possible to keep reasonably active to prevent this happening. When the supported muscles around the spine are weakened the strain is taken by the joint and ligaments themselves, and this often serves to exacerbate the back pain where the joints are already inflamed.

Corsets and collars

In much the same way that other disorders of the moving parts of the skeleton can settle when restricted in movement, the application of corsets around the lumbar spine and collars around the neck can ease discomfort and allow muscle spasm to settle. Their use also serves to diminish movement and where pressure on nerves exists, for example from slipped discs, this can prevent further damage.

Patient education

Back pain is very often linked to lifestyle and it is well known that anybody with a weak or deconditioned back is more likely to suffer from recurrences. Learning about the anatomy of the spine as well as the physiology and psychology of back pain helps you avoid problems in the future through the development of an increased level of fitness and a greater awareness of musculoskeletal injuries.

Physical therapy

The correction of poor movement patterns and lifting techniques means that future strains and stresses may be avoided. The use of supportive and ergonomically designed seating, both at home and in the office, is important. Physical treatments using ultrasound, electrical stimulation, heat or ice, mobilisation, acupuncture, hydrotherapy, massage and stretching may all be carried out by physiotherapists and all have a place.

Osteopathy and chiropractic

Physical manipulation of the spine in the early stages of back pain have been shown in scientific studies to be superior to conventional means of treatment when compared to standard treatment given in hospital outpatient departments. A visit to these practitioners of manipulative medicine is therefore often very well worthwhile and your GP may be able to recommend a reputable local osteopath or chiropractor to you.

PAIN RELIEF

Standard medications include analgesics and anti-inflammatories, although muscle relaxants such as diazepam are sometimes used in conjunction with them. Doctors are reluctant to use powerful painkillers as these are more likely to induce side effects and lead to addiction if used in the long term. Local injections may be used if the pain is sufficiently localised, but often this is not the case. Epidural anaesthesia can be very successful when used appropriately, either when employed as a diagnostic technique or following the use of investigative scans which strongly suggest that pressure on spinal nerves is the cause of the discomfort. New techniques involving sclerosant injections into the lumbar facet joints have had an increasing success rate in recent years, and selective nerve root blocks are also available for people suffering nerve entrapment or irritation. Certain more invasive therapies such as spinal cord stimulation and programmable intrathecal pumps (which inject long-acting anaesthesia around the spinal cord) are also available in certain cases of severe pain and leg pain that are resistant to all other treatments.

SURGERY

Surgical techniques are rarely considered these days apart from in exceptional circumstances. Surgery would be needed for the removal of slipped discs causing either nerve root damage and muscle wasting, or any interference with bowel or bladder function. In other circumstances we know that slipped discs often dry out and shrink of their own accord given time, and many experts have reported equal or superior success with the treatment of back pain without recourse to invasive surgery which can induce serious complications. In fact, much controversy exists over whether an operation to remove a slipped disc (laminectomy) represents a useful treatment as can be seen from the fact that the laminectomy rate varies by tenfold in different European countries. If removal of a slipped disc needs to be carried out, the newer technique of microdiscectomy, which involves the sucking out of the prolapsed tissue through a fine needle, is well worth investigating as the procedure is much less invasive. Where abnormal front to back movement occurs between two vertebrae, however, spinal fusion to prevent further slipping of one vertebra on another becomes necessary, and clearly in these situations a good rapport between the patient and surgeon is imperative.

OTHER TREATMENTS

There are so many different causes of backache that not all treatments could be considered here. Where secondary deposits from malignancy elsewhere in the body have occurred in the spine, radiotherapy or chemotherapy may be used. For many people only a combination of the above treatments will help, and even then, they may be left with some degree of ongoing discomfort. In summary, a good logical approach to the management of back pain is vital and this is summarised in the box below.

INTEGRATED APPROACH

1. Rapid access to professional help.
2. A comprehensive assessment.
3. Appropriate treatment based on a full clinical history and examination.
4. Thorough investigation.
5. Quick referral to a specialist if appropriate.
6. Access to an acute back pain clinic.
7. Active rehabilitation to increase muscle strength and flexibility.
8. Back education, relaxation training and stress management.

❧ Bereavement

Twenty years ago, Edith had a stillborn child. She was extremely distressed at the time and her GP prescribed Valium for her. She took it for many years and fairly recently became medication free. Three or four months ago, the daughter of a friend had a stillborn baby and since that time Edith has been tearful, restless, irritable and ruminating on her own loss in a way she was never able to do at the time. Her husband can't understand why after all these years she is behaving in this way since they now have two lovely sons and the event was so long ago. Edith is suffering from a delayed grief reaction.

When somebody loses a person who is close to them and is bereaved, they experience a number of painful emotions as part of the normal grieving process. Initially, after the shock and denial that this person has actually died, pangs of acute distress and anxiety occur. Yearning and searching for the person who has been lost is quite normal and understandably this takes precedence over all other activities. It is easy for someone who is bereaved to then become physically restless and to go over and over again in their minds the events leading up to the tragedy as if hopelessly trying to remedy the situation or pretend that it has not really happened. Some people find they actually see or hear the dead person. They may experience a feeling of anger towards the deceased, blaming them for not taking more care of themselves, or for leaving them prematurely and rendering them lost and alone. This is really just another common expression of intense grief but because it is illogical and puzzling, it can often lead later to a sense of shame and guilt that these feelings could ever be harboured and in turn this can occasionally bring about depression.

For a time, a bereaved person will feel lost and lacking any sense of purpose. They may lose their appetite, lose weight and find it difficult to sleep. Interest in the outside world is abandoned and friends and other social contacts are shunned.

In some cultures the expression of grief is much more overt than in others, with highly ritualised or organised communal mourning, and rigorous encouragement of public displays of emotion. In other societies, the British included, grieving remains a particularly private matter from which anybody but the very closest relatives is excluded. Normally, however, sooner or later, the pangs of grief become less frequent, less intense and shorter-lasting, and interest in the outside world is re-established. Recovery from the psychological and physical symptoms gradually occurs but is punctuated by acute recurrences at particularly significant times such as anniversaries and birthdays.

David, 57, answered his front door to a policewoman who had the unenviable duty of having to inform him that his wife had been involved in a car accident and had died on her way to hospital. David next saw his wife's body in the hospital mortuary and the shock of the whole affair was too much for him. His surprising level of calm and self-control continued for several days during which he refused all offers of help and counselling. Six days later he was admitted to hospital himself, having taken an overdose of sleeping tablets.

Abnormal grief

Grief may be considered to be chronic or abnormal when severe emotional distress continues well beyond the time when it would be expected to have been resolved. This might happen, say, if a spouse lost a partner on whom they were particularly dependent and it also frequently happens when a bereavement is totally unexpected or traumatic. Children of pre-school age who lose a parent and young parents who lose a child are especially prone to chronic grief. These groups of people particularly need help but everyone who suffers from the trauma of bereavement can benefit from understanding and support.

Conventional Treatment

The most important support for a bereaved person generally comes from other members of the close family unit, but often this may not be available. Doctors can take over this role to some extent or add to it by listening sympathetically and encouraging the person concerned to talk frankly and openly about their loss. One of the most valuable things we, the authors, have discovered that a doctor can do, if they are the family's usual doctor, is to express their own feelings of fondness, respect and care for the person who has died. Families may respond to this very positively and often feel that however awful the events of the death may be, at least their medical attention at that time was warm, caring and sympathetic.

In abnormal or chronic grief there is often a prolonged denial of the loss and a strong repression of the natural expression of emotion. People may say they feel unable to cry or that they find it difficult to believe that their loved one has really gone. In this situation they may respond well to guided mourning whereby they are actively encouraged to make the loss more real by, say, visiting the grave, reviewing possessions and photographs of the deceased, and changing the contents and arrangements of the house. Psychotherapy to build confidence and self-esteem is important too so that the bereaved can feel more optimistic about continuing a changed yet meaningful and fulfilling life in the future. Sometimes the grieving may need their doctor to give 'permission' for the period of grief to stop.

Toni's husband left her 2 years ago and is living with another woman. She could neither eat, sleep nor work for a long time, feeling shocked and unable to believe that he had really gone. She then became very angry with him and his new girlfriend. She eventually settled into a new routine but she feels lost and depressed, cries most nights and feels it would be less painful if he had actually died. Toni is suffering grief at the loss of her marriage.

As far as drugs are concerned, the use of sedatives and tranquillisers is usually discouraged unless anxiety symptoms and distress are so severe that to withhold a small dose for a short period of time seems cruel or unreasonable. Numbing emotional reaction by prescribing these types of drugs merely blunts and postpones the normal grieving process, and should be avoided if at all possible. If severe anxiety or depression sets in at a later date as a consequence of chronic grief, that is a different matter and medication may then prove to be more appropriate.

Doctors are also aware that after bereavement, changes in a person's physical health can occur too, so symptoms such as breathlessness, chest pain and joint problems should certainly be reported by the patient and enquired about by the doctors looking after them.

Counselling is an important part of the treatment of grief and abnormal grief, and may be provided either by the GP and professional counsellors or by voluntary organisations such as CRUSE. Apart from offering support and sympathy, counselling can also monitor susceptible patients for the occasional development of severe depression and any risk of suicide. Hopefully it will ultimately result in the social and emotional rehabilitation of the bereaved so that once again they can face the future with renewed enthusiasm and vigour and lead normal independent lives.

Mary, 43, had a mastectomy operation for cancer of the breast within 2 months of its initial diagnosis. Having been focused on the enormity of her cancer, she woke from her anaesthetic not wanting to live or face the world again. As far as she was concerned she had lost her femininity as well as her sexuality and could not see that she had any value in anyone else's life anymore. Mary is suffering from a bereavement reaction to the loss of a very important part of her body.

Nutritional Healing

Although the last thing you may want to think about is food, you really do need to have a nutritious diet right now. In some cultures, friends, relatives and neighbours bring tempting food to the grieving, to show their love, to help and also to tempt the flagging appetite with good things. If you know of someone who is grieving, this would be a loving thing to do for them. A little of what you fancy should be the rule here and no amount of preaching about what you *should* eat will help. Sometimes, those who are in the midst of grief simply forget to eat, but will do so when food is actually put in front of them. Food that is nutritious, attractive but easy to digest would be good.

Vitamins and Supplements

Because eating is sometimes a problem and appetite is poor, supplements are particularly useful at this time. Fatigue is a feature of the grieving process and in any case those who have lost loved ones often enter the process already feeling exhausted from weeks or even months of heavy physical and emotional work, their resources drained. Building up with a good vitamin and mineral supplement is essential. Try to ensure that you get proper rest. Some chamomile tea at night would help and kava tea through the day will relax you, but ration yourself to perhaps 3 cups a day. You can sweeten it with orange juice if you wish.

Exercise and Lifestyle

Exercise is good and walking, yoga or swimming are perhaps the best kinds. Slowly swimming alone in a quiet pool with the silence and gentle massage of the water can allow you to heal in a way that may be difficult at other times. However, be sensible and make sure that someone is with you close by and will check on you at regular intervals. Some people on the other hand need some aggressive exercise to get rid of the anger they feel at being left.

Complementary Therapies

Aromatherapy for your bath, room or massage might include rose oil for your heart chakra and bergamot for your depression. Melissa (lemon balm) is also soothing when used as a massage oil and particularly for burning in the house. As always, an aromatherapist would blend some oils for you if you ask. Some aromatherapists will come to your home, and a massage in the evening would probably help to unwind you before bedtime, as would writing a journal so that you can externalise all the thoughts that go around in your head and prevent you from settling down.

The classical homeopathic treatment for grief is Ignatia. Arnica would be good for the shock of a sudden death or separation. Aconite may help if there is accompanying fear, anxiety or violent shock. If your grief seems stuck, talk to a homeopath and have something prescribed for you. Rescue Remedy, a Bach Flower Remedy, would be useful to carry with you and take when necessary, although there may be other essences that would also help.

Your immune system will be depressed and you're more susceptible to infections so take good care of yourself. If necessary, take some echinacea for a few days to boost your immunity.

Emotional and Spiritual Healing

Grief tends to result in closing down of the heart chakra and tender care will help it to open again. In helping others, touch, be it holding a hand, putting a comforting arm around a shoulder, hugging or massage, will often set flowing a stream of healing tears. However, make sure that if you do this with a friend or loved one, you have permission to do so and that you choose an appropriate time and place. You would be doing no favours to a work colleague to help them tip into much needed crying in the middle of the office! If you are grieving don't be afraid to ask someone to hold you if that's what you need.

Undoubtedly you will want to talk about your loved one. Sadly many of us have forgotten how to do this and friends may appear embarrassed at the mention of the person and try to change the subject. But you do need someone to talk to and a professional bereavement counsellor might be the person. Conversely some people who are grieving refuse to talk and become agitated or angry if the person who is gone is mentioned. This person also needs to be encouraged to talk and probably needs professional help. You may feel angry with God or conversely feel a sudden need to look toward a religion or spirituality you may have neglected for years. Sometimes talking to someone from your local church or synagogue will help even if you have never been an active member before.

Patricia Davis in her lovely book *Subtle Aromatherapy* suggests a wonderful meditation for the friends who are grieving. There is also a grief meditation you might like to use in *The Rainbow Journey* (Brenda Davies). Sharing with others who are grieving can be very healing. If you think this could be so for you, call CRUSE (see Useful Addresses) and ask where there are groups in your area. The book, *A Grief Remembered* by C.S. Lewis, sharing his thoughts and experiences on the death of his wife, is a touching account which may help you feel less isolated in your grief. *The Tibetan Book of Living and Dying* by Sogyal Rinpoche (Rider, 1998) is also wonderful and answers many questions about the meaning of life and what happens after death.

Whatever you do, don't let anyone hurry you in your healing. Grief usually takes about two years to resolve, although by the first anniversary of the death things may be much easier to bear. In former times, and still in some cultures, mourning was marked by the wearing of black. Until the first anniversary there would be full mourning which was not only a sign of respect for the dead but also a signal that the person was fragile and grieving. After the first anniversary there would be a change to black armbands, women also having a black hat or headscarf and men a black tie. Only after the second anniversary were normal clothes worn again as a sign that mourning was complete. Although we have lost that tradition, the timescale has not changed. Should you still be stuck in your grief after this period, however, perhaps you should be considering professional help.

If your loved one has died without you being able to say all you needed to say, then often writing a letter to them, even though you cannot send it, can help. Even years after someone has died or left you, this technique can have enormous benefits in healing the past. If grief remains unresolved and is getting in the way of your moving on with your life, you may like to consider a tie-cutting ceremony. This is a ceremony in which, guided by a healer, you visualise the bonds that still hold you to the person who has gone, and then sever them after a meditation in which you affirm that you are doing this for your own good as well as that of the person who has left, to allow both of you to be free. We usually advise that a letter is written ahead of the tie-cutting ceremony to ensure that all has been said, although cutting the ties does not mean that you cannot write later if you so desire.

Whatever, be gentle on yourself and be aware that all your sensory thresholds are likely to be depressed so that you feel irritated by sound, by light, by touch, etc. Talking of sound, music can be one of the most healing and yet exquisitely painful things at this time. If your grief is stuck, music can often access it.

If you know someone who has lost a dear one, try to remember that often in the first few weeks there is much activity – preparing a funeral, writing letters, dealing with solicitors, etc. It is often months later that the bereft person will need continuing support, when friends and even family have moved on and the true loneliness and grief sets in. A bunch of flowers, a phone call or an invitation to supper could make all the difference to the person starting to live once again.

If you are someone who works with the dying, don't forget your own needs. Although you may have a very good understanding of death and feel comfortable with the process, you're only human. Don't neglect yourself. Sometimes it isn't the dealing with the dying, but dealing with the bereft that takes its toll. Have some support for yourself.

Integrated approach

1. You should never have to cope with bereavement on your own.
2. Your family and friends have the most important role to play overall.
3. Abnormal grief requires urgent and vigorous treatment.

4. Professional bereavement counsellors, Macmillan nurses, family doctors and voluntary organisations such as CRUSE can also help you.
5. The Church and its religious advisers can greatly contribute if you have a faith.
6. Specific ceremonies can help you move on with your life.
7. Never neglect your own health. A positive and healthy lifestyle and a doctor's check-up are important.

Blood Disorders

Normal Functions of the Blood

Healthy blood has 3 main functions:

1. It is a transport system to transfer gases such as oxygen and carbon dioxide to and from the body, but it also transports glucose, protein, fat, salts and minerals as well.
2. Another function is to act as a defence against infection and inflammation including cancer. For this it relies on the white blood cells and on antibodies in the plasma.
3. Its third main role is to allow the blood to clot effectively when there has been an injury. The bone marrow constantly produces new blood cells to replace those whose lifespan has expired.

The average healthy adult has about 5 litres of blood in total and nearly the same amount is pumped around the body by the heart each minute. During exercise, when more oxygen is required by the tissues, this amount can increase to 30 litres a minute with the heart rate increasing proportionately in order to achieve this. The blood consists of roughly 50 per cent cells and 50 per cent plasma. The red blood cells contain haemoglobin which is a pigmented protein containing iron which binds to oxygen and carries it from the lungs around the body. The white blood cells help fight infection and are important in the immune response, and the platelets (which are much smaller fragments of other cells in the bone marrow) are important in the blood clotting process. The plasma is a straw-coloured fluid consisting of 95 per cent water although its salt content is very similar to that of sea water and this transports all the nutrients that the body requires, along with hormones and waste products of metabolism, for excretion through the bowel or kidneys.

Blood Disorders

The commonest types of blood disorders include anaemia, leukaemia and abnormal bruising. These warrant a more detailed description, although there are many other blood disorders that should not be forgotten. Just as the blood can be too 'thin' as in anaemia, the blood can become too 'thick' when too many red blood cells are produced by the bone marrow, resulting in a condition known as polycythaemia. The thicker blood results in headaches, high blood pressure, flushed skin and widespread itching. Thrombosis or the formation of blood clots is another common blood disorder which is a major threat, particularly to women, as this condition is more likely if you take the oral contraceptive pill or are pregnant. Smoking also leads to thrombosis which can occur in the deep veins of the legs (deep vein thrombosis, or DVT) or travel through the circulation to the lungs. Here, it causes a bloodstained cough and shortness of breath in mild cases, or collapse and a life-threatening situation in severe cases (pulmonary embolus).

There may also be a genetic disorder of the blood where there is an inherited abnormality in the production of certain blood components. In thalassaemia and sickle cell anaemia, abnormal kinds of haemoglobin make the red blood cells very fragile so that at certain times they break down leading to anaemia and blockages within blood vessels. Haemophiliacs fail to manufacture enough of the blood clotting factors which enable their blood to clot properly, resulting in uncontrolled bleeding if not treated. Blood poisoning due to the large numbers of bacteria in the blood is known as septicaemia and is a life-threatening complication of diseases such as meningitis or peritonitis. Other types of blood infections include malaria, where a parasite invades the blood cells themselves at a particular stage in their life cycle. Blood is also susceptible to poisoning from substances such as lead and carbon monoxide, a toxic ingredient of car exhaust fumes. Blood disorders may also arise from exposure to radiation or the presence of liver or kidney disease. We will only look in detail at the commonest blood disorders: anaemia, leukaemia and abnormal bruising.

Anaemia

Mabel, who lives alone in the country, simply cannot understand why she feels so exhausted. She has had a little nagging indigestion of late, but gardening makes her unduly breathless and she has experienced some chest pain when climbing the stairs. In fact Mabel has been losing blood internally as a result of a stomach ulcer and has gradually become severely anaemic. Her shortness of breath and chest pain are directly related to this underlying disorder.

Anaemia is a condition where the oxygen-carrying capacity of the blood is reduced. This can happen for a number of reasons although the commonest worldwide is a deficiency of iron in the diet. This reduces the amount of haemoglobin in the red blood cells which cannot therefore bind to enough oxygen in the lungs. However, anaemia can also result from a decreased production of red cells in the bone marrow, or a deficiency of other nutrients such as Vitamin B_{12} or folic acid (folate). There may also be a decreased survival rate of red cells in the blood for a variety of reasons. Sometimes the blood itself is made normally and in sufficient quantities, but blood is lost through chronic bleeding. This might happen in a menopausal woman with heavy persistent periods or in someone with a bleeding stomach ulcer, for example.

Symptoms, Diagnosis and Treatment

Symptoms include tiredness and lethargy, breathlessness on exertion, palpitations and pallor of the skin. Angina or chest pain occasionally occurs in people who have a degree of previously undetected coronary heart disease. The diagnosis is suggested by the patient's symptoms and is confirmed through blood tests. Treatment depends on the type of anaemia from which the patient is suffering, but necessitates correcting the disease responsible for the anaemia and then making sure that the number and quality of the red blood cells in the circulation is adequate.

LEUKAEMIA

Jimmy was 8 when he first started feeling unwell. He had several throat infections in close succession and generally looked pale and tired. One weekend his father took him swimming and noticed he was covered in bruises. Jimmy's doctor did a blood test which showed abnormally high numbers of white blood cells, a low platelet count and anaemia. Jimmy has acute leukaemia.

Leukaemia is a form of cancer where a disorganised proliferation of white blood cells in the bone marrow occurs. As the bone marrow becomes replaced with these abnormal white cells, normal white and red cells and platelets are squeezed out and their numbers in the circulation may drop to alarming levels. Consequently bruising, anaemia and frequent infections are among the commonest symptoms of the various types of leukaemia. In addition other organs such as the lymph glands, liver and spleen can be taken over by abnormal cells. There are two main types of leukaemia, namely acute and chronic, depending on how quickly they develop. Further classification depends on the exact type of the white cell that is proliferating so fast. Every year there are some 5000 new cases of leukaemia diagnosed in Britain.

Symptoms, Diagnosis and Treatment

Symptoms of the acute leukaemias generally include anaemia, frequent infections and bruising, whereas the chronic leukaemias may often develop slowly over many years and are sometimes discovered by chance when a blood test is performed for some other reason. Symptoms of the chronic leukaemias include tiredness, night sweats, fever and weight loss as well as enlargement of organs such as the liver and spleen. The diagnosis of leukaemia is generally suggested by the characteristic nature of the symptoms and confirmed by blood tests which analyse the quantity and quality of the various blood cell components in the sample. Sometimes a bone marrow test is also performed to more accurately assess the exact type of leukaemia present. Treatment of the acute leukaemias involves transfusions of blood and platelets to boost the numbers of cells that have been depleted and the use of anticancer drugs to kill the leukaemic cells themselves. Antibiotics are often required to deal with any infection that arises, and radiotherapy and anti-cancer drug treatment of the cerebrospinal fluid are also both used in an attempt to eradicate all abnormal cells. Remission is said to be present when there is no evidence of leukaemic cells in the blood or the bone marrow. Because relapses take place, however, a number of drugs are usually continued for several weeks after remission in the hope of achieving a cure. After several relapses a bone marrow transplant may be considered although increasingly the bone marrow transplantation is offered during the first remission to guard against any relapse taking place.

The chronic leukaemias also require anti-cancer drugs, radiotherapy and antibiotics, although immunoglobulin injections to boost the patient's immune system may additionally be offered. Bone marrow transplants are also used in these chronic leukaemias in an attempt to achieve a cure while the patient is still in the chronic stage, before the disease transfers into the more difficult-to-treat acute phase. Generally the chronic leukaemias have a better outlook than the acute leukaemias, although survival rates have improved across the board in recent years as a result of better medical treatment.

The Outlook

The survival rate from leukaemia varies, depending on the exact type of leukaemia and the age of the patient. With the advent of bone marrow transplantation, the outcome has improved considerably and some less aggressive forms of leukaemia may now be cured when detected early on.

A large part of orthodox treatment is directed at supporting the psychological needs of the patient as well as the physical ones, as the side effects of chemotherapy and radiotherapy can be hard to endure. By and large, orthodox medicine achieves this very well with dedicated units able to forge excellent doctor/patient relationships in specialised but friendly units where the leukaemia patients themselves become almost as expert about their condition as the professional experts themselves. Treatment may include steroids, immunosuppressant medications or plasmaphoresis. In the latter, blood is removed allowing plasma to be 'cleaned' and modified. The way that platelet deficiency is treated depends on the underlying cause although top-up transfusions of platelets alone can always be given. Where the body is destroying its own platelets because of abnormal antibodies in the bloodstream, steroids may be used, although removal of the spleen through surgical means is sometimes also carried out.

Abnormal Bruising

Christine came home from work one day and was horrified to find a number of unexplained bruises on her arms and legs. She has been feeling under the weather recently anyway and she soon convinced herself she was suffering from a serious blood disorder like leukaemia. In fact, the only abnormality in her blood proved to be a deficiency of platelets. This was merely a temporary response to a recent viral infection in her throat.

Bruising occurs whenever there is leakage of blood from a damaged blood vessel. Where bleeding occurs in the absence of any injury or where it is abnormally prolonged and excessive after an injury, a bleeding disorder is said to be present. These bleeding disorders may be the result of a blood clotting disorder (coagulation defect), a defect in the blood vessel itself or a reduced number of platelets in the circulation – a situation that might arise as a result of something as simple as a viral infection or, equally of something as serious as leukaemia. A vast number of conditions may lead to bleeding disorders, some of which are congenital, such as haemophilia; some are acquired as a result of infection or an overdose of anticoagulant drugs, and some may be brought on by the side effects of therapeutic drugs such as steroids which thin the walls of blood vessels allowing them to rupture and leak more easily. The diagnosis is almost always made through blood tests and treatment obviously depends on the underlying cause.

Nutritional Healing

Whatever the cause of your blood disorder, you should look very seriously at your nutrition. Whether your anaemia is due to blood loss, acute or chronic, blood cell destruction or deficiency of nutrients, you need to replace what you don't have and what you need to be well. Make sure that you have a proper diagnosis before you cover up any signs with heroic dietary measures or take supplements. However, eating better is a must. The basic eating plan on p. 5 will give you all you need for maintenance, but you need to look also at what you are deficient in now and replace it. Your doctor will be keeping an eye on your haemoglobin and Vitamin B_{12} and folic acid (folate) levels, but you will be able to monitor yourself in terms of your energy etc. It's worth remembering that if you eat a strictly vegetarian or vegan diet, nutritional deficiencies may take 3 or 4 years or even longer to manifest themselves.

Be aware of times when you need more and should supplement your diet. Growing children and adolescents, pregnant and nursing mothers, those doing strong physical work or playing sports and those ill or recovering from trauma or illness are depleting their resources and probably need supplements. If you're constantly tired, have recurrent colds, can't do the things that your peers do with ease, get up in the morning feeling tired and irritable and feel that life is one long hard struggle, then you may well be labouring under a nutritional deficiency even if it hasn't yet manifested clinically. Time to eat more healthily!

If you are iron-deficient, then add beetroot (and beet greens), spinach, watercress, parsley, raisins, prunes, asparagus, pumpkin seeds and soya products. Eat plenty of dark green leafy vegetables and ideally also add meat, chicken and liver to your diet. You need Vitamin C to help with the absorption of iron so eat strawberries, citrus fruit, peppers and kiwi fruit.

If you're deficient in Vitamin B_{12}, add soya products, yogurt, cottage cheese, eggs, mackerel and salmon.

For folic acid (folate) deficiency you need to add peas (including black-eye peas) and beans, orange juice and other fruit juices, oats, cereals, lentils, spinach, beet, broccoli, Brussels sprouts, mushrooms and canteloupe melons. Poultry and tuna are valuable sources of folic acid.

Also keep up your protein by adding grains, soya and beans as well as fish and animal protein. You may find that you need to eat every few hours, small but highly nutritious snacks such as nuts or protein bars, with some fruit juice or milk.

Vitamins and Supplements

These depend upon the type of blood disorder you have. However, start with a good multivitamin and multimineral and add whatever else you need. Vitamins C and E may need to be taken at well above the recommended daily dosage. Higher than usual doses of Vitamin A are also fine in the short term, say for about 3 weeks, but if taken for longer at high doses they may start to depress your immune function. Once your diagnosis has been made, your doctor may prescribe iron, Vitamin B_{12} or folic acid (folate).

If heavy periods are the cause of the problem (which may in turn be due to stress, fibroids, endometriosis etc., see p. 379), a low-fat diet high in complex carbohydrates for at least 3 months will lower your oestrogen levels a little and help ease the situation.

Bee products such as propolis, pollen and royal jelly are not only potent natural sources of vitamins and minerals but have additional benefits. Royal jelly, the substance fed to the queen bee to help her grow bigger and live much longer than the other bees, is a great food. It's best taken at the turn of the season: around March or April and again in September. It's available in vials, capsules or fresh. Begin with a vial every morning for 10 days, then take one capsule each morning for 30 days and then stop. It will boost your energy, clear your complexion, help you sleep and improve your vitality. Propolis and pollen are available in capsule form. Spirulina will provide you with masses of of Vitamin B_{12}, and folic acid (folate) is available on its own or as an ingredient in a strong Vitamin B complex tablet which we would highly recommend. Taken at bedtime it will help you relax and sleep better. Don't be concerned about the fact that it will turn your urine a delightful shade of yellow!

Herbs that you would find useful include dandelion, alfalfa and parsley, while golden seal will help digestion and absorption and don quai will boost your energy.

Complementary Therapies

A visit to a Traditional Chinese Medicine practitioner would yield great benefits. Acupuncture is useful to help unblock the meridians and help absorption and you may also be prescribed herbs. Reflexology can be beneficial. Since the problem may well be linked to a second chakra block (see below), some art therapy could be very healing. Lavender aromatherapy oil would be soothing in your room or your bath. Massage would help as would creative visualisation. Take time to relax and meditate and see your body getting back in balance.

Emotional and Spiritual Healing

Blood and its circulation is governed by the second, the sacral, chakra and it is here that any healing needs to be concentrated. In many people with such disorders, especially women, there are unresolved issues regarding sexuality and the willingness and ability to flow with life and become less rigid in our bodies, our thinking, our attitude and our spirituality. If there has been some trauma between the ages of 5 and 8, it will manifest in this chakra and blocks here stunt our creativity as well as our ability to relate well to others and have relationships that are equal, deep and long-lasting. Since this chakra also has a special connection with the throat chakra, we may find difficulty in being self-assertive and communicating our true feelings and needs. If any of this sounds familiar, then do seek some help and/or begin to do some work to clear your chakras and ease the flow of all the fluid systems of your body. You may find that any period problems settle down and you will find yourself flowing through life with ease instead of rigidly holding the controls and bumping up against the same problems again and again. Why not make a date with yourself to do something creative such as painting, drawing, doing some craft as well as meditating and treating yourself to some gentle rituals involving water?

Integrated approach

1. Ensure plenty of iron, folic acid (folate) and Vitamin B_{12} in your diet to help prevent anaemia.
2. Report symptoms of fatigue, pallor, prolonged infections or bruising as soon as possible.
3. Seek as much information about the diagnosis as possible.
4. Ask about all the different treatment options for leukaemia including new techniques such as bone marrow transplantation.
5. Find out about the side effects of treatments too.
6. Don't be afraid of specialised hospital units – modern ones are very friendly and welcoming as well as offering you the best chance of a cure.
7. Treat yourself to some complementary therapy – but always check with your specialist first.

Cancer

What is it?

Cancer occurs when an abnormal cell grows and multiplies in a disorderly and uncontrolled way. As this chaotic growth continues, healthy surrounding cells and organs become damaged. The initial stimulus for these events is in the original cell, which escapes from the normal control mechanisms and passes this autonomy or freedom from control on to each of its daughter cells. The genes within a cell that control its growth and multiplication are called oncogenes, and they become damaged and no longer function normally because they are altered and damaged by carcinogens in the environment.

Cancer cells not only grow faster and behave differently to other cells, but they fail to perform the normal functions of the original cells from which they arise. They are to this extent parasites in the human body, contributing nothing to it as a whole but at the same time absorbing nutrients and being nourished by it. The rate of growth of a cancer depends very much on its cell type and its location, but it is not uncommon for cancers to be present for several years before they ever cause symptoms. During this time, the cancer cells can spread to distant organs such as the liver, lungs, bones and brain, and it is for this reason that even when the main cancer is discovered, curative treatment is sometimes not possible as the cancer has already spread to numerous other organs.

Cancer is known by many other names and euphemisms, many of which are frequently used by doctors in the presence of patients in an effort to soften the blow of the diagnosis and to avoid that frightening 'C' word. The words neoplasm, mitosis and carcinoma are all good examples. The word growth is sometimes also used although growths may be benign as well as malignant. Unlike benign growths, however, malignant ones are capable of infiltrating the tissues around them as well as spreading to distant sites around the body, and they can cause localised symptoms as a result of blocking passageways, eroding bone and destroying nerves. Malignant growths or tumours are often life-threatening whereas benign tumours rarely are, and even then only when in a location that would make treatment exceedingly difficult in terms of access.

Mary, 48, was relaxing in a hot bath when she idly felt a distinct lump in the upper right-hand part of her right breast. She was used to performing a gentle self-examination every now and again as she has been advised to do by the practice nurse, but this was something quite unaccustomed and new. Her doctor was attentive and efficient and confirmed the abnormal lump the same day. A mammogram also located the growth and a biopsy revealed that the cells were cancerous. But this happened 8 years ago. Mary had a mastectomy at the time and although she still takes Tamoxifen as a kind of insurance policy against any recurrence, she remains fit and well and is, to all intents and purposes, probably cured.

Which Areas of the Body are most Affected?

Any part of the body can be affected by cancer, but those organs consisting of constantly dividing and regenerating tissue are most vulnerable to malignant change. These include the lung, breast, intestine, skin, stomach and pancreas along with the bone marrow and lymph glands. The testes and ovaries not uncommonly give rise to cancer, and any parts of the soft tissues of the body, the muscles, lips and tongue for example, are no exception. Those parts of the body which do not divide rapidly (such as nervous tissue and the brain itself) seldom give rise to malignancy although they may well represent sites of development of secondary cancer due to spread from some more distant location. Cancers are often therefore referred to as 'primary' or 'secondary' depending on whether they started in the organ in which they develop or whether they developed there as a secondary result of cancer elsewhere. Brain tumours, as we have described, are mainly secondary.

How Common is Cancer?

Because we hear so much about it, it must seem to many people in this day and age that cancer is a modern epidemic. In fact cancer has been present since time immemorial and does not affect just humans but domestic and farm animals, sea creatures and birds alike. Also as people live longer they become increasingly likely to die from cancer than from anything else because so many other disorders are now treatable. Cancer certainly becomes more prevalent as people grow older, but even then it still only accounts for a fifth of the total number of deaths. In total it affects more than 25 per cent of people in Britain at some stage in their lives and remains the second commonest cause of death after heart disease.

Statistically it seems that cancer tends to be commonest either in childhood or in the older age groups, one explanation being that the immune system that helps to fight the development of cancer is less efficient at these two chronological extremes. Between the ages of 20 and 30, a person is very unlikely to develop cancer, but the risk more or less doubles between 30 and 40, and then doubles again for every syc-ceeding decade. Post-mortems on people who die in their nineties often reveal a previously undetected cancer, and in men of this age group in particular, the discovery of a developing cancer of the prostate, for example, is almost predictable.

What Causes Cancer?

There is no doubt that a person's risk of developing cancer is partly determined by their genetic make-up. But there are also environmental triggers that can bring about cancerous changes in susceptible people. We know that smoking undoubtedly contributes to cancer of the lung, mouth, larynx, bladder, pancreas and kidney. We know that excessive exposure to the sun contributes to skin cancer. We know that a high-fat, low-fibre diet contributes to malignancy in the bowel and that a high-fat diet is thought to account for up to 35 per cent of cancer deaths overall. We know that chronic liver damage caused by infections such as some types of hepatitis may contribute to liver cancer, and that HIV infection leads to AIDS-related cancer, and that human papilloma virus infection of the cervix is a factor in the development of cancer of the cervix. Radiation and other occupational hazards are also well-known trigger factors for the development of malignant growths. However, the genetic susceptibility of any one person to cancer modifies the impact of these environmental factors. A woman may avoid a high-fat, low-fibre diet, not smoke and keep extremely fit all her life, but if she has more than two first-degree relatives (mother, sister or grandmother) with cancer of the breast or ovaries, her chances of developing a similar cancer are quite definitely increased.

Ned, a smoker for as long as he could remember, developed a chest infection and was surprised to see quite a lot of blood mixed up with the phlegm he was coughing up. When it happened a second and then a third time, and especially when the infection failed to clear up with the usual antibiotics, he became rather concerned. A chest X-ray revealed an obvious star-shaped shadow at the centre of his left lung. Unfortunately this proved to be cancer.

Signs and Symptoms

The variety and severity of the symptoms and signs that cancer produces are enormous. Much depends on the location of the cancer, the tissue in which it originated and the rate of growth. Some cancers arise with obvious and visible symptoms such as lumps, bumps or skin changes. Or it may be that patients have unexplained bleeding such as when they notice blood in the urine, blood mixed with the bowel motions or bloodstained sputum when coughing. Sometimes an obstruction of a passageway may occur, such as in the intestine, leading to pain and altered bowel function. Alternatively pain may be the predominant symptom as an enlarging growth presses against sensitive nerves. Occasionally tumour cells can produce hormones, giving rise to effects in far distant parts of the body and of course generalised features such as weight loss, anaemia and fatigue are common to many different types of cancer. There are, however, a number of classic warning signs of cancer which everybody should understand and be aware of and these are listed in the box below. Any of these occurring at any age should be regarded as suspicious and brought to the urgent attention of your doctor.

CANCER WARNING SIGNS

1. Rapid and unexplained weight loss.
2. Any scab or ulcer on the skin which fails to heal within 3 weeks.
3. Any mole on the skin which gets bigger, itches, bleeds or changes colour.
4. Hoarseness lasting more than 3 weeks.
5. Coughing up blood.
6. Lumps or changes in the breast shape.
7. Bleeding or discharge from the nipple.
8. Vaginal bleeding between periods or after the menopause.
9. Any persistent change in regular bowel habit.
10. Blood in the urine when there is no pain.
11. Change in the shape or size of the testicles.
12. Persistent unexplained abdominal pain for more than a few days.
13. Increasing difficulty in swallowing.
14. Severe or recurrent headache particularly when present in the morning or which wakes the patient up.

Diagnosis

The diagnosis of cancer is achieved in a number of ways. Symptoms alone may suggest the underlying problem but the doctor will examine the patient and microscopic examination of tissue cells can be obtained through a biopsy. Often scanning and imaging techniques will also be employed to provide further information while at the same time sparing the patient any discomfort. The box below describes the commonest type of tests used.

INVESTIGATIONS FOR THE DIAGNOSIS OF CANCER

Cytology tests: These, like cervical smear tests, look at abnormal cells arising from the surface of the tumour itself. In the smear test, cells are scraped from the neck of the womb and examined microscopically to detect any early pre-cancerous change. With urine cytology, cells that have been passed from the bladder are examined for abnormality. Cells aspirated through a needle into a syringe from a swollen abdomen may reveal the presence of cancer cells in cases of bowel cancer.

Biochemical tests: These show the presence of enzymes or hormones indicative of cancer. High levels of 'prostate specific antigen' indicate cancer of the prostate, and persistently large amounts of blood in the faeces can indicate bowel cancer.

Direct inspection: Endoscopy, involving the use of a narrow flexible tube attached to a viewing lens, is frequently used to examine the state of health of hollow organs such as the colon, gullet and stomach, and bronchial tubes. While the tissue is being directly observed, a tissue sample can also be obtained through a biopsy for microscopic examination.

Imaging techniques: These are usually non-invasive but extremely valuable techniques whereby the structure of internal organs can be seen in detail without the need to operate. Examples include mammography (a low-dose X-ray technique carried out as part of screening for breast cancer), ultrasound screening using high frequency sound waves, and MRI and CAT scans which are used increasingly frequently as these provide excellent 3-D images of the internal anatomy of the body.

Modern diagnostic techniques have meant that cancer is diagnosed much earlier than it has been in the past allowing treatments to achieve a better cure and survival rate. Screening tests have undoubtedly reduced mortality as well.

Treatment of Cancer

The aim of cancer treatment is to achieve a cure if at all possible. Surgical excision of a tumour that has been detected early offers the best chance of this happening. However, even small cancers can sometimes have undetectable seedlings that spread by the time an operation is carried out, so surgery is often combined with radiotherapy and the use of anti-cancer drugs as a kind of insurance against recurrence. This three-pronged attack on cancer is designed to kill off any tumour cells remaining after surgery. Unfortunately chemotherapeutic agents (anti-cancer drugs) are not entirely specific to tumour cells and can damage and interfere with normal cells at the same time. This results in the well-known side effects that patients experience such as hair loss, nausea, loss of appetite and anaemia. The benefits of using such treatments must always therefore be weighed against any adverse effects and the decision as to what treatment is used and for how long is one in which both the doctor and patient should be involved.

The Outlook

Contrary to popular belief up to half of all cancers diagnosed today are completely cured, and even the survival rates in the years following the diagnosis of cancer have improved dramatically in recent years. The fear and uncertainty faced by patients is something that all orthodox doctors should address, as emotional needs are just as important a part of the treatment as physical ones. As doctors who have worked on radiotherapy and leukaemia wards, we know that the battle against cancer for doctor and patient alike is so very worthwhile. At best a successful outcome is reached; at worst, the patient is helped to achieve not only a better quality of life, but also much calm and spiritual peace.

Ray, 24, was curious when his girlfriend mentioned that she thought he had a lump on one of his testicles. It did not hurt and to be honest, Ray could not really tell for sure whether it had always been there or not. He was not in the habit of checking although he had read that some men routinely did.

Deciding to have a check-up with the doctor, he was stunned when he heard the news. He had a testicular cancer that warranted urgent treatment.

Nutritional Healing

Eating a healthy diet can do much to prevent cancer, possibly even reverse some pre-cancerous changes and help build your immune system to fight any cancer already in existence. But eating healthily will also make you feel better by giving you more energy to exercise, another major way of helping you cope and fight cancerous change. A good book to read on the subject would be *Food For Life* by Oliver Gillie in association with the World Cancer Research Fund (Hodder & Stoughton, 1998) which explains which kind of foods can help in preventing cancer.

Apart from the basics (see p. 5) there are plenty of specifics for you to consider. Diets high in fish have been linked with a reduced risk of breast cancer, heart disease and rheumatoid arthritis due to the omega-3 fatty acids they contain. If you feel you cannot eat fish, flax seed (linseed) oil is a good alternative. Phytochemicals are substances found in plants that help them to survive environmental threat. What's really exciting is that they have also been shown to be useful in humans to help fight chronic diseases such as cancer. There is still much work to be done in this exciting new field; however, you can start to help yourself now by adding to your diet natural foods that have been found to be treasure houses of protective substances. Soya is one such food. It contains isoflavones which act like oestrogens, slowing and preventing prostate and breast cancer while reducing the effect of the body's own sexual hormones. In fact Japanese women have a much lower risk of breast cancer, partly due to the high amounts of soya and fish in their diet, and the words 'hot flushes' are barely recognised as menopausal symptoms hardly exist.

GARLIC

This amazing foodstuff can reduce cancer of the digestive tract, scavenge free radicals and destroy *Helicobacter pylori* which is implicated in the formation of stomach ulcers and possibly stomach cancer. It also boosts the immune system and stimulates lymphocyte production. Diallyl trisulphide (DATS), a compound found in garlic oil, can destroy or slow down the growth of cancer cells in laboratory tests at a rate comparable with some chemotherapy (5-flourouracil) but without the toxicity. Two other garlic constituents, S-allylcysteine (SAC) and diallyl disulphide (DADS), also kill cancer cells, reducing tumour size by 50 to 75 per cent. These figures have been duplicated at two centres in the USA (Pennsylvania State Department of Nutrition and the University of Texas). It is thought that garlic may be especially useful in oesophageal, breast, colon and skin cancers.

Tea

The national drink turns out to be full of antioxidants (see p. 163) and it does not matter whether you drink it hot as we like it in the UK or cold as the Americans prefer, the benefits remain the same. Research from China shows that tea drinkers have 60 per cent less cancer of the oesophagus than others, while in the USA fewer kidney, bladder, colon, oesophagus and skin cancers are reported in tea drinkers. It is more potent than Vitamin C or E as an antioxidant and reduces the risk of heart attack. Women at risk of breast cancer should drink 3–4 cups of tea a day. Green tea may be more effective than ordinary tea, although that isn't clear yet.

Grapes

Grapeseed extract can slow the growth of and kill cancer cells, fighting DNA damage caused by free radicals twice as effectively as Vitamin E. It appears to work best on breast, lung and stomach cancer cells while simultaneously promoting the growth of healthy cells and protecting them from damage caused by pollutants such as cigarette smoke. Resveratrol, a substance found in the skin of grapes, may also inhibit initiation of tumour growth and may possibly return pre-cancerous cells to their normal state.

WHOLE GRAINS

Inositol hexaphosphate (IP6), found in wheat, rice, maize and oats, acts like an antioxidant and slows the rapid multiplication of cancer cells especially in the breast, colon and prostate. In animals it also has a protective action and can reduce the size of existing tumours.

ANTIOXIDANTS

Carotenoids found in colourful vegetables and flavinoids found in brightly coloured fruits are highly protective against cancer, being powerful antioxidants. Lycopene in tomatoes is especially good for prostate cancer (eat some every day!) while the cruciferous vegetables (cabbage and kale, for example) contain phyto-oestrogens that reduce the risk of breast and prostate cancer in animal studies. Chilli peppers contain capsaicin which has been shown to fight off stomach cancer, while quercitin in onions and broccoli slows development of cancer cells. Make all of these regular additions to your diet.

Vitamins and Supplements

Although you should get a lot of antioxidants from your diet, if you are at risk or already have cancer, then supplements are worth considering. However, don't take antioxidants while actually undergoing chemotherapy without first discussing this with your consultant. Part of the function of anti-cancer drugs is to form free radicals which then attack cancer cells, so you may be working against your therapy if you take antioxidant supplements. The exceptions to this rule are milk thistle and CoEnzyme Q10 (CoQ10) which protect the heart and liver and won't interfere with chemotherapy, and Vitamins C and E which may actually assist chemotherapy.

Antioxidants are best taken in groups so that they synergise and protect each other, rather like an army. For example, Vitamins C and E are best taken together since alone they can be disarmed by the free radicals they have scavenged.

Propolis, a bee product, contains caffeic acid which appears to have the ability to prevent the development of cancer and can kill liver and lung cancer cells in the laboratory.

Hyperacin, the active ingredient of St John's Wort, may be toxic to cancer cells and some viruses.

There is some fascinating work on gingko biloba and its use to help heal chromosome damage. Thirty workers from the Chernobyl disaster took 120 mg of gingko biloba extract daily and after 2 months their chromosomes were almost back to normal. Benefits were still evident a year after the supplement was stopped, although the chromosome damage then started to reappear indicating that perhaps it needs to be taken for longer. There is reason to think, therefore, that this powerful antioxidant can reverse radiation damage caused by radiation therapies as well as by nuclear accidents.

French maritime pine bark helps Vitamin E in its antioxidant capacity and also regulates the body's nitrous oxide levels. Nitrous oxide is useful to maintain the muscle tone of blood vessels, but it can also act as a free radical and result in chronic inflammation which can cause cancer. Milk thistle protects the liver from free radical damage and boosts the immune system. Selenium reduces the risk of all kinds of cancers especially prostate, colorectal and lung. Vitamin A may not only prevent but reverse oral cancer.

Complementary Therapies

If you are undergoing chemotherapy for cancer there are therapies such as acupuncture, acupressure and massage that will help with side effects such as nausea, vomiting and fatigue. The Royal Marsden Hospital offers acupuncture to relieve breathing difficulties and emotional distress in those suffering from cancer while the Women's and Infants' Hospital in Rhode Island, USA offers those undergoing chemotherapy simple foot massages and the opportunity of having a pet with them during treatment. Of those receiving foot massage, 93 per cent have reduced side effects from chemotherapy and 84 per cent of those on the animal companion programme are soothed by the presence of a pet. A hospital in Texas offers yoga classes, massage therapies, support groups and Internet courses with great benefit to their patients. Bristol Cancer Help Care offer similar support to patients in Britain (see

Useful Addresses). The herb astragalus can boost the immune system by protecting bone marrow. And reishi mushrooms are said to inhibit tumour growth. Maitake mushrooms are also useful in that they are antiviral, fight cancer and can enhance immunity.

Exercise and Lifestyle

Obviously for all of us, to live in a pollution-free world would be wonderful, although this is probably almost impossible in the modern world. However, being aware and steering clear of such things as cigarette smoke, toxic diesel fumes, pesticides and other noxious substances is only common sense. Exercise doesn't have to be vigorous to be useful, but if you can manage some aerobic exercise 3 or 4 times a week that's great. Walking still remains the best, although it needs to be more than a gentle stroll if possible. Yoga, T'ai chi and Chi gong yield spiritual and emotional as well as physical benefits and a weekly class would also give you companionship and support. Talk to the teacher about any particular difficulties you may have and these will almost certainly be accommodated. You'll be amazed at the difference exercise will make to how you feel. Try it.

Emotional and Spiritual Healing

To have cancer diagnosed is the most frightening prospect for the majority of people, setting them apart and leaving them feeling isolated and often without much hope. How someone feels emotionally and spiritually affects their recovery and is therefore extremely important. We talked fairly recently to a woman who had survived breast cancer for just over 5 years so far and yet she was still aware every day of the possibility of the illness returning, but even more afraid of expressing that fear. She understood that a positive attitude was of the utmost importance. But it is OK, even necessary, for sufferers to express the fear that this illness strikes into the heart of most people. This beautiful woman had been suppressing her fear and anger for all these years, smiling and saying that she was fine, while being brittle and shut off from the support and love she needed. We are sure that this has been much more detrimental to her than being able to share her feelings. The fear of dying, of leaving your children, the anxiety about living after mastectomy, how that will affect not only you but your relationships with others, still waiting for the axe to fall and wondering how long you'll survive – are naturally frightening issues. Having named the fear, addressed the anger and asked the inevitable 'Why me?' we can often move on to have a more positive attitude and adopt a more defiant stance which gives us a much better chance not only of survival but of good quality of life. For some this can become a life better than it was before, and free of the negative outlook that was probably in part responsible for the illness in the first place.

In 1985 a study by Pettingale and colleagues looked at women with breast cancer and divided them into groups according to their psychological coping styles. They found that 80 per cent of those women with a fighting spirit were alive after 5 years. Those who accepted the illness stoically fared less well with 50 per cent surviving for 5 years. But of those women who saw themselves as hopeless and helpless victims, only 20 per cent survived. There are other traits associated with a cancer-prone personality. Those who suppress their emotions, allow anger to build up, withdraw and feel hopeless and helpless and have a history that includes a troubled childhood are more likely to suffer cancer. If instead you can let go of negative thoughts and feelings and concentrate on the positive aspects, freely express your emotions and actively live your life, then your likelihood of developing this disease is greatly reduced. Conflicts that can be resolved need to be confronted, but try to become aware of what you can't change and let those things go. Remaining angry about things long gone helps nothing and you only hurt yourself. Are there things it's time to forgive and just let go? Are there things that you constantly try to change and can't? Let them go too. The basic rule is that 'the only thing I can change is me'. Other people, the past, the weather or the fact that I'm sitting in a traffic jam are beyond my control and I'll be much happier and healthier if I recognise that and smile.

Spiritual healing will always help, even if it's only in allowing you some peace and letting your whole system benefit from the circulation of loving energy. There's much you can do alone, although having someone guide you would always be good. You can learn to visualise your healthy cells growing, surrounding and then eventually eradicating unhealthy cells; you can visualise tumors getting smaller, with healing light coming in to cleanse you of illness and disease. You might be amazed at the power of the connection between your mind, body and spirit.

Human touch is one of the most healing things, so have a massage, let your friends give you a hug, enjoy someone holding your hand. You'll be amazed at the difference it will make to the quality of your life. If hugging is new to you, buy yourself *The Little Book of Hugs* and learn. Take some time out to meditate and know that it's never too late to change, to learn to enjoy being of service to others and to develop a new way of life. The benefits are enormous. And don't forget prayer! At the Baylor University Medical Center in the USA, founded almost 100 years ago, the doctors, numbering about 100 in all, uninhibitedly and unashamedly pray with their patients.

PREVENTION – 50–90 PER CENT OF CANCERS CAN BE PREVENTED

1. Consume plenty of fruit and vegetables especially dark green leafy ones and the cruciferous group – broccoli, cauliflower and cabbage.
2. Eat citrus fruits which are also full of antioxidants.
3. Choose the leanest cuts of red meat.
4. Boost your intake of fish and fish oils.
5. Use only monounsaturated fats, olive oil preferably. Eat a low-fat diet.
6. Reduce obesity. This is important even for children for their future health and reduction in risk of developing cancer.
7. Take Vitamin C and E supplements – it's almost impossible to get enough in your diet.

8. Vitamin D can lower the risk of breast cancer so we need at least a little sun to help us manufacture it.
9. Stop smoking and move out of smoke-filled atmospheres and strongly object to others smoking in your space.
10. Minimise your use of alcohol.
11. Boost your exercise programme.
12. Eat plenty of fibre – fruits, grains, rice (brown), beans, legumes, wholemeal bread, potatoes, pasta, etc.
13. Avoid food cooked at very high temperatures, especially charred food.
14. Limit the salt in your diet.
15. Get regular physical examinations from your GP.
16. Check if you live in a radon area and if so have your home assessed for levels of this colourless, odourless gas which leaks into buildings from geological formations.
17. Look into ways of reducing geopathic stress (see p. 9).
18. Check your home and workplace for asbestos, radiation and arsenic as well as other pollutants.
19. Take a folic acid (folate) supplement.
20. Protect yourself with sunscreen and examine your skin once a month.
21. Do a breast exam yourself once a month.
22. Protect yourself from the Human Papilloma Virus by using condoms during sexual activity and being discriminating about the number of sexual partners you have.
23. Men should eat tomatoes which protect against prostate cancer.
24. Ninety per cent of cancer is due to the effects of environmental carcinogens, combined with poor nutrition, and lowered function of the immune system and detoxification processes. Detoxifying your liver (see Detoxification, p. 7) can increase enormously its ability to complete the liver's primary function of filtering out toxic waste.

SPECIFIC CANCERS

Lung Cancer

Lung cancer remains the commonest type of cancer in Britain, and although men are affected more than women, the incidence in women is gradually catching up, as their smoking habits in recent years have reached a par with men's. The peak age for a diagnosis of lung cancer is about 70, and without doubt, smoking remains the main culprit in its development. The more cigarettes a person smokes per day, and the younger they were when they started, the bigger the risk they carry of developing lung cancer. Although there are different types of lung cancer, all of them are strongly linked to smoking tobacco.

SYMPTOMS

The commonest symptom is a cough. This is present in more than three quarters of patients with lung cancer. Unfortunately, because so many heavy smokers develop a morning cough anyway, this often masks any additional stimulus for coughing caused by the cancer. Patients also sometimes complain of bloodstained phlegm, shortness of breath, wheezing or chest discomfort. Lung cancer often spreads to other sites in the body, particularly the liver, brain and bones. Generalised weakness, tiredness and weight loss are also common and doctors may suspect the diagnosis when a heavy smoker develops a chest infection which proves unresponsive to antibiotics or which becomes recurrent. If the cancer affects the surface of the lung (the pleura), a build-up of fluid known as an effusion can arise between the lung and the chest wall.

DIAGNOSIS

Any of the above symptoms may suggest the diagnosis, although a chest X-ray usually shows a typical shadow where the cancer lies. Cytology can identify cancerous cells in the sputum, and these are present when the cells are shed into the airways and are then brought up with the phlegm. A flexible telescopic viewing instrument known as a bronchoscope is often passed down into the lungs under local anaesthetic enabling a biopsy to be taken for microscopic analysis. This may confirm the presence of a cancer while at the same time identifying the exact cell type, a characteristic useful in determining the optimum treatment.

Conventional treatment

In the early stages, removal of part or all of the lung may be performed. This offers the best chance of a cure. In later stages, however, the cancer has often spread beyond the lung tissue or the patient's general condition may not be healthy enough to survive this type of major surgery. In these instances the treatment of choice is chemotherapy and radiotherapy to destroy as many cancerous cells as possible and to limit their spread.

Future prospects

The outlook for patients with lung cancer is generally very serious. Less than 10 per cent survive for 5 years after the initial diagnosis although those having surgery because they have been detected early and where the cancer has not yet obviously spread can look forward to a 15–30 per cent five-year survival.

It remains clear that the best chance we have of cutting the death rate from lung cancer is to employ better preventative measures. The single most important thing you can do for yourself is never to start smoking in the first place or to stop as soon as possible. In particular the one group of people who currently have not shown an improvement in smoking habits are female teenagers in whom the incidence of lung cancer in the future will almost certainly increase as a result.

Breast Cancer

This remains the commonest cancer in women with 1 in every 12 developing the condition at some stage in their lives. There are estimated to be around 15,000 deaths every year as a result of breast cancer, and although it can occasionally affect men, these represent a mere 1 per cent of the total. Most people who die from breast cancer do so because the cancer has already spread beyond the breast to more distant sites in the body when the diagnosis is first made. Factors which increase the likelihood of developing breast cancer include a hereditary susceptibility, being childless or having the first pregnancy at an older age, having previous benign tumours of the breast, and enjoying a diet rich in saturated fat together with regular heavy alcohol intake. Speculation that hormone replacement therapy taken for many years might increase the risk of breast cancer can be put into perspective with the following facts. A woman taking HRT for 5 years is estimated to have a 2 in 1000 extra chance of developing breast cancer over the following 20 years. If she has taken it for 10 years, it is a 6 in 1000 extra chance, and for 15 years, a 12 in 1000 chance. However, the risk returns to normal within 2 years of stopping HRT, and research has shown that breast cancers developing in women who take HRT are easier to detect and treat. Also, it is important to realise that taking HRT confers protection against osteoporosis and heart disease. All in all, the safety profile of HRT is extremely good and the benefits far outweigh the risks provided it is used appropriately.

In terms of the family history, two recently indentified genes called BRAC1 and BRAC2 mean that a woman who has breast or ovarian cancer in a close family member (sister, mother or daughter) is at increased risk of developing either of these two types of cancer in the future. This is especially so if the breast cancer was in both breasts or was diagnosed at a young age. Identification of these genes in 'at risk' families is useful in that it allows such women to be counselled about regular screening in the future and even to consider the possibility of having a prophylactic mastectomy on both sides before any cancer begins so they may enjoy a worry-free life. Although this sounds very drastic only 5–10 per cent of breast cancers have a hereditary basis and among the women in this predicament there are still a minority who would prefer to undergo this procedure rather than face a future of fear and uncertainty.

Symptoms

Symptoms include a bloodstained discharge from the nipple, inversion of the nipple, a lump which is usually not painful and dimpling or creasing of the skin.

Diagnosis

Changes in the breast may be detected by the woman herself when she conducts an occasional self-examination, or the lump may be noticed during routine examination by the doctor as part of a screening procedure. When a lump is found a special X-ray of the breast (mammography) is carried out in women over 35 (breast tissue in younger women is too dense for this X-ray to be useful) and if any suspicion of malignancy is present, a needle operation or biopsy is carried out for microscopic examination of cells. It should be remembered that 9 out of 10 breast lumps are benign, and these are particularly noticeable in the premenstrual period when fluid retention commonly occurs. Ultrasound tests are also used increasingly frequently, especially to distinguish between cysts and solid lumps.

Conventional treatment

Despite the spectre of fear that haunts the subject of breast cancer, surgical removal of the tumour achieves a cure in a third of women with early breast cancer. These days simple removal of the lump rather than of the whole breast is usually performed with equally good results. Often this simple 'lumpectomy' is combined with radiotherapy and anti-cancer drugs as a form of insurance against any recurrence. Treatment, however, depends on the age of the patient, the size of the tumour, whether there are any signs that it has spread to the lymph glands under the arm, and the sensitivity of the tumour cells to hormones. This can be determined by laboratory investigations known as oestrogen receptor tests. If the breast cancer has already spread to other sites in the body, anti-cancer drugs and hormones are used.

FUTURE PROSPECTS

A cure can be achieved if the cancer is treated early enough. Even then regular check-ups are required. Regular self-examination of the breast and mammograms should be carried out, and should the cancer recur, hormonal treatment, radiotherapy and chemotherapy can relieve symptoms and prolong life.

SKIN CANCER

In Britain the incidence of newly diagnosed skin cancer appears to be doubling every 10 years and there were more than 40,000 new cases diagnosed in 1998 alone. There are three major types of skin cancer, namely malignant melanoma, basal cell carcinoma (also known as rodent ulcer) and squamous cell carcinoma. All three types are increasingly common in white-skinned people the nearer they live to the equator where ultraviolet radiation is more intense, and we know that childhood sun exposure involving severe sunburn considerably increases the risk of melanoma as an adult.

Malignant Melanoma

This skin cancer begins in the cells that make the pigment in the skin. It is the rarest form of skin cancer but can be very aggressive with a high tendency to spread to distant parts of the body. It also occurs in younger people which means that whole families can be devastated if it is not caught early enough. It is curable when detected and treated early, although its behaviour is often very difficult to predict and it can recur many years after the first abnormal area of skin is removed. The key to its prevention is the use of sunblock creams and the avoidance of sunburn and deep tanning, as radiation from sunlight is a major contributory factor.

SYMPTOMS

Many people have large numbers of moles or freckles on their skin, and these are normal. Warning signs that a mole or melanoma has turned malignant, however, include the following:

a new mole that is coloured blue-black or is patchilly coloured with brown-black and purplish areas within it, changes to an existing mole such as enlargment, bleeding or itching, and satellite lesions around an existing mole. As a general rule, moles are more of a concern when they are larger than the blunt end of a pencil.

Conventional treatment

Surgery offers the best chance of a cure and is the usual treatment. The extent of the surgery will depend on the size, position and depth of the melanoma. Where the melanoma has already spread, radiotherapy and chemotherapy are sometimes used, although stimulating the immune system using biological agents such as interleukin 2 or tumour vaccines may be employed with variable results. Occasionally chemotherapy is given exclusively to the area involved, a technique known as isolated limb perfusion. This concentrates powerful anti-cancer drugs to the required area while minimising the side effects on the rest of the body.

Basal Cell Carcinoma (BCC)

This type of skin cancer occurs almost exclusively on the face or neck and is also known as a rodent ulcer. It is the commonest type of skin cancer in Britain with about 30,000 cases diagnosed per year. Fair-skinned people over 50 are most at risk, and direct skin damage caused by exposure to sunlight is the predominant cause.

Symptoms

BCC starts as a tiny flat nodule which grows very slowly, eventually forming a shallow ulcer with raised edges. People often believe that they have been bitten by an insect and that the initial bite has failed to heal. A crust forms which drops off only to re-form again repeating the same cycle. Without treatment, however, the ulcer gradually invades the deeper tissues of the skin, although they never behave like other malignant skin cancers by spreading to distant sites in the body. BCCs are therefore relatively benign and harmless.

CONVENTIONAL TREATMENT

Surgical removal is usually employed in younger people whereas radiotherapy is usually used in older people. Either results in a complete cure although patients who have been affected should be monitored regularly to see if any other BCCs are developing in the facial area.

Squamous Cell Carcinoma (SCC)

Again, this skin cancer is commonest in fair-skinned, fair-haired people over the age of 60 and is caused by exposure to strong sunlight over many years.

SYMPTOMS

This cancer starts as a small, hard painless lump on an exposed area of skin, gradually enlarging until it resembles a wart or an ulcer. If left untreated it will eventually spread to other areas of the body.

CONVENTIONAL TREATMENT

After a skin biopsy to determine the type of cells responsible for the symptoms, treatment is carried out using either surgery or radiotherapy. If there is any evidence that the cancer has spread, then anti-cancer drugs will be used in addition. There will usually be follow-up examinations to monitor any recurrence.

In all cases of skin cancer, prevention is the key. Ways of decreasing the risk of developing skin cancer are shown in the box below.

PREVENTION OF SKIN CANCER

1. Skin damage from the sun is most dangerous at a young age so the most important time to protect against sunburn is in childhood.
2. Fair-skinned, red-haired individuals are at most risk as they have less protective skin pigment, melanin.
3. Avoid the sun during the hottest times of the day between 11 a.m. and 4 p.m. and stay in the shade during those hours.

4. Always use a sunblock with a minimum sun protection factor of SPF15. Ensure the cream used protects against both UVA and UVB types of radiation.
5. Wear shirts and wide-brimmed hats to increase protection and remember that good sunglasses protect against eye damage as well.
6. Remember the famous Australian slogan that has been so successful in preventing skin cancer in that very hot part of the world: 'Slip, Slap, Slop'. Slip on a T-shirt, Slap on a hat and Slop on the sunblock.
7. Not even sunbeds are entirely safe. Any exposure to ultraviolet radiation is potentially hazardous.

CANCER OF THE BOWEL, STOMACH AND PANCREAS

Freda, 61, had vaguely noticed that her perenially 'slow' bowels had become even slower in recent weeks and that eating more dietary fibre in an attempt to rectify the situation only produced abdominal cramps. When she passed some jelly-like material into the loo and noticed that the colour of her motions resembled that of tar, she visited her doctor. The GP felt a definite firm lump on the left-hand side of Freda's abdomen quite low down and suspected diverticulitis. As it turned out, tests the following week revealed a tumour in the large intestine. Freda has cancer of the colon.

Cancer of the bowel, stomach and pancreas are common in Britain, with cancer of the colon, the large intestine, accounting for 20 per cent of all cancers in this part of the world. Each year, 25,000 cases of cancer of the colon are diagnosed with one third of them being located in the last part of the colon, the rectum. In addition there are 13,000 deaths each year from stomach cancer and 7000 diagnosed cases of pancreatic cancer in Britain. Stomach cancer seems to be becoming less common while pancreatic cancer is becoming more so, but all of these types of cancer appear more frequently in the age group over 50.

Diet seems to contribute to the cause in many instances: a diet rich in saturated fat is responsible for concentrating carcinogenic toxins within the lining of the bowel, and a lack of fibre is responsible for slow bowel movement, which in turn effectively allows any environmental pollutants to linger longer within the intestine. Heavy smoking and a high intake of alcohol are also thought to be contributary factors in stomach and pancreatic cancer.

SYMPTOMS

Any alteration in normal bowel habit lasting more than 10 days or so in someone over the age of 50 should be regarded as a potentially sinister warning sign and reported to a doctor. Alternating diarrhoea and constipation is frequently reported but it is the permanent change in what is normal for you, the individual, that is important. The presence of blood mixed with the motions is another important sign, although sometimes the amounts may be so microscopic that they can only be picked up on laboratory testing. There may be pain or discomfort in the abdomen and the presence of a lump can sometimes be detected by the doctor on examination. Occasionally the patient develops sudden obstruction of the bowel leading to an emergency admission to hospital with intense pain.

Stomach cancer produces symptoms almost indistinguishable from a stomach ulcer. There is pain in the upper abdomen and there is also weight loss, decreased appetite, nausea and vomiting, and a sensation of fullness after even small meals. The symptoms of pancreatic cancer are similar, with pain in the upper abdomen, although in this condition pain is also felt in the back. Symptoms common to cancers of both the stomach and the pancreas include considerable tiredness, weakness, loss of weight, loss of appetite, and in pancreatic cancer, jaundice is frequently seen.

DIAGNOSIS

The diagnosis of these conditions can be achieved in a number of ways. Bowel cancer may be picked up on screening tests where microscopic traces of blood are detected in the stool (occult blood). Barium X-rays can reveal cancers of the bowel or stomach. Endoscopy, whereby a narrow flexible viewing instrument is passed into the relevant organ, is effective in directly observing a tumour or allowing a biopsy to be taken from it. (For bowel symptoms a sigmoidoscopy or colonoscopy is carried out, and for stomach symptoms a gastroscopy would be the appropriate procedure.) Endoscopic techniques may also be used to diagnose pancreatic cancer, although ultrasound tests and CT scans are more likely to be used as they confer just as much if not more information and are considerably less invasive.

CONVENTIONAL TREATMENTS AND OUTLOOK

The key in all these cancers is to detect the cancer as early as possible to give the best chance of a cure. Thanks to screening procedures, the outlook for bowel cancer has improved enormously with 50 per cent of patients surviving for more than 5 years after surgical treatment. Treatment usually involves a partial colectomy (removal of part of the colon) with the diseased portion of the gut being removed and the cut ends of the healthy bowel being sewn back together to restore normal function. In cases where the diagnosis is made later, when the cancer has already spread, palliative therapy to prolong life and relieve symptoms is achieved using medication. Stomach cancer has the worst outlook with only those whose cancers are diagnosed extremely early surviving. Treatment in these cases would be removal of the entire stomach, total gastrectomy, followed by radiotherapy and anti-cancer drugs, although only a fifth of such patients are fit enough to withstand such surgery at the outset. In cases diagnosed later than this, there is a survival rate of less than 10 per cent for 5 years. Pancreatic cancer has the worst outlook of all as it spreads very rapidly to other parts of the body and the only chance of a cure is very early diagnosis with a pancreatectomy (removal of the entire pancreas) followed by radiotherapy and chemotherapy. In other cases, pain relief is given and surgery performed to bypass any tissue that may be responsible for jaundice or bowel obstruction, although only 10 per cent of patients survive for a year after diagnosis.

OVARIAN CANCER

This type of cancer is commonest in women over the age of 50. Around 5000 cases are diagnosed in Britain every year, and it appears commoner in women who have never had children, but less common in women who have taken the oral contraceptive pill. In British women, ovarian cancer is the fifth leading cause of death from cancer.

SYMPTOMS

Unfortunately this cancer rarely causes symptoms until it has become widespread. Vague abdominal discomfort and swelling are often the first signs, although nausea, abnormal vaginal bleeding and bloating may be reported.

DIAGNOSIS

Ultrasound tests and direct viewing of the ovary, either through a viewing instrument (laparoscopy) or through an exploratory surgical operation (laparotomy), are usually performed. A biopsy using either of these last two methods confirms the diagnosis on a cellular level.

CONVENTIONAL TREATMENT

Treatment is designed to remove malignant tissue surgically and often this means removing both ovaries and fallopian tubes, and performing a hysterectomy at the same time. Radiotherapy and chemotherapy is generally carried out to prevent any recurrence of the tumour in the future.

FUTURE PROSPECTS

When the cancer is confined to the ovaries, the outlook means that up to 70 per cent of patients survive for at least 5 years. However, when it has already spread to distant parts of the body this is reduced to about 15 per cent. The outlook is likely to improve with the increased use of ultrasonic screening tests for more and more women, particularly those with a family history, and the development of new and better combinations of anti-cancer drugs.

Testicular Cancer

This cancer affects about 1200 men each year in Britain and is mostly seen in those between 20 and 35. Men who have had an untreated undescended testicle are particularly at risk. There are two main types, namely seminomas and teratomas, although symptoms and treatment are generally very similar.

Symptoms

The usual symptom is simply a firm painless swelling of one testicle, although occasionally discomfort and inflammation may be present. Because of this, self-examination of the testicle is recommended in order to detect a tumour early enough to achieve a cure. The entire surface of both testicles should be felt, and although one testicle is normally larger than the other and may lie slightly higher or lower than its partner, the significant finding is a discrete, non-tender, firm lump which is different from the rest of the smooth, regular contour of the testicle.

Diagnosis

The essential step in reaching a diagnosis is to remove the tumour and with it the testicle on that side (orchidectomy) for examination under the microscope. Other tests include blood tests to detect cell markers which are useful in providing a reliable measure of how much cancer there is in the rest of the body and whether the treatment is working. The two most commonly detected markers are AFP (alpha feto protein) and beta HCG (human chorionic gonadotrophin). In addition, other tests may be carried out to see if the cancer has spread elsewhere and these may include X-rays of the chest and kidneys and CT scanning.

CONVENTIONAL TREATMENT

In the early stages an orchidectomy may be sufficient to achieve a cure. However, where there is a high risk that spread has occurred, preventative treatment follows using anti-cancer drugs and radiotherapy.

FUTURE PROSPECTS

The cure rate for early testicular cancer is 95–100 per cent, only dropping to 80–90 per cent for advanced disease. Furthermore, when the remaining testicle is healthy, fertility is usually preserved even when chemotherapy and radiotherapy are used.

CANCER OF THE LYMPH GLANDS

Cancers of lymphoid tissue, comprising mainly the lymph glands and the spleen, are known as lymphomas. There are two main types, Hodgkin's disease and non-Hodgkin's disease, and although they behave in very similar ways, their cellular characteristics are different. Lymphomas account for some 7000 new diagnoses every year in Britain and they appear to be most commonly seen in the age groups between 20 and 30, and then again over 50.

SYMPTOMS

Painless enlargement of one or more groups of lymph nodes in the neck or groin is the commonest symptom. There is impairment of the body's immune system, a general feeling of malaise, a low-grade temperature and loss of appetite and weight. Night sweats are frequently reported, and sometimes itching or pain after drinking alcohol may be experienced. Sometimes breathlessness can occur if the lungs are involved and a variety of recurrent infections are commonly seen.

DIAGNOSIS

Biopsy specimens taken from the enlarged glands can identify the characteristic cells which in turn may help determine the chances of a cure. The extent of the illness (its 'staging') is assessed using other tests including chest X-rays, CT scanning and a bone marrow biopsy. Sometimes a surgical exploration of the abdomen (laparotomy) is carried out, and a liver biopsy, X-rays of the lymphatic system or surgical removal of the spleen may be recommended.

Conventional treatment

This largely depends on the stage of the disease. Detected early, localised lymphomas can be cured by radiotherapy alone. Otherwise, anti-cancer drugs can be used in addition to radiotherapy.

Future prospects

The outlook depends very largely on the cell characteristics of the tumour and on the spread of the disease. Up to 80 per cent of patients survive for at least 5 years and an absolute curc can be achieved in many of the cases which are detected early. (For information on cancer of the prostate, see the section on prostate problems, p. 417. For information on leukaemia, see the section on blood disorders, p. 144.)

Integrated approach

1. Avoid smoking and an excessive alcohol intake.
2. Protect yourself from sunburn.
3. Eat a high-fibre, low-fat diet and take antioxidant supplements.
4. Be aware of any family history of cancer.
5. Avail yourself of all relevant and appropriate medical screening procedures.
6. Familiarise yourself with the classic warning signs of the commonest forms of cancer.
7. If in doubt, talk to your doctor about your worries anyway.
8. If cancer is suspected, ask to be referred to a specialist centre rather than just to the local surgeon.
9. Express your fears and emotions openly.

10. Try to obtain a precise tissue diagnosis based on microscopic analysis.
11. Find out about all treatment options and what they involve.
12. If unsure consider a second opinion.
13. Once decided, consider complementary therapy but only with your doctor's consent and NEVER as an alternative to conventional treatment.

Chest Problems

Apart from asthma and heart disease which are dealt with elsewhere in the book, the commonest chest problems encountered include acute and chronic bronchitis, emphysema and pneumonia. Despite advances in immune protection through vaccination and the development of more powerful and broader-spectrum antibiotics, these conditions remain a major cause of death and disability in Britain.

Bronchitis

James, a carpenter, has smoked 25 cigarettes a day for just over 40 years and develops at least two fairly incapacitating chest infections each winter. He coughs for an hour or two every morning bringing up creamy or green-coloured phlegm and increasingly suffers from breathlessness on exertion. He has developed chronic bronchitis.

Bronchitis is an inflammation of the bronchi, the large airways that connect the windpipe to the lung. Acute bronchitis comes on suddenly and generally lasts a few days, whereas chronic bronchitis lasts for several weeks at a time and recurs over several years. Both types are much more common in smokers and in parts of the country where there is significant atmospheric pollution. Both types are more of a problem in the winter months and the most susceptible people are smokers, the elderly, people who have reduced immunity and babies.

Symptoms

The underlying characteristic of bronchitis is inflammation of the lining of the bronchi resulting in swelling, congestion and mucus production. In acute bronchitis the main symptoms include shortness of breath, a productive cough with yellow or green sputum and wheezing. Sometimes there may be a raised temperature and pain behind the breastbone on coughing. In chronic bronchitis the symptoms are very similar but much more persistent. Because it is also recurrent, damage to the air passages gradually leads to narrowing of the tubes and obstruction. Chronic bronchitis often develops further resulting in emphysema (see below) and these two when present together are sometimes referred to as chronic obstructive airways disease (COAD).

Causes

Without doubt smoking is the major cause of chronic bronchitis. Smoking leads to the production of mucus in the lining of the bronchi which clings to the muscular walls of the tubes, leading to narrowing. Vulnerability to infection and atmospheric pollution also contributes, which is why these diseases are much more common in industrial cities. Britain has the worst rate of COAD anywhere in the world, and it is the major cause of work absences in Britain, accounting for up to 30 million working days lost annually. In all, something like 3 million people in the UK suffer from chronic bronchitis, mostly men and mostly over 40.

Complications

As chronic bronchitis worsens over the years in conjunction with the development of emphysema, the lungs become stiffer and more resistant to the flow of blood within them. The heart then has to work harder to pump the blood through. Increasing breathlessness occurs and eventually heart failure results with the patient suffering from a bluish complexion, a build-up of fluid around the ankles, feet and lower legs, and occasionally bloodstained phlegm. At this point the possibility of lung cancer needs to be excluded using X-rays. Other tests often used include blood tests, lung function tests, tests on the sputum to look for abnormal cells or any potentially harmful micro-organisms.

EMPHYSEMA

The tiny air sacs within the lungs which allow oxygen and carbon dioxide to be exchanged between the blood and the air we breathe are called alveoli. When their fragile walls become damaged these sacs burst and larger but less efficient sacs are formed which are less able to allow the transfer of respiratory gases. The lungs also become stiffer and less elastic leading to increased resistance of bloodflow through the lungs and the likelihood of heart failure. Atmospheric pollution and smoking are predominant predisposing factors. An enzyme known as alpha-antitrypsin protects the alveoli against damage but some people inherit a deficiency of this chemical which makes them more susceptible to smoking-related illnesses. Emphysema usually accompanies chronic bronchitis but despite the fact that it has become less fashionable to talk about chronic lung disease these days, up to 20,000 men and 10,000 women perish every year in England and Wales from chronic obstructive pulmonary disease. Around 25 per cent of these deaths are due to emphysema alone.

Cyril is a retired miner who is red-faced, barrel-chested and constantly out of puff. Constant exposure to coal dust in the past undoubtedly damaged his lungs, a situation made drastically worse by his smoking. A recent cold went straight to his chest and Cyril became so breathless that he needed to breathe oxygen through a mask for several hours a day to fight it off. He has emphysema.

Symptoms and Diagnosis

Shortness of breath, particularly on exertion, is usually the first symptom. As the person affected has to work harder to breathe normally, a barrel-shaped chest gradually develops, together with a chronic cough and perhaps a slight wheeze. Blueness of the face and fluid retention around the feet and legs occurs as a result of impending heart failure. The diagnosis is reached by a combination of the patient's symptoms, the doctor's examination and respiratory function tests.

PNEUMONIA

Pneumonia is an inflammation of the lungs and is due to infection from any one of a number of potentially infectious organisms. The symptoms, treatment and progress of pneumonia depend on the cause and the general health of the patient. Pneumonia is a frequent complication of any serious disease, and as such, is the certified cause of death in around 30,000 cases every year in Britain. The most susceptible people seem to be men, babies and the elderly, and all those with damaged immunity such as AIDS sufferers or alcoholics.

Doctors tend to talk about two major varieties, 'lobar' pneumonia where only part of a lung is affected, and broncho pneumonia where the infection starts in the respiratory passageways (the bronchi and bronchioles) and then spreads to affect widespread patches of tissue in one or both lungs. A number of different viruses and bacteria may be responsible, and the identification of these bugs is important in determining the best treatment.

Maureen, 43, had a heavy cold a fortnight ago which has left her absolutely drained and physically exhausted. She has no strength, has lost her appetite and has a slight fever and a mild cough. Her doctor listened to her chest with his stethoscope, tapped one finger over another on her ribcage to hear the sound made and confirmed his clinical diagnosis with an X-ray. Maureen has lobar pneumonia.

Symptoms and Diagnosis

These include shortness of breath, a cough with yellow/green or even bloodstained phlegm, fever and chest pain. When pain is sharp and sudden and brought about by breathing deeply, it is usually due to infection on the surface of the lung, a condition known as pleurisy. The diagnosis is reached via the symptoms, the doctor's examination with a stethoscope, a chest X-ray and a culture of the causative microorganisms in the sputum.

Conventional Treatment of Chest Problems

Steam inhalations can be helpful in getting rid of mucus in acute bronchitis, but in the chronic form, bronchodilator drugs are usually helpful to widen the calibre of those bronchi that are not too damaged to respond. Antibiotics help to prevent and to treat bacterial lung infections, and oxygen therapy using cylinders or concentraters kept at home are sometimes employed. Heart failure is treated with diuretics (water tablets) and medication to increase the efficiency of the heart.

Regrettably emphysema is irreversible and incurable. Stopping smoking is the single most important measure a patient can take. Treatment involves bronchodilator drugs, steroids to reduce inflammation in the lungs, diuretics to reduce fluid retention in the lungs and legs, and oxygen therapy if required. As disabling lung and heart failure are often the end result of this serious disease, it is important to encourage the patient to remain as positive as possible and to live within the limits of their condition.

Mild cases of pneumonia can be treated at home with antibiotics, analgesics and plenty of fluids but in severe cases hospitalisation may be necessary, particularly in the frail and the elderly. Physiotherapy to help expectorate tenacious phlegm, oxygen therapy and artificial ventilation are sometimes needed. Most people make a full recovery if they are generally healthy, but patients with pre-existing respiratory or cardiac disease are obviously more at risk.

Nutritional Healing

The basic eating plan on p. 5 gives you a good balance of all the nutrients essential for a healthy immune system and a healthy body. However, if you are prone to chest problems, then you might like to make a few adjustments.

Your need for Vitamin C is increased so add some extra citrus fruit, kiwis or peppers. Complex carbohydrates such as pasta and rice with an increased fibre intake are useful with whole grains, extra fruit and vegetables. Raw or lightly cooked foods will retain the vitamins and minerals you need. Onions and garlic are essential and radish, horseradish and ginger are all healing to the respiratory tract. Chlorophyll-containing foodstuffs are cleansing both to your lungs and your blood, enabling the easier transport and exchange of oxygen across the cell walls, so green leafy vegetables, parsley, celery, coriander leaves and other salad greens would help. If you can get some wheatgrass juice it is particularly cleansing. Try having a regular curry, or a Thai or Mexican dish at least a couple of times a week, since most of the ingredients – cayenne, cardamom, cumin, clove, coriander, ginger and of course garlic and onions – are all good for those with chest problems. You can take some of them as supplements if you don't like them in cooking. Perhaps the most important is cayenne. A good morning tonic is to add a teaspoonful of virgin olive oil (cold pressed) and a teaspoonful of lemon juice to a cup of hot water. It will not only soothe your chest but also help detoxify your liver. Check for any possible food allergies (see low allergy diet p. 74) and take plenty of fluids – water, fruit and vegetable juices (freshly squeezed if possible), tea, herb teas and soup. If you have a chronic or recurrent chest problem such as chronic bronchitis or emphysema, do invest in a juicer. It will be worth its weight in gold! A last word: try having small nutritious meals every few hours rather than a larger meal two or three times a day. You'll have less discomfort as your chest and abdomen fight for available space and less oxygen will be needed for the digestive process.

Vitamins and Supplements

As always it's best to get all that you can from your diet, but sometimes you need to supplement your diet no matter how good it is. If you have a chest problem, this is one of those times. Despite taking extra fruit and vegetables, you may want to top up your Vitamin C even further and if so take a time-release supplement. Start this as soon as you're aware of the problem, and if it is chronic, then make this a part of your daily routine. Remember that chest problems can be life-threatening in the very young and the very old, and Vitamin C can reverse chest illness or reduce its severity fairly quickly. In the short term, the addition of bioflavinoids, Vitamin A, beta carotene and zinc will help combat even the most stubborn infections. Bromelain (from pineapple) will help break down mucus making it easier to get rid of and thereby reduce congestion. Bee products such as propolis and honey are both soothing and healing, and CoEnzyme Q10, oil of evening primrose and borage oil would all be worth considering.

Exercise and Lifestyle

Although exercise of your whole body is essential, breathing exercises are of major importance if you have a chronic problem. Learning to use your breath to your best advantage will not only make you feel better but will reduce fatigue and help you conserve your strength. Doing some stretching both before and after postural drainage would be helpful. Yoga will help your breathing while calming your mind and exercising your body. If you have emphysema, then walking, even if very slowly, will help, but stop whenever you need to and learn to attack stairs or other obstacles resting as you breathe in and moving when you breathe out. Wear loose clothing so that your chest is restricted as little as possible. If you smoke, hypnotherapy could help. Even using a patch or inhaler would be much less harmful than continuing to burn your airways. Also look at stress reduction techniques such as meditation and relaxation.

Complementary Therapies

HERBS

There are many herbs that are good for the respiratory tract so you could either see a herbalist or choose from the list below. For clearing congestion and loosening and dislodging mucus, any of the following: horehound, elecampane, mullein or hyssop. For soothing inflammation: plantain, liquorice, marshmallow, lavender or peppermint. If there is infection you may need antibiotics (check with your doctor), but there are some natural agents for clearing infection which include thyme, eucalyptus and garlic. Tea tree oil would be good to vaporise and inhale or put in your bath, but don't take internally except under supervision.

For boosting your immune system so that you can fight your illness more efficiently try Siberian ginseng or echinacea (take 4 days on and 4 days off). And finally to help stimulate your cough reflex to get rid of a tight, heavy chest, try gumweed or wild cherry bark.

AROMATHERAPY

All the herbs mentioned above can be used as oils either for massage or for vaporising in your room. Since moist air is beneficial, if you can obtain a steam machine you could add to it a mixture of eucalyptus, thyme and lavender. A boiling kettle would serve the same purpose but don't leave it unattended or let it boil dry.

BACH FLOWER ESSENCES

Easter lily, white pine and spruce are useful.

HOMEOPATHY

A homeopath will assess the complete picture, but if you want to try some remedies yourself, then Belladonna may alleviate your breathing problems, Adrealinum open your airways and Nat sulph ease a rattling chest that feels worse in damp weather. If you have violent cough, Ipecac should help.

CREATIVE VISUALISATION

This can be a very powerful technique which effectively uses the power of your mind to bring about changes in your body. The old adage that whatever the mind can conceive, the body can achieve remains as true today. Seeing yourself getting well, and your cells becoming stronger and healthier, can make an enormous difference to your physical health. That is not to say that permanent damage can be reversed, although in some cases it appears to be so, but it does give you the power to add to the rest of your regime, your own intention to heal. We would highly recommend Dossey Achterberg's book *Rituals of Healing: Using Imagery for Health and Wellness*, (Bantam 1994). What have you got to lose by trying?

MASSAGE

Whether soft and gentle or firm and accompanied by hot compresses to break up mucous plugs before postural drainage, massage is a very effective tool in dealing with chest problems. Combining it with an oil such as lavender or ylang-ylang with help you relax, ease stress, and can help to slow down and regularise your breathing which is sometimes chaotic in those with chest problems. A different style of massage can help you to cough and dislodge phlegm. Either way you benefit from the healing power of human touch so you can't lose! You can also do it yourself, of course. Self-massage is very nurturing and makes you take time for yourself. You may like to try Shiatsu massage as an alternative.

REFLEXOLOGY

You may be amazed at how effective this ancient method of healing is. You can massage the reflex points on your own hands and feet or, better still, go to a professional.

HYPNOSIS

This may help your breathing considerably. Ask to be taught self-hypnosis which you can practise at home using some vivid imagery about your chest becoming clear and your breathing easier.

HOW TO USE HERBS

Most herbs can be made into a tea by steeping a couple of spoonfuls in hot water, leaving this to stand for a few minutes, straining and drinking the liquid. Many herbs can be bought in pre-prepared tea bags. If you go to a herbalist or Traditional Chinese Medicine establishment, they will give you instructions. Sometimes a tincture is available which you can put in water or fruit juice. Some herbs are available as cough drops, syrups, cough mixtures, sweets, etc., and inhaling the active ingredients is often useful. This can be achieved by putting either the oil or fresh herbs in hot water and inhaling the steam with a towel over your head. **Don't take herbs when pregnant or breastfeeding except under supervision.**

Emotional and Spiritual Healing

Being ill can be a spiritual experience if you use it well. It's a time for reflection, for taking care of ourselves, nourishing our minds and spirits as well as our bodies. But chest problems are especially poignant because they call us to be aware of the function of breathing which we usually take for granted, despite the fact that it is one of the few functions of the body that can be either automatic or fully conscious. Breathing is the very essence of life and when it is threatened, we are brought face to face with our mortality. Often we are also forced to confront what we have done to ourselves. There is often a good deal of anger and sometimes guilt, remorse and grief as we confront the self-inflicted nature of some chronic illness. Not only that but we may also have to suffer the anger or resentment of partners or family members, or even medical staff who have warned us over the years of the consequences of our actions. Although grief for what we once were or what we used to be able to do is natural, once it has been confronted it is better to accept and move on. For whatever reason, this has been your life and having a chronic illness may be part of it. In a spiritual sense, see what there is to learn from it.

The respiratory system is the province of the heart chakra and doing some work to heal this area will help. If there are things you need to forgive, this is the time. If your heart has become as rigid as your lungs, try to let go of whatever you have been carrying and open yourself to love and be loved. Having some psychotherapy may help and finding a spiritual healer who is also experienced in psychotherapy will help you release the past, heal you and help your breathing at the same time.

INTEGRATED APPROACH

1. Stop smoking.
2. Avoid atmospheric pollution wherever possible.
3. Practise breathing exercises alone or with a physiotherapy or yoga teacher.

4. Eat healthily and consider taking nutritional supplements.
5. Keep physically active to keep the heart/lung unit in prime condition.
6. Use steam inhalations and aromatherapy for acute conditions.
7. Consider bronchodilators, oxygen therapy, diuretics and steroids for chronic conditions.
8. Use antibiotics only when appropriate and preferably where micro-organism sensitivity is known.
9. Try hypnotherapy and other useful forms of complementary therapy.

Depression

Michael, a 54-year-old director of a road haulage business, was devastated by the threatened failure of his business. He could not sleep, lacked concentration at work and felt constantly exhausted. His GP's check-up revealed no abnormalities, but when the same doctor was called to see Michael at home two weeks later, he had lost weight, become permanently tearful, had not been into work, opened letters or answered telephone calls, and his wife reported him saying that he would be 'better off dead'. He told his GP that he felt a complete failure, was a burden on his family, and to cap it all was racked with numerous physical symptoms that just would not go away. Michael is in the midst of a severe depressive illness.

The word depression can mean different things to different people. Everyone can feel 'down', sad, tearful or uninterested in life at certain times and many people can be emotionally fragile when things do not always go right for them in their daily life. But medically speaking a true clinical depression exists when those feelings are deep and persistent with no let-up in the symptoms. A depressed patient is devoid of moments of optimism and cheerfulness, and their physical wellbeing, general demeanour and behaviour are also affected.

Depression is the most common of all psychiatric illnesses and up to 15 per cent of people will suffer from it at some time in their lives. All age groups are affected but because the elderly often suffer from social isolation, physical ailments and reduced mental abilities, they remain particularly vulnerable to this condition.

SYMPTOMS OF DEPRESSION

feelings of hopelessness and despair
bouts of crying
anxiety

mood swings
loss of appetite
insomnia
social withdrawal
loss of interest in hobbies
fatigue
poor concentration
guilt and suicidal thoughts

Someone who is depressed can experience all or many of the symptoms listed above and often the depression fluctuates in severity. Classically it is more severe at night or first thing in the morning and eases off slightly as the day goes on. Gradually, however, unless recognised and treated, the depression can worsen with the sufferer eventually withdrawing totally from social activities and walling themselves off emotionally from the outside world. A terrible but not uncommon consequence of severe neglected depression is suicide.

Lydia sat facing the doctor wringing her hands and crying. She could not understand why she felt so desperate. She has lovely children, a marvellous husband, a beautiful home and financial security. But still she felt profoundly depressed and had even contemplated taking an overdose of sleeping tablets to put herself out of her misery. She felt guilty about being so ungrateful for everything good in her life and genuinely believed her family would be better off without her. The doctor noticed, she had lost several pounds in weight since her last visit several months before for a well-woman examination, and had totally changed in outlook and demeanour. Lydia has a typical endogenous (biological) depression.

Causes

There is no single cause of depression. It is a complex and often perplexing illness but one which lends itself extremely well to an holistic and integrated 'body and soul' medical approach. Every person requires such individual therapy. Depression can be triggered by certain events such as bereavement, social rejection, dysfunctional relationships, sexual or psychological abuse and other stressful life events, but it can also result from physical illnesses such as viral infections like ME, as a side effect of drugs or medications, as a consequence of light deprivation as in seasonal affective disorder (SAD), or as a result of hormonal fluctuations as seen premenstrually and post-natally or as a result of taking the oral contraceptive pill. You are also more at risk of becoming depressed if your mother or father suffered from depression, although by no means necessarily so.

As often as not, however, no identifiable trigger factor can be determined. The illness just seems to descend on the individual – however cheerful and bubbly their personality may have seemed in the past – totally out of the blue and for no obvious reason. This form of depression, known as endogenous depression (in other words, from within), is often the most difficult form to treat. There are other types of depression that may form part of a more complex disorder, for example in association with ME, Parkinson's disease or multiple sclerosis. Also, depression can fluctuate with bursts of euphoria and an excessively elevated mood, as in the so-called 'bipolar affective disorder' known as manic depression.

Larry is suffering from a recurrence of his depressive illness only weeks after having a 'high' that led to his having to be admitted to hospital. At that time he thought that he was invincible. His bubbly good humour quickly gave way to irritability and he was up most of the night calling his friends and making outrageous plans. He spent a lot of money he could ill afford and needed medication to help stabilise him. Now he feels slowed down and withdrawn and wants to die. His aunt and his mother also suffered from depression and a great-uncle committed suicide 30 years ago. Larry suffers from bipolar affective disorder (manic depressive illness).

The Outlook

Early recognition and treatment of depression is vital if suffering is to be avoided. There still remains a deep-seated stigma associated with depression, and this has to be overcome by an ignorant and judgemental public if the situation is to improve. All of us would do well to remember that this condition could just as easily befall us at some time in the future in which case the understanding and support of others will be essential.

As suicide is the greatest danger of all in depressed people, and 80 per cent of all suicides are related to depression, everybody concerned with caring for someone who is affected should keep a close and careful eye at all times on how they are feeling and coping. Also, since many of the difficulties faced by depressed people are related to financial, relationship and accommodation matters, the intervention of effective community services such as housing departments, employment agencies, self-help groups and other social services are all extremely important.

Sam was brought to the surgery by her husband who was worried that she was tearful and sad much of the time, she wasn't sleeping and she wasn't taking care of herself, the home or their children as usual. Normally bouncy, Sam could now neither concentrate to read, enjoy TV nor talk about their shared dreams for the future. With eyes downcast and monotone voice, she said that she felt worthless and hopeless and that everyone would be better off if she was no longer there. She'd had thoughts of killing herself but couldn't think of how to do it. Although a few weeks ago she had some relief in the evenings when her mood seemed to lift for a few hours, now the depression was pervasive and unremitting. She was depressed previously in her early twenties, although it wasn't as severe as this. Sam is suffering from unipolar affective disorder, or depressive illness.

Conventional Treatment

Broadly speaking there are three main conventional types of treatment for depression and the one chosen generally depends on the nature and severity of the illness.

Psychotherapy

This basically involves talking and listening to relieve specific symptoms and to help people adjust to and cope with the problems of everyday life. Consequently it is sometimes referred to as supportive psychotherapy or dynamic psychotherapy.

Psychoanalysis is a more intensive form of dynamic psychotherapy which involves extensive exploration of a person's behaviour and psychological functioning, and which often requires treatment over a period of many years.

Cognitive psychotherapy involves changing a person's responses to situations so that negative ways of thinking which lead to the depression can be avoided.

Behavioural psychotherapy aims to improve a patient's emotional wellbeing and success in life by effecting a positive change in their behaviour.

2. Medication

The second major kind of treatment for depression relies on medication and this is generally most successful where physical symptoms are dominant. The majority of patients respond to antidepressant drugs of one kind or another, provided that the drug selection is appropriate to the symptoms and that the medication is given in sufficient dosage and for long enough. The treatment should always be carefully monitored while the recipient is kept under close supervision, but these days modern antidepressant treatment is much safer in cases of accidental or deliberate overdose and is relatively free from unpleasant side effects. Furthermore, contemporary antidepressant drugs are non-addictive. Their main problem is that relapses are always possible if the drugs are not continued for long enough.

3. Electroconvulsive therapy

The third type of treatment for depression consists of electroconvulsive therapy although this is now reserved for a very small minority of severely depressed people in whom the other two less invasive methods have not worked. Despite popular misgivings about ECT among the general population, appropriately employed ECT given under general anaesthetic is effective and safe and may even be life-saving for those whose depression and associated delusions appear intractable.

Very frequently a combination of the first two methods of treatment are used to help those with the commonest forms of depression, with the vast majority making a full recovery within a few weeks or months. Thereafter, early recognition of any similar symptoms is important as in some people there is a tendency for depression to recur.

Emotional and Spiritual Healing

The good news is that you should eventually recover from depression and feel as well as you ever have, or with good therapy, even better. Depression need leave no scar on you or your personality and in later times you may actually be able to see it as a gift that changed your life. If you're grieving, then you may be feeling angry with God or whatever you see as the supreme force. Or it may be that the present situation helps open your spirituality as you look for some way to make sense of what has happened. Depression almost always gives us a chance to see the world differently. In trying to determine what you need to do for yourself right now, perhaps you could think about what advice you would give to your best friend if he or she were in the same situation, then take it for yourself.

Perhaps one of the questions you could ask yourself is why are you staying in your current situation? What are you still gaining from being there? For instance, is it easier to stay in your depression than to take the courage to do whatever you need to do to make a change in your life? Do you gain attention from being where you are that you felt you wouldn't gain if you were well? Have you been in a similar place before and if so, why have you found yourself there again? What can you learn from the pattern so that you don't have to revisit it? Are you holding onto some anger or resentment that's eating away at you? Is there someone you need to forgive? What one small change could you make to get yourself out of the depressed rut you're in and start to get your life moving again? It might help to take some time and write out what you feel your problem to be. Keeping a journal, writing out the pros and cons of the situation may give you some clarity and help you see a way forward.

Spiritual healing, either with the help of a healer as a guide or doing the work yourself, can help you understand and let go of the past and heal the present while giving you a more realistic outlook for the future. There *is* a biochemical basis for much depressive illness, and a biochemical imbalance usually requires a biochemical solution, i.e. antidepressants; and we're not suggesting you give up your antidepressant if you're taking one. But some work on your aching heart chakra will yield great benefits of which you may hardly be aware at present. Buy yourself some rose quartz and keep it with you. Having a rose quartz pendant over your heart will be soothing. Though the results may appear subtle they will nonetheless be there. Guided imagery may be part of the healing session helping you use the power of your mind to lift your spirits and heal body as well as mind. A healer will also teach you to protect yourself from allowing your energy to be drained away by picking up negative energy from those around you. Most of all, we hope you will learn to truly love yourself which is an essential prerequisite for happiness and peace of mind. And lastly, let go of any guilt about being depressed. It is not your fault, nor does it indicate that you have not tried hard enough or done something wrong. Be gentle with yourself.

Nutritional Healing

Levels of omega-3 fatty acids are found to be 40 per cent lower in patients suffering from depression (*Biological Psychiatry*, 1 March 1998). Whether this is a cause of depression or the result of it isn't clear, but the bottom line is that if you add these substances to your diet, you'll feel better. Oily fish such as salmon, herrings, sardines, tuna and mackerel are the best natural sources (see Basics, p. 4) although flax seed (linseed) oil is perhaps the most concentrated source.

Complex carbohydrates have a direct effect upon serotonin production so adding plenty of these will help, while foods laden with Vitamin C such as kiwis, peppers and citrus fruits are also necessary for the production of your own internal antidepressants.

Cutting out coffee and other caffeine-containing drinks as well as chocolate will help in the long run, although you may have a withdrawal headache for a few days if your consumption was high. Alcohol may seem to help, but is actually a depressant and even its sedative action is short lived. Although it may help you to go to sleep initially, you may wake up after only a few hours feeling even worse. Best to stay away from it. If you eat meat, try having turkey regularly. It's low fat and contains L-tryptophan which is a natural antidepressant and also has a mildly sedative action (no wonder we feel happy and fall asleep after Christmas dinner!). Warm milk has the same ingredient which is why it's good as a bedtime drink. Sugar in large quantities in drinks, sweets, biscuits and cakes can also add to your depression, but don't get hypoglycaemic (low blood sugar) because that can lower your mood also. Eating may be the last thing you want to think about, but small nutritious meals will help you recover, not only by helping you feel nurtured, but by giving you the essentials to manufacture what you need to bolster your mood and get you back to normal as quickly as possible.

Vitamins and Supplements

If your appetite is very poor, and certainly this is so in many forms of depression, then at least make sure that you get essential nutrients in the form of supplements. These do not replace normal food, however! Vitamins B, C and E are essential for the manufacture of neurotransmitters which are often depleted in depression. Vitamin B will also help you deal with stress and improve your drive and motivation. A tablespoonful of flax seed (linseed) oil will give you your daily quota of omega-3 and omega-6 fatty acids. St John's Wort has been used for centuries for mild to moderate depression. It acts like a selective serotonin re-uptake inhibitor (SSRI), of which one example is Prozac, and it doesn't affect REM (rapid eye movement) sleep – that deep sleep necessary for total relaxation and repair. There are many studies on its effectiveness and although it may take 6 to 8 weeks to start to work, it's worth persevering. However, 6–8 weeks is a very long time if you're severely depressed in which case you may need a more traditional antidepressant. Importantly, you shouldn't take both St John's Wort and an antidepressant together without professional supervision, so discuss the situation with your GP before making a decision. Side effects of St John's Wort may include stomach upsets and mild headache, tiredness and dizziness. Also be careful in the sun as it can cause hypersensitivity and you may get sunburn.

Sometimes one of the features of severe depression is that people deny just how ill they are. It's important therefore that a proper assessment is made since, sadly, many people who are severely depressed, particularly older men, take their own lives because they feel hopeless and despairing of ever being well again.

Kava in the form of tea will have a calming and mildly antidepressant effect and will help a little with agitation. However, if agitation is a major feature of depression, you may need traditional orthodox treatment. Gingko biloba will help with your thinking, improve concentration and memory, and will also gently lift your mood.

Exercise and Lifestyle

Keeping going, having a routine and structuring your time are all helpful in getting you back to normal as soon as possible. However, your body and mind (and spirit!) are telling you to slow down and take care of yourself and you need to heed this. Exercise taken out in the fresh air will help. Walks, especially in nice natural surroundings, will lift your spirits while the natural light will help, particularly if there tends to be a seasonal pattern to your illness. Movement, whether a good workout in the gym, dancing, yoga or swimming, will help you feel refreshed and keep you in shape while also prompting the secretion of endorphins, your own natural antidepressants. Dancing is especially good since it improves posture, poise, balance and rhythm but it also helps release your spiritual energy in a way that other exercise sometimes fails to do. You don't need to be good at it. Just let your body do what it was meant to do, move. You might find yourself meditating to the music or just letting it flow through you. You may find that it precipitates much-needed crying. That's OK. Tears bathe the soul, so if you need to cry, go ahead. If you do have a partner with whom you can dance at home, you may find that your flagging libido begins to re-emerge and this intimate activity can become a prelude to the more intimate activity of making love. Make sure that you are in control of that situation, however, by discussing it beforehand. You may want only to be held and cuddled and your partner needs to be aware of this and be willing to proceed at your pace.

If you suffer from seasonal affective disorder (SAD), you may like to invest in a SAD lamp which you can switch on in your bedroom for 20 minutes in the morning to feel as though the sun just came out. You don't need to sit in front of it, although you may. If you do, protect your eyes as you would in the sun. It's very easy to use. Just pop on the lamp and potter around getting ready as usual while your room is filled with the same frequency of light as sunshine. Also spend as much time outdoors as possible and think of taking your holiday in the winter, going somewhere where you can be in the sun. Pine forests, waterfalls and the sea are particularly healing, the negative ions having a remarkable effect upon your aura and your energy in general.

Keeping busy, but not too busy, will usually help and volunteering to do charity work may be a way of doing this while getting your own worries into perspective and often being inspired by others. It will also give you a sense of belonging and achievement, both of which will help your energy and self-esteem to rise. If you need a mantra for when you're down, perhaps you could say 'This too will pass' whenever you remember to do so. However disempowered you may feel right now, you have all the answers within you and the power to do whatever you wish. A tiny word of caution, however. This may not be the best time for making major changes. Very often we've had people come along who think they should leave their marriage, sell their business or retire, but when the depression is resolved, they often wish someone had stopped them. Take your time. There are changes for you to make, and if your depression was caused by someone mistreating you physically or emotionally, then perhaps it is the time to go, but in general, think carefully and talk it over with someone whose judgement you can trust at a time when your own may be impaired.

If you use alcohol or any recreational drugs, they could be contributing to your depression so think carefully about getting rid of them, and get some help if you need it (see the section on addictions). A last word. Even if you don't feel like it – SMILE! There's evidence that smiling (and better still, laughing) actually has a direct effect on your brain and helps lift your mood. Raising your arms adds to the effect. Waving your hands increases if further. If you feel really stupid doing that when you feel so down, lock yourself in the bathroom and experiment. If you let yourself, you'll have to acknowledge that something feels lighter and better.

Complementary Therapies

Bach Flower Remedies can be a gentle but powerful remedy for mild to moderate depression. Larch will help rebuild your self-confidence and improve your faith in your own ability. White chestnut will help calm you. Wild rose will help you adjust to whatever change in circumstance you're having difficulty with. Carry some Rescue Remedy with you and use it when you're feeling particularly vulnerable and stressed or in shock.

Several aromatherapy oils are helpful in depression, including geranium, which helps relieve mood swings and creates mental harmony and peace. Chamomile has a similar effect. Rose also helps with melancholy and will gently uplift you. Neroli, grapefruit, jasmine and bergamot are among our favourites for depression. As a special mood-lifting treat full of antioxidants and other goodies, brew a pot of tea with equal parts of Earl Grey (flavoured with bergamot) and Assam and sit down quietly to relax with a piece of gentle music.

Of the herbs, St John's Wort, mentioned above, performs even better when partnered with gingko biloba. Kava with its anxiety-relieving properties is also helpful in mild depression.

Cayenne, which encourages the production of endorphins, can be helpful even for debilitating depression. Use it in cooking and also as a supplement, gradually increasing the dose. If you haven't heard of 'chilli eater's high', try eating a chilli regularly and you might find out!

Acupressure and acupuncture can be useful, as can massage. Get a friend to rub between your shoulder blades at the level of your heart. Not only will there be stimulation of the heart chakra, but it is also a major acupressure point. Homeopathic remedies include Sepia if you're weepy, irritable and with poor libido; Ignatia where there is also an element of loss or grief; Natrum mur where there is bereavement and distress, and Pulsatilla if you crave attention and reassurance.

Integrated approach

1. Remember that depression is both common and treatable. You will get better.
2. There are many different types of depression so the treatment must be carefully chosen for you.
3. Emotional support and spiritual therapy is a vital first step.
4. A healthy diet and regular exercise helps greatly.
5. Avoid alcohol and other recreational drugs which can compound depression and interfere with sleep.
6. Experiment with gentle complementary therapies.
7. In severe depression, with dramatic and severe fluctuations of mood, a combination of psychotherapy and modern medication will improve symptoms enormously.
8. A sympathetic, patient and understanding therapist is vital. If you think your therapist fails to fulfil these criteria, move on if you can and find one who does.

Diabetes Mellitus

Diabetes is a disorder caused by insufficient or absent production of the hormone insulin by the pancreas gland or by an increased resistance to the action of insulin by the body's tissues. In this situation glucose in the bloodstream cannot be absorbed into the cells which require it for energy, nor into the liver and fat cells which require it for energy storage. Glucose therefore accumulates in the bloodstream leading to the cardinal symptoms of diabetes which include polydipsia (excess thirst), polyuria (passing large amounts of urine), weight loss, hunger and fatigue.

Diabetes is a potentially devastating illness that is constantly on the increase. Poorly controlled, it is the leading cause of blindness and amputations and it is a major cause of nervous system damage. Diabetics are four times more likely than others to develop stroke or heart disease. However, there's much that can be done to alleviate the condition itself and to minimise complications.

Charlie, at 52, had never felt so weary in his life. He simply had no energy to do anything. He knew he was overweight and unfit, but he had not felt his normal self for some time. He had had a number of skin infections and was perpetually thirsty and this is what finally prompted him to see his doctor. A urine test showed sugar in his urine and a blood test confirmed that he had developed Type II diabetes mellitus.

There are two main types of diabetes: Type I which is more severe and sudden in onset, usually occurs in younger people and requires insulin to treat it; and Type II which comes on gradually and generally affects people over the age of 40. In the latter type, dietary adjustments, weight reduction and tablets are usually enough to keep the disorder under control.

Causes

A genetic predisposition is certainly present in diabetes, particularly in the Type II variety, although in this type, being overweight and enjoying a sugary, fat-loaded diet is usually the critical trigger factor in its development. 'Latent' diabetes can be revealed by other factors such as taking diuretic or steroid drugs, pregnancy and pancreatitis, an inflammation of the pancreas gland itself.

Diagnosis

For every diabetic who already knows about their condition there is another who remains blissfully unaware that they are developing it. Symptoms may forewarn the person that something is wrong but in Type II diabetes, where the onset is gradual, that person may go for years living with high blood glucose without ever being treated for it. During this time, however, significant damage is being done to many of the cells and tissues of the body including the eyes, the heart, the kidneys and the nervous system. This is why heart attacks, strokes, blindness and kidney failure are all more common among diabetics. Routine and regular screening for glucose in the urine is therefore essential for everyone to detect diabetes early and prevent such long-term complications occurring. A good family doctor will be doing this anyway when any opportunity arises.

If glucose is detected in the urine, blood tests can confirm the presence of diabetes and its severity.

Treatment

The aim of treatment is to keep blood glucose levels as near to normal as possible, to relieve symptoms and to prevent any long-term complications. The more the person can understand and look after the disorder themselves, the better the treatment is likely to be. This requires keeping their weight under control, enjoying regular exercise, eating the right foods and balancing their blood sugar by use of medication.

John was losing a lot of weight. As he was just 6 this was obviously of great concern to his parents. Then he started weeing much more frequently and drinking pints and pints of orange squash. One morning he simply could not get out of bed and was rushed to hospital just in time to prevent him going into a coma. John is now a Type I diabetic who will require insulin injections for the rest of his life.

TYPE I

Type I diabetics always require regular daily self-injections of insulin of either animal or human type although the latter is now synthesised by genetic engineering. Most people now use handy, disposable lightweight insulin pens with refill cartridges which allow for immediate adjustment of insulin dosage whenever necessary. The aim is to keep the blood glucose level as normal as possible by timing the injections to coincide with mealtimes, avoiding dramatic rises and falls in these levels (which can happen when relatively too much insulin is given).

Glucose intake and insulin dosage must be carefully balanced so that symptoms of excess glucose in the blood (hyperglycaemia) and too little glucose in the blood (hypoglycaemia) do not occur. The symptoms of hyperglycaemia are those of untreated diabetes and those of hypoglycaemia are confusion, sweating, weakness, aggressive or altered behaviour, dizziness and, if extreme, convulsions and coma. The best possible way to achieve good diabetic control is for patients to use modern do-it-yourself testing kits such as Boehringher's Softclix II near-painless finger pricking device and their Glucotrend II blood glucose monitoring device. These enable an accurate reading of the blood glucose at a precise moment and within seconds of the blood being taken. Carrying such an easily portable item around at all times as well as a sugary snack in case of low blood sugar symptoms means diabetic equilibrium can be attained, theoretically at least, at all times.

TYPE II

Type II diabetics may be able to control their disorder by dietary adjustment alone. This requires regulating their carbohydrate intake more carefully and losing weight. Others need hypoglycaemic tablets as well to lower blood glucose levels and a minority may at some stage require small doses of insulin to achieve adequate control.

Diabetic Care

All diabetics require regular check-ups to monitor progress and to avoid or detect any complications. Damage to the blood vessels at the back of the eye can be corrected using laser therapy to prevent blindness, and kidney dialysis or transplantation is a solution for end-stage kidney failure. Other risk factors for heart disease can be identified and treated, and much good advice can be obtained from GPs, diabetologists and diabetic practice nurses with a view to the diabetic themselves leading as healthy a lifestyle as possible. Stopping smoking, cutting back on fat in the diet and taking daily physical exercise is merely a starting point.

The Outlook

These days there is no reason why almost all diabetics cannot expect to enjoy a normal lifespan despite the inconvenience of their condition. But in order to achieve this, regular medical check-ups and efficient self-monitoring of blood glucose is essential.

Nutritional Healing

For most diabetics diet is of the utmost importance. The aim is a low-fat, high-fibre diet with as much as possible of the energy-providing foods coming in the form of complex carbohydrates. These foods, like bread, cereals, pasta, potatoes, rice and fruit, release their glucose content slowly and avoid causing the rapid peaks of blood sugar levels that can be damaging. Sweets, cakes, confectionery, jams and other sugary foodstuffs are all best kept to a minimum or avoided altogether. A dietitian or nutritionist can easily supply you with a suitable diabetic diet. These days, this is not restrictive; occasional treats are allowed and the diabetic diet itself is healthy and can be followed quite easily by the entire family.

Try to eat organic produce as far as possible and have plenty of raw vegetables. It's worth noting that onions can lower blood sugar and may be useful in diabetes, as may cucumber. Alpha lipoic acid is a potent antioxidant which can normalise blood sugar levels in diabetes. It can also help relieve the symptoms of nerve damage and help reduce complications such as blindness. The richest natural sources are broccoli, spinach, heart, liver, Brussels sprouts, tomatoes and garden peas. Salmon, herrings, tuna and mackerel are rich sources of omega-3 fatty acids, although remember to watch your calorie intake. Ginger, onions, alfalfa sprouts and cranberries will stimulate your pancreas to produce more insulin. Small meals taken often are far better for you than a couple of large meals each day. If you're trying to lose weight do it gradually by changing your eating habits rather than by crash diets that will only upset your delicate balance and set off a pattern of yo-yoing weight which will destabilise you further. Fads and fasting are not for you. Add garlic to your cooking wherever you can.

Vitamins and Supplements

Niacin (Vitamin B_3) has been found to prevent or slow down vascular disease including damage to the retina. Large doses are needed (2000 to 3000 mg daily) so please use only under medical supervision. Vitamins C and E are also useful supplements for macular degeneration (see visual problems, p. 525) along with carotenoids, in particular lutein and zeaxanthin. Vitamin E also slows down the development of atherosclerosis. Chromium, essential in the metabolism of glucose, helps reduce blood sugar and in addition can reduce the risk of retinopathy (damage to the retina of the eye). Damage to the retina and heart in diabetes may be associated with magnesium deficiency. Taken as a supplement it will also help reduce irritability and give you more energy. Calcium, magnesium, potassium and zinc also need be kept in balance so have your levels checked from time to time. If you have to take a calcium or magnesium supplement, ensure that you look on the label for the citrate salt which is readily absorbed. The magnesium dose should ideally be half that of the calcium dose for it to be in balance. Since maintenance of the delicate insulin/glucose balance is essential, please check regularly with your doctor since you may find that your needs will change as you get better. Aloe vera juice taken internally can help peripheral vascular problems such as leg ulcers, hopefully avoiding such complications and reducing the necessity for amputation.

Exercise and Lifestyle

Exercise is a must since it tones the whole body including the heart and vascular system, helping prevent heart disease and stroke. It lowers cholesterol which in turn has the effect of lowering triglyceride levels and reduces insulin requirements. It can help you lose weight and reduce the absorption of foodstuffs. Even 10 to 20 minutes daily will help reduce insulin requirements, but do check first with your doctor especially if your diabetes is difficult to control, and of course always have available a carbohydrate snack or a glucose drink. Try to get into the habit of carefully washing, drying and inspecting your feet every day – if you do have some nerve damage (neuropathy), you may be unaware of small wounds that could become infected or refuse to heal because of compromised circulation. Wear socks or stockings and well-fitting shoes and try to avoid footwear such as sandals that do not protect your feet well. Barefoot walks are out! Avoid very hot baths and saunas. Since stress can destabilise your insulin requirement, do adopt a lifestyle that suits your personality and leaves you feeling good. Take some relaxation every day and see the section on meditation (p. 10).

Complementary Therapies

Ayurvedic medicine recommends the use of turmeric and neem which help to normalise blood sugar and reduce the need for insulin in insulin-dependent diabetics. There are many herbs that stimulate the pancreas such as aloe, golden seal, kelp, blueberry and juniper berry, all of which are safe while taking other medication. Gingko biloba, by helping the circulation, can cut the risk of ulcers, poor circulation and retinopathy. Dandelion and eyebright would help detox the liver and kidneys respectively. Do see a good herbalist rather than prescribe for yourself. The homeopathic remedy Mucokehl may be useful for retinopathy.

Emotional and Spiritual Healing

Having an illness that has such potentially damaging effects on the body long term is not a very cheerful prospect and it's not surprising therefore that depression may be concurrent. Where the illness occurs in childhood there are the added complications of children having to learn to inject themselves, being set apart from their friends as a result. Often parents feel overprotective which sets the child apart even further. But with good understanding and confidence, a diabetic can lead as normal a life as the next person. Steven Redgrave, an insulin-dependent diabetic, has already won four Olympic gold medals in rowing for Britain, and if he gets his way a fifth is shortly going to be added to the collection. Getting the balance right can be tricky, but it is essential to normalise things as much as possible while being sensible. Seeing a healer regularly can help reduce stress and bring things back into balance while also helping the body stay well, and of course the benefits are endless in terms of mobilising the spiritual aspects of yourself to help heal your physical condition. Meditation and creative visualisation are helpful. Having a regular massage, especially with essential oils, helps your circulation, prevents the development of ulcers and also improves your mood and spirits. Sometimes there is a lot of anger associated with this illness which you experience on a daily basis, and psychotherapy or counselling will help you accept the situation and focus on the good things you have in your life. Should there be clinical depression or anxiety, do ask for a referral to a psychiatrist to assess your needs.

INTEGRATED APPROACH

1. Be aware of any family history of diabetes.
2. Report urgently excessive thirst, frequency of urination and tiredness.
3. Have your urine checked for glucose at least annually to test for undiagnosed diabetes.
4. When diabetes is diagnosed, remember you can still lead a normal life.
5. Gather as much information about the disease as you can.
6. Adjust your lifestyle, your diet, your exercise levels and, if needed, your weight.
7. Monitor your blood sugar level closely and every day if your diabetes is Type I.
8. Have regular diabetic specialist check-ups to identify complications early.
9. Experiment with nutritional adjustment and vitamin supplementation.
10. Deal with any unresolved emotional feelings appropriately.

Digestive Disorders

The alimentary canal runs the length of the digestive system and consists of the mouth, gullet, stomach and intestine. In this chapter, disorders of all these parts of the gastrointestinal tract are included as well as conditions affecting the liver and gall bladder, as these two organs affect the functions and health of the rest of the bowel.

The basic function of the digestive system is to break down food and water from the diet and absorb them into the bloodstream. Disorders of the alimentary canal are many and varied, so we focus here on the conventional approach to treatment of the commonest disorders experienced by the majority of people at some stage in their lives.

Nausea and Vomiting

Nausea and vomiting are extremely common symptoms which can have a huge number of potential causes. Simple overindulgence in food or alcohol, short-lived food poisoning or early pregnancy are often responsible, but equally they can be a side effect of drugs or the consequence of serious disease such as ulcers, appendicitis, bowel obstruction or pancreatitis. Equally, the condition responsible may not lie within the gastrointestinal tract at all. A head injury can result in vomiting, as can a brain tumour or meningitis. Disorders of the middle ear can produce symptoms similar to motion sickness, and travel sickness itself can also cause nausea and vomiting. These symptoms are common in early pregnancy too, and may occur in poorly controlled diabetes. Vomiting may also be brought about deliberately by a patient suffering from an eating disorder such as bulimia or anorexia nervosa. The symptoms of nausea and vomiting are usually short lived and transient (lasting 2 to 3 days or so) and the underlying cause is generally not serious. Persistent vomiting and nausea, on the other hand, require investigation to determine the cause.

It is wise for the patient not to take anything other than sips of water while symptoms continue and doctors sometimes prescribe anti-sickness (anti-emetic) drugs if symptoms are severe. Ultimately treatment depends on the underlying cause.

Self-Help Measures

Christine felt terribly sick for days although to begin with, she just had a little bit of nausea and was off her food. Initially she put it down to the sinusitis she had been suffering from and the mucus she had been swallowing in the night. The real cause of her nausea, however, was the antibiotic, doxycycline, which her doctor had put her on to combat the infection while forgetting to advise her to take it only with or after meals.

Replace lost fluids with drinks that are not too cold or they will further shock your already delicate stomach. Water or clear fluids would be best although ginger tea (made with ginger root in hot water, sweetened with a little honey if you wish) may help settle things. Alternatively, put a couple of drops of peppermint oil in a glass of pure cool water and sip it. You can replace electrolytes (body salts and sugars) by drinking apple or cranberry juice, adding a little salt and sugar to each glass (less than a quarter of a teaspoon). Your urine should be a pale straw colour so if it's deeper than that, you're not drinking enough and are getting dehydrated. However, as with diarrhoea, vomiting may well be your body's brave defence to rid you of something it really doesn't want, and therefore letting it run its course may be the best thing to do. You can ease the nausea by using an acupressure technique. Apply deep pressure to the web between your thumb and index finger and massage the area for a few minutes. The same applies to the area between the tendons of your second and third toes.

Taking no solid food whatsoever is best when nausea and vomiting are experienced as the process of digestion may stimulate further gastric irritation and intestinal motility. Also, because gastro-enteritis (food poisoning) can temporarily deplete levels of the digestive enzyme lactase in the bowel, dairy products are best avoided for a week or so to prevent undigested lactose sugars in dairy produce causing further diarrhoea and abdominal cramp.

When you do start to eat solids again, try jelly, dry toast or crackers and keep off fat for a few days at least. If you feel hungry as well as nauseous, add just a pinch of nutmeg, cumin or cardamom to about 2 fluid ounces (60 millilitres) of yogurt or warm milk which will satisfy your hunger while acting as an anti-nauseant.

One of the best homeopathic remedies to try is Ipecac.

INDIGESTION, HEARTBURN AND DYSPEPSIA

These interchangeable terms refer to discomfort in the upper abdomen which may be associated with belching, acid reflux into the gullet and abdominal pain. Treatment in the first instance involves the avoidance of foods and situations that seem to trigger the symptoms and taking small but regular meals throughout the day. Avoiding smoking and excessive alcohol is also recommended. Occasionally antacid drugs are prescribed to neutralise the erosive effect of strong acid within the stomach. When antacids fail to work or when the symptoms arise in somebody over the age of 40, where there is an increased suspicion of more serious pathology, further investigation is required.

Not uncommonly, further tests will reveal the presence of a hiatus hernia. This is a condition where the upper part of the stomach pushes upwards through the opening in the diaphragm (the sheet of muscle separating the chest from the abdomen) allowing acid to reflux from the stomach up into the back of the throat. This condition is commoner in those who are overweight, who smoke and who have physically demanding occupations. Symptoms include heartburn which is made worse by stooping forwards or bending over. The diagnosis is confirmed either through oesophagoscopy (where a viewing instrument is passed down the throat into the gullet to take a direct look) or by a barium X-ray examination with manometry (where pressure measurements between gullet and stomach can be taken).

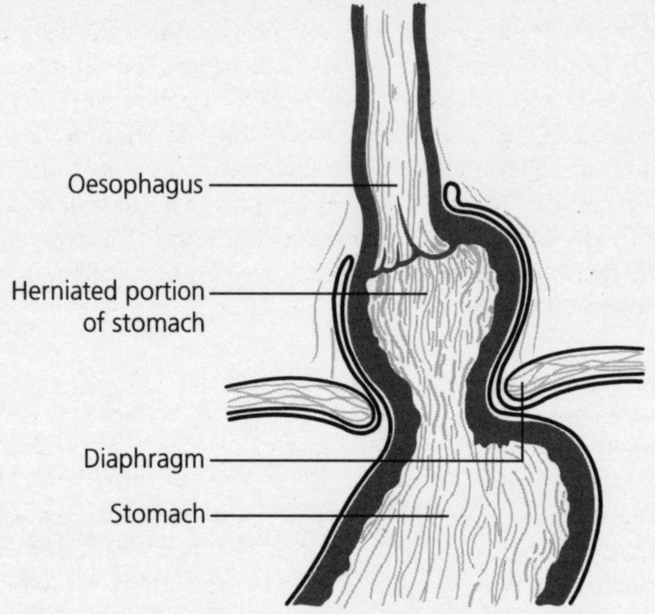

Common Type of Hiatus Hernia

Treatment

Eating little and often, and raising the head of the bed to prevent acid reflux, are all helpful. Losing weight and stopping smoking are important, and a variety of different types of antacid drugs may be recommended. In severe cases surgery may be required, although an operation is generally avoided if at all possible as access to this part of the body is difficult. A technique called fundoplication is a simpler, less drastic form of the operation, where the herniated part of the stomach is surgically folded back into place. It is suitable for slimmer, younger patients with a hiatus hernia.

Bruce has had terrible indigestion and heartburn for weeks. He has lost about a stone (6 kg) in weight during this period and his appetite has all but disappeared. Sometimes he wakes in the early hours of the night with a sharp, penetrating pain just below his breastbone which he could relieve within an hour or two by drinking a glass of milk and taking an antacid. Bruce has a duodenal ulcer.

A common finding when indigestion is investigated is an ulcer. Ulcers in the stomach or in the first part of the intestine, the duodenum, result from erosion of the lining of these structures, known as the mucosa. The ulcers may be shallow or deep, benign or malignant, and can cause abdominal pain and often loss of weight. Duodenal ulcers tend to be quite well localised to the extent that the sufferer can point to the area of pain with their finger. Classically the pain is worse in the early hours of the morning when acid secretion is at its strongest.

Treatment

We now know that the bacterium *Helicobacter pylori* is responsible for ulcers in the vast majority of cases and 'triple therapy' is now used more and more to eradicate the symptoms. Triple therapy consists of two different antibiotics and an agent called a proton pump inhibitor which helps to protect the lining of the stomach and small intestine. Antacid medication is also used and some of the most powerful types work by blocking the effects of histamine, which in turn reduces the secretion of acid from the stomach and helps promote the healing of ulcers. These days surgery is generally restricted to deep penetrating ulcers which perforate and cause heavy bleeding.

Self-Help Measures

If indigestion *is* due to hyperacidity, adding bananas to your diet can help. They are high in potassium which combats hyperacidity and they also promote the secretion of mucus which coats and protects the stomach lining. Low levels of pancreatic protease enzymes can leave protein molecules impossible to digest. These can then become toxic in the gut, producing symptoms that include indigestion, bloating and gas, as the body signals its intolerance. Papaya is very useful here, aiding the digestion not only of proteins but also of carbohydrates and fat.

Milk thistle, an ancient herb used in Europe since the 1500s, stimulates the production of bile which is essential to proper digestion. Turmeric will also stimulate bile flow and helps break down fat. It is an ancient treatment for obesity. Fennel is useful for flatulence and indigestion. Ginger begins its action by stimulating saliva in the mouth which aids peristalsis in the gut and can break down protein molecules that could otherwise cause inflammation.

A recent study in the journal *Cancer* suggests that Vitamin C reduces the risk of both stomach cancer and ulcers. It has been shown to prevent the growth of *Helicobacter pylori*, both in laboratory cultures and in animals, and to slow down the growth of *Campylobacter jejuni* (another micro-organism which can abnormally colonise the bowel). Bromelain, a constituent of pineapple, is also useful here, limiting inflammation and reducing swelling, acidity and pain. Peppermint soothes ulcers, while liquorice is anti-inflammatory and extremely healing for the whole digestive tract, especially the stomach. It can relieve the pain of heartburn, prevent ulcers from forming and has also been said to be an anti-cancer agent.

Irritable Bowel Syndrome

Chloe, 27, is hardly ever free of cramping abdominal pain, a feeling of bloatedness, wind and alternating diarrhoea or constipation. It gets her down and seemingly the more stressed and frustrated it makes her, the worse her symptoms seem to be. She has tried a variety of diets to no avail and all the medical tests have proved negative. Like thousands of others, she has irritable bowel syndrome.

This is one of the commonest disorders of all affecting the intestine. It brings about abdominal cramps which come and go, an unpredictable bowel habit varying from constipation to diarrhoea, bloating of the abdomen and wind. The only good thing about it is that it is not connected with any other identifiable disease process. The symptoms, however, are unfortunately recurrent throughout the sufferer's life, and it can seriously affect their quality of life. Irritable bowel syndrome is basically due to an oversensitivity of the muscular wall of the large intestine, and certainly seems to be made worse by stress and worry. The disorder is twice as common in women, and usually starts in early adulthood. The diagnosis is confirmed when all the usual X-ray and endoscopic tests (see below) have excluded more severe and serious conditions.

Treatment

Medical recommendations include a high-fibre diet, although patients should be warned that symptoms are quite likely to get worse for a few weeks before they improve as the intestine adjusts to the greater volume of food residue. Sometimes anti-diarrhoeal drugs are prescribed when diarrhoea is particularly troublesome and persistent, and anti-spasmodic drugs may be prescribed to ease abdominal cramps. Much success has been had in certain gastroenterology units with the use of hypnosis, but although patients may notice an improvement in their symptoms, IBS cannot in itself be 'cured'.

Self-Help Measures

Aloe vera soothes the whole intestinal tract, helping not only the irritable bowel but indigestion and malabsorption too. Colonics (gentle washing of the bowel by inserting a tube into the anus and instilling fluid), using a range of gentle oils such as chamomile, are healing. Of course, chamomile can also be taken internally as a tea, calming the mind and spirit as well as the body.

Crohn's Disease and Ulcerative Colitis

Both these conditions are chronic inflammatory diseases that can produce ulceration of parts of the gut and intestine. In ulcerative colitis this is restricted to the colon and rectum, but Crohn's disease can lead to problems anywhere along the gastrointestinal tract, from the mouth right down to the anal canal. The causes of each disease remain unknown, although an abnormal sensitivity or an allergic reaction to something in the diet or environment may well be responsible.

In ulcerative colitis the predominant symptoms are bloody diarrhoea and the passage of mucus with the stool. Sometimes abdominal pain and tenderness can occur and the patient can feel generally unwell and feverish. Anaemia often ensues as a result of the chronic loss of blood, and sometimes the condition is associated with arthritis, rashes on the skin and inflammation of the eye. Where the disorder has been present for more than 10 years or so, there is also an increased risk of developing cancer of the colon, so screening for this should be part of the ongoing medical management. Diagnosis is made using special viewing instruments called endoscopes and barium X-rays.

In Crohn's disease, because the whole of the bowel may be affected, albeit in scattered patches, symptoms include pain, diarrhoea, sickness, loss of appetite, anaemia and weight loss. Other parts of the body may be affected, leading to arthritis, inflammation of the spine (ankylosing spondylitis) and skin disorders such as psoriasis. Diagnosis again relies on direct viewing of the bowel using endoscopic tubes and barium X-rays, in order to distinguish Crohn's disease from ulcerative colitis.

Treatment of Ulcerative Colitis

Medical treatment consists of steroids and the drug sulfasalazine. Surgical removal of the colon (colectomy) is sometimes needed when inflammation is severe and extensive. Although this sounds like a terrible price to pay, the patient's health usually improves dramatically following the procedure, and living with an ileostomy (an opening on the surface of the abdomen through which waste products are passed) is these days much more convenient and tolerable than it has been in the past.

Treatment of Crohn's Disease

Treatment consists of sulfasalazine and steroids, but when symptoms can not be controlled, admission to hospital is often required for blood transfusion and intravenous feeding. Occasionally, because deep ulcers can cause scarring or thickening of the intestinal wall, obstruction of the intestine may occur, requiring surgery. Fistulas (abnormal hollow connections between loops of intestine) may develop in about 30 per cent of patients, and these will also need surgery. The severity and persistence of the disease varies enormously in individual patients. Dietary modification is generally of little value, although a high-vitamin and low-fibre diet is probably best. Sometimes surgery to remove the worst affected portions of the intestine can lead to a good improvement, although it is not usually as permanently successful as it is in ulcerative colitis, as the condition is not restricted to any single part of the alimentary canal. Crohn's disease can therefore recur after surgery.

Self-Help Measures

It is important that you destress your life as much as possible (see p. 481). Many of the problems associated with the gastro-intestinal tract have a psychosomatic basis, whereby they are physical manifestations of a more emotional or psychological problem. Rooting out the cause with some therapy would be useful. Spiritually, healing would help and as always there is much you can do yourself. The intestinal tract is the province of the solar plexus chakra. Unresolved feelings of anger, resentment, bitterness or hatred will cause blocks here, as will any trauma that happened to you between the ages of 8 to 12. If you are aware that something there needs to be addressed, it would be good for you to do some healing exercises yourself, to do your best to forgive and let go of the past. If necessary find a healer who will help you with some chakra clearing.

DIVERTICULITIS

Many people develop small sacs or pouches in the lining of the wall of the large intestine as the years go by, particularly if their diet provides insufficient fibre to promote a regular bowel habit. This condition is known as diverticulosis. When these sacs or diverticulae become inflamed, a condition known as 'diverticulitis' occurs. Symptoms include abdominal cramps (particularly on the lower left side) and vomiting. In severe cases an abscess may be felt by the doctor as a lump, and there may be bleeding from the rectum as a result of intestinal haemorrhage. Unusually, perforation of a diverticulum or abscess can occur leading to peritonitis (inflammation of the surface lining of the abdomen itself), or a stricture (narrowing) or fistula may be produced.

Treatment

Treatment with bedrest and antibiotics usually resolves symptoms but in more severe cases a liquid diet or intravenous infusion may be necessary. Surgical intervention is usually only needed in cases of abscess or peritonitis or if bleeding is heavy and persistent. A temporary colostomy is sometimes performed to rest the most severely inflamed part of the bowel. This involves a procedure whereby the colon is diverted to the front of the abdominal wall to form an opening for the discharge of waste products until the diseased part of the bowel settles down.

Self-Help Measures

Diverticulosis can be prevented by keeping the gut working smoothly, avoiding constipation by eating a high-fibre diet, avoiding coffee (which is constipating) and taking exercise – which tones the muscles of your colon as well as everything else. Drinking lots of liquids (preferably fresh water) and taking time to go to the toilet and relax will help as will cutting out smoking, reducing your alcohol intake to one unit daily and eating unprocessed foods where possible. When diverticulitis is present, usually medical intervention is necessary. But you can help yourself by resting, taking lots of water and other clear fluids such as juices, and supporting your immune system (see p. 536).

Gallstones

Gallstones are solid lumps, round and smooth or multi-sided in shape, which form in the gall bladder and which may or may not give rise to symptoms. They consist mainly of cholesterol but bile pigments (which are the breakdown products of red blood cells) also make up part of their chemical composition. Where they exist they only cause problems in about 20 per cent of cases, which normally happens when one such gallstone becomes stuck in the bile duct (the tube from the gall bladder leading to the bowel). Symptoms include pain (usually in the upper right-hand side of the abdomen) and flatulence. The patient may also feel sick and suffer from indigestion. The attack often follows a fatty meal because the gall bladder contracts in order to release fat-digesting enzymes. Sometimes the gall bladder itself becomes infected (cholecystitis), or the bile duct becomes obstructed, leading to jaundice with its characteristic yellowing of the skin and eyes. Diagnosis is confirmed using ultrasound scans capable of detecting stones in 95 per cent of cases, although sometimes special X-rays are carried out. Stones that do not cause trouble are generally left alone, but when symptoms are severe and recurrent, surgical removal of the gall bladder (cholecystectomy) is recommended which cures the problem in the vast majority of cases. These days the operation is often done through keyhole surgery which leaves merely a tiny scar.

Self-Help Measures

The old adage of the 5 Fs still holds for the development of gallstones: they are most common in females who are fair, fertile, fat and fortyish. However, those who are sedentary, overweight and who have had them before are also at risk, as are those of native American descent. Losing weight quickly can cause stones and smoking is a risk factor. More than 30 per cent of all gallstones in men are preventable by 30 minutes of exercise 5 times a week. This interferes with the metabolic process that gives rise to gallstones. Peppermint stimulates the gall bladder to contract and release bile and can also alleviate cramps. The homeopathic remedy Calc carb is useful especially if there is pain after eating fatty food.

Liver Problems

All the blood from your intestine goes through your liver and if this major organ isn't working well, toxic substances cannot be removed nor the digestive process completed. Common symptoms of liver dysfunction from infection (hepatitis A, B or C) or from scarring (cirrhosis) includes jaundice, dark urine, fatigue, nausea and vomiting, loss of appetite and muscle and joint pains. Both are potentially serious problems requiring specific treatments and prevention is far preferable in this situation to cure. Regular detoxification of the liver is therefore a good discipline. For 2 weeks eliminate red meat, dairy produce, fried foods, sugar, caffeine and preservatives, while increasing your fruit and vegetable intake and drinking at least 8 glasses of water daily. Juices are a good addition to your usual regime, apple and beetroot juice or carrot juice with ginger being excellent. It would help the detox if you were to increase your level of exercise and take a sauna once a week. Supplements of milk thistle, Vitamin C and flax seed (linseed) oil would help. You will see the difference in 2 weeks in terms of your energy, the condition of your skin, hair, etc. (Milk thistle is an antioxidant that promotes regeneration of the liver cells and is good for hepatitis and cirrhosis.)

CONSTIPATION AND PILES

Constipation means different things to different people. It is as normal for somebody to empty their bowels once a week, if they have always done so, as it is for someone else to do so 3 times a day. The critical factor is any change in your normal bowel habit and the presence of discomfort and pain when passing hard, dry motions. Sometimes unaccustomed constipation can be an underlying symptom of something more serious, so any persistent change in bowel habit should certainly be brought to the attention of a doctor. The vast majority of cases arise because of insufficient fibre in the diet. Poor toilet training in childhood and persistently ignoring the urge to evacuate the bowel can lead to a 'lazy' intestine where the muscles of the intestine walls cease to effectively push waste products along the digestive canal. The symptom occurs commonly in irritable bowel syndrome, in people with an underactive thyroid and, rarely, in cancer of the colon where there is some degree of obstruction. It is a feature of diverticulitis too. Doctors should always treat constipation sympathetically and carefully as the patient is often distressed, and should remember that there may be a more serious problem underlying it. The practice of abusing laxatives should be strongly discouraged, and patients are advised to adopt simple self-help measures such as drinking plenty of fluids. Investigations using flexible telescopic viewing instruments and barium X-rays may be advisable.

Haemorrhoids or piles often coincide with constipation, as the straining to pass hard motions leads to congestion in the veins within the lower part of the rectum, which can then prolapse through the muscular ring of the anus, causing swelling, pain and itching. Initial treatment consists of suppositories and creams, although in more severe cases surgical procedures may be required to permanently remove the congested veins.

Self-Help Measures

Other than gradually introducing more fibre-rich foods into the diet, one of the most pleasant remedies for constipation is to take 3 fruits (for example, a peach, a banana and a pear, although any combination will do), add half a glass of orange juice, half a teaspoon of chopped ginger root (you can buy this ready chopped in a jar if you like) and half a glass of pure water, and blend them all together. This will release nutrients and enzymes which are beneficial to the digestive process. These enzymes are often not available because chewing your food simply cannot achieve the degree of cellular breakdown necessary to release them from our food. Drink it fresh in the morning or last thing at night. Flax seed (linseed) or psyllium are helpful. It might be worth having your magnesium level checked either by your doctor or dietitian since sometimes there just isn't enough of this essential element (which aids peristalsis) in our diet.

Nutritional Healing

A high-fibre diet has a beneficial action throughout the intestinal tract. Fibre, the material that plant cell walls are made of, is indigestible. It moves quickly through the body without being altered but carrying debris with it and it acts as a gentle abrasive to cleanse the bowel wall as it goes. Not only does it relieve constipation and mop up toxins, but it dramatically reduces the risk of colon cancer. It also reduces the risk of haemorrhoids and diverticulosis. It is a good nutrient for the friendly intestinal bacteria that eliminate toxins and stabilise the environment of the bowel. However, taking more fibre means that you must drink more water, since fibre absorbs water from the intestine, increasing the bulk of your stool. The fibre in apples, pears and wheat bran (lignin) can protect against gallstones. Fibre in vegetables helps everything move more quickly through the gut, relieving constipation. Cellulose, found mainly in lettuce, can help prevent haemorrhoids and constipation.

Soluble fibre acts differently. Pectin, found in apples, oranges, peaches and carrots, slows down the absorption of food after eating, thereby helping maintain a steady blood sugar level. This makes it invaluable for diabetics and those trying to reduce their weight. Gums are soluble fibres found in oats, peas and beans. These also regulate blood sugar and reduce cholesterol. Guar gum helps control blood fats. Glucomannan combines with fat in the intestine helping in the treatment of obesity, as does chitosan which is made from the shells of crustaceans. Whole grains including oatmeal, whole grain bread, whole grain pasta, cereals, brown rice, fruit, nuts, salads and vegetables should give you enough fibre but if necessary you could add wheat bran or take a supplement.

There are millions of friendly bacteria in your gut that aid digestion and maintain the equilibrium of gut flora, preventing overgrowth of other gut residents such as candida albicans. Antibiotics can kill off the intestinal flora and create problems. Lactobacillus acidophyllus, found in live yogurt, can restore the number of friendly bacteria, as can tempeh and the sugars found in fruit, particularly ripe bananas.

Try to avoid using a microwave for cooking. It changes the cellular structure of food and a friend of ours who is a powerful healer claims that it robs food of much of its nutritional value. Steaming vegetables helps preserve their vitamin content better than boiling.

Chew slowly since digestion actually starts in your mouth.

Drink before or after your meal, rather than with your food, since liquid will dilute both stomach acid and enzymes and hinder digestion. Eating in a relaxed atmosphere, not in front of the TV, where your concentration is on something other than your food, and where your emotions may be being stirred by what you are watching, will also help. Having your tummy tied in knots by a suspense thriller or your heart torn apart by some drama will not aid digestion!

Other herbs for the digestive tract

Diarrhoea – nettles
'Nervous stomach' – oats
Excess gas – dill, fennel, peppermint
Halitosis – cardamom, peppermint, fennel
Heartburn – angelica, chamomile, peppermint
Hepatitis – dandelion, milk thistle, turmeric
Indigestion – chamomile, ginger, peppermint
Constipation – flax seed (linseed), plantain, senna, cascara sagrada

Integrated approach

1. Combat symptoms with an adjustment of lifestyle.
2. Relieve stress, curb your smoking and alcohol consumption, eat fibre-rich foods and exercise regularly.
3. Drink plenty of water.
4. Have persistent or 'unaccustomed' symptoms properly investigated.
5. Never assume a diagnosis without tests, especially if you are over 40.
6. Use nutritional healing and detoxification regimes regularly.
7. Remember that prescribed medication or surgery can be dramatically effective in severe and appropriate cases.
8. The National Association for Colitis and Crohn's Disease are well worth joining if you are sufferer.

Ear, Nose and Throat (ENT)

Martin has been off school 7 times in the last year with tonsillitis. Not only is he very poorly each time he comes down with the infection but his education is inevitably suffering. His mother feels worried by the amount of antibiotics he is being prescribed and she wonders about the benefits of a possible operation to have his tonsils removed.

The anatomical structures and tissues which make up the ear, nose and throat are delicate and complex, and they can be affected and upset by a large number of genetic and environmental factors. Little wonder that maladies and malfunctions of this part of the body are among the commonest of all the reasons why people consult their doctor.

Of all the symptoms most often reported to the GP, earache, sore throats, nasal congestion, sinusitis, tinnitus and deafness are the commonest. They are also among the commonest symptoms least satisfactorily dealt with by conventional doctors as growing waiting lists, official complaints statistics and legions of unsatisfied customers will testify.

The Conventional Approach to Common ENT Problems

Earache

Few children escape earache. It is usually due to an infection of the middle ear cavity, when it is known as acute otitis media. This is a frequent problem in young children and a common reason for parents requesting a house call from the doctor when their offspring are crying and distressed in the small hours of the morning, pulling at their ear and exhibiting a moderately high temperature. During daylight hours, children may not respond to their parents' conversation because of loss of hearing, and sometimes the eardrum may even burst producing a discharge of fluid from the ear canal. Although this looks alarming as well as messy, it serves to relieve the pressure on the eardrum and represents nature's way of relieving the problem.

Other sources of earache include inflammation of the skin within the ear canal itself. This is known as otitis externa and may be due to infection, or to inflammation such as that caused by constant moisture, seen in people who swim frequently or who do not dry their ears after showering. Pain may also follow infection with the shingles virus, or even be referred pain from other structures in the head such as the teeth or tonsils. Conventional treatment relies on pain relief in the form of paracetamol, aspirin or ibuprofen (although aspirin is not recommended for children under 12), and antibiotics where infection is present. Resistance to the inappropriate overprescribing of antibiotics is to be welcomed but where the delicate structures within the ear are significantly inflamed and where there is a risk of permanent hearing loss if treatment is delayed, broad-spectrum antibiotics are still strongly recommended. Whenever middle ear infections are diagnosed, a follow-up appointment should always be made to ensure that the situation has fully resolved. If there should be fluid or pus present behind the eardrum despite treatment with antibiotics and antihistamines, an operation known as a myringotomy may be necessary to allow the escape of such material, and sometimes a tiny hollow dumb-bell shaped device called a grommet is inserted into the hole made in the eardrum to dry out the middle ear cavity over a period of months so that hearing may be preserved long term. Growing interest in allergy as a possible cause of chronic middle ear infections (glue ear) is encouraging many patients to experiment with supplements and dietary restriction in an attempt to avoid recurrent problems.

Nasal Congestion

Nasal congestion is also common and results from swelling of the sensitive lining of the nose, the mucous membrane. When it swells, it tends to leak more fluid so that a thick nasal mucus is produced which further gets in the way of breathing. Causes range from the common cold to allergies like hay fever, deviation of the nasal septum and previous injury right through to chronic sinusitis and nasal polyps. These are pear-shaped growths emanating from the mucous membrane itself.

The traditional approach to treating nasal congestion is to identify the underlying cause and either to avoid the trigger factor or treat the resulting symptoms. Steam inhalations can loosen nasal mucus so it can be expelled through vigorous nose blowing, and decongestant sprays and drops can shrink the mucous membrane, opening up the airway and reducing the leakage of fluid. However, these should not be used for more than a maximum of 2 weeks at any time because ultimately the blood vessels become resistant to their action, and permanent exacerbation of the symptoms may result.

If short-term measures such as these have failed, investigation by the doctor to identify sinusitis, polyps or persistent allergy is required. There is no doubt that avoiding the inhalation of cigarette smoke, keeping out of the way of environmental pollution and reducing the number of house dust mites in the household would solve a large number of problems. If chronic sinusitis and polyps are discovered, surgical procedures to drain fluid from the sinuses and to strip away chronically swollen mucous membrane in the sinuses or nasal cavities can be performed.

TONSILS AND ADENOIDS

Although these glands, situated as they are at the back of the throat and nose, tend to be regarded as something of a nuisance, they are actually one of the body's first lines of defence against invading micro-organisms. As such they have an important function. As they do battle with viruses and bacteria, they swell and become inflamed, causing pain and discomfort. Removing them without good reason through a surgical procedure exposes the individual to the risk of general anaesthesia, will not prevent future sore throats and only means that the second line of defence against infection, namely the glands each side of the neck, are called on to respond instead. Consequently any operation on the tonsils and adenoids is now restricted to those situations where to leave them would be detrimental to health.

Children suffer most up to the age of about 7 when their immune system becomes more fully mature and able to deal with invading bacteria and viruses and when their growth rate is such that their nose and throat passages become wider and less vulnerable to obstructive symptoms. The conventional approach to tonsillitis and adenoid enlargement is to assess the frequency and severity of infections in the child as well as the degree of time lost from school and any interference with sleep. When the child is frequently ill with high temperature, very inflamed glands, difficulty swallowing, weight loss and nasal obstruction as a result of tonsillar and adenoidal enlargement, an operation to remove these structures is seriously considered. In most cases, however, sore throats are due to viral infections which will not respond to antibiotics and which are of short duration anyway. The GP is expertly placed to advise patients accordingly on the best course of action in their individual circumstances.

Chloe is fed up to the back teeth with nasal congestion. She snores at night, much to the irritation of her partner, she cannot smell or taste properly and her voice has taken on this unattractive nasal tone as well. Sometimes it is so bad she feels she cannot breathe. Chloe has a moderately severe nasal allergy.

TINNITUS

This refers to a hissing, ringing or whistling sound in the ear when no external noise actually exists. For reasons not fully understood, the hearing nerve transmits signals to the brain which interprets the messages as background noise. There is often some hearing loss which accompanies the tinnitus and this may be associated with exposure to loud noise in the past or to disorders of the inner, middle or outer ear or even to the side effects of certain drugs such as aspirin or quinine. Many people can experience tinnitus to some degree if they listen hard enough to the sound of silence, but in some people the tinnitus is extreme and they suffer such distress they may even be driven to contemplate suicide. The conventional approach to treatment is unsatisfactory to say the least as no cure is possible and sufferers are merely advised to block out the noise by overriding it with other sounds such as from the radio or hi-fi. Some ear, nose and throat specialists, however, recommend a tinnitus 'masker', very much like headphones, which transmits a random mixture of sounds from a broad range of frequencies to drown out the abnormally generated sound from within the ear itself.

DEAFNESS

There are many forms of deafness and many of them result from problems either in the nerve of hearing itself or in the structures that transmit sound from the outside through the ear cavities to the sensory apparatus of hearing itself, deep within the skull. Infection, injury, deterioration due to age and congenital problems may all prove to be the underlying cause. The conventional approach to deafness is first of all to reach a diagnosis and then to treat it accordingly.

Children who are born deaf will clearly have special needs and will need to undergo the long and difficult process of learning to communicate effectively with those around them. Children who become deaf as a result of chronic middle ear infection (glue ear) may require an operation known as a myringotomy to drain fluid from the middle ear cavity and dry out the cells lining it. Where wax in the outer ear is a problem it may be syringed away with warm water by your GP or the practice nurse. Perforated eardrum as a result of loud noise or rapid changes in air pressure may either heal spontaneously or require a surgical procedure known as a tympanoplasty to cover the defect. In cases of deafness due to otosclerosis, where the tiny bones within the middle ear cavity fail to move normally in relation to one another in response to external sound, a stapedectomy operation to insert an artificial stapes bone is effective.

Hearing aids are recommended where it is necessary to increase the volume of sound reaching the inner ear, and for this purpose they contain an amplifier and an earphone that fits into the outer ear. Modern digital hearing aids are so tiny that they fit into the ear canal themselves and are hardly visible to other people. They can improve hearing loss dramatically by enhancing certain frequencies of sound while cutting out others. When the central apparatus for hearing within the skull is severely damaged, a new operation known as a cochlear implant is now being performed which creates new hope for people who are profoundly deaf, even those who have been deaf from birth.

Ellen came to a healing workshop complaining of tinnitus and recurrent sore throats that did not respond to orthodox medicine. From time to time she also suffered from sinusitis, having pain in her face with associated headache. She is gentle and rather shy and admitted that she had difficulty with self-assertion. She enjoys her work where she is fairly popular and efficient as the deputy coordinator of a child welfare team. About 6 years ago she witnessed something which she knew she should have reported but had not the courage to do so. Although it constantly worried her that the professional in question was still working in a situation where other children could be damaged, Ellen said nothing and tried to avoid the nagging feeling that she had compromised her integrity and failed to speak the truth. Ellen has a blocked throat chakra.

THE COMPLEMENTARY APPROACH

For Sinusitis

NUTRITIONAL HEALING

Check whether you suffer from any food sensitivities since these can cause a chronic problem that appears to be unresponsive to any intervention. Dairy produce in particular can cause you to produce so much mucus that the sinuses become full. Completely eliminating foods to which you are either intolerant or allergic may have apparently miraculous effects. (If you cut out dairy produce, do substitute other calcium-rich foods such as sesame seeds or broccoli, or take a good calcium supplement.)

Vitamins and supplements

Vitamin C will support your immune system while Vitamin A will also be helpful, although check this with your doctor if you're pregnant. Echinacea is also useful in the short term in acute sinusitis.

Complementary therapies

Where orthodox medicine may have little to offer the chronic sinusitis sufferer, complementary therapy can be very useful. The *Lancet* recently published research on the use of homeopathic remedies in sinusitis and found them effective, especially in acute sinusitis where they were found to reduce the frequency and severity of attacks. Your homeopath may give you a constitutional remedy, although Arsenicum may help when there is throbbing pain aggravated by light, noise and movement, where the pain is aggravated by anxiety and exertion and if you feel better in a darkened room. Belladonna is indicated if your head feels full and as though it could burst and if the pain is located mainly around your forehead and eyes, being worse on bending forward, lying flat or when touched. If you feel worse lying down or sitting in a warm room and better in cool air, then you might like to try Pulsatilla. Agaricum is useful when the headache is persistent and severe.

Chamomile and peppermint oil mixed in equal parts and used in a vaporiser will relieve inflammation and relax the passages leading to increased air flow. Rosemary, juniper, bergamot and hyssop may also be useful. Tea tree oil is a natural antiseptic and antibiotic and would be good to vaporise along with eucalyptus and lavender to help boost your immunity and to clear and protect your sinuses. While out and about why not have some on a handkerchief or tissue.

For Earache and Ear Infections

If you have ruled out any serious cause for the pain, acupuncture, healing or aromatherapy may help. Oils that may be particularly useful are rosemary, lavender and tea tree. Garlic, echinacea and mullein are worth a try although the response will depend upon the cause. Homeopathic Lycopodium may help if the infection is first on the right, then on the left, and Lachesis if there is an accompanying fever with the infection beginning first on the left and then on the right. Kalium bichromicum, Apis, Pulsatilla, Graphites and Belladonna may be useful, but ideally consult a professional and have the appropriate remedy tailored especially for you.

For Influenza

Echinacea can inhibit viruses such as influenza (and herpes) while also having the capacity to relieve other complicating upper respiratory tract infections. However, if your immune system is already compromised, for example if you have AIDS, or if you have an allergy to daisies, then this is not for you. In any case use for a maximum of 8 weeks, then stop. Taking it for 4 days, then stopping for 4 days and repeating will increase its effectiveness.

For Hearing Problems (Including Tinnitus)

NUTRITIONAL HEALING

The *Journal of the International Academy of Preventive Medicine* reported improvement in 90 per cent cases of tinnitus treated by improved diet, exercise and stress reduction programmes alone, while the *Lancet* in 1986 suggested that omega-3 fatty acids in fish oils may be useful. There is a link between blood sugar levels and tinnitus, so reducing dietary sugar intake is helpful. Reducing fat and cholesterol can help, as can giving up smoking and reducing alcohol intake

VITAMINS AND SUPPLEMENTS

Low levels of Vitamin A have been associated with hearing loss (*Archives of Otorhinolaryngology*, 1982) and many elderly patients with progressive hearing loss have low levels of zinc. A supplement will often help. Some tinnitus sufferers also have zinc deficiency and it is well worth asking your doctor to check your blood for zinc levels. There have been cases reported where symptoms have cleared completely with zinc supplementation. Magnesium, potassium and sodium are also worth checking. Gingko biloba may be helpful by improving circulation. There is also a German enzyme product available (a mixture of trypsin, chymotrypsin, bromelain, papain and pancreatin with the riboflavinoid rutin) which helps the body fight inflammation.

Complementary therapies

Current treatments for tinnitus include masking the noise with a sound that is more tolerable. Hypnosis may also be of benefit. However, chronic inflammation is often the cause of tinnitus in a large proportion of cases. Other important things to remember are to protect yourself from loud noise and various pollutants such as aluminium and lead. Gingko biloba may help by increasing the circulation. Acupuncture may also help.

Emotional and spiritual healing

As we saw with Ellen, problems in this area are often due to blocks or other dysfunctions of the throat chakra and work on this area may bring you relief. Healing and cleansing of the whole chakra system is usually necessary, but starting to own your truth, seeing it as an entity that needs to be constantly updated in the light of new information and having the courage to speak out whenever your integrity is compromised, can have amazing benefits on chronic ear, nose and throat problems. Ask yourself if there's something you are trying not to hear, something you are afraid to say or some area in which you do not have the courage of your convictions. You may need some help to clear this area since the blocks may go back to the time of its development in your late teens and early adulthood, especially around the age of 16 to 21. If you had some trauma then, or even earlier, then have a look at Brenda's book *The Rainbow Journey* and do the meditations and exercises to clear this area. You may need the help of a healer or psychotherapist.

Integrated approach

1. Ear, nose and throat problems are very common and many defy conventional medical treatment.
2. Ear infections are probably still best treated with antibiotics to reduce the possibility of permanent hearing loss.
3. Tonsillectomy and adenoidectomy are now generally reserved only for very severe cases.
4. Modern treatment for deafness, by contrast, continues to improve. Find out about the latest technology.
5. Nutritional, homeopathic and other complementary therapies are all worth experimenting with, especially for chronic symptoms with an allergic basis.

Eating Disorders

There are tens of thousands of people in Britain who suffer from eating disorders and many feel stuck and trapped by them. Contrary to popular belief it is not just the rich and famous who suffer from them – they can affect anyone of either sex and a few people even die from them. They create a huge amount of misery and suffering for the patients themselves and a great deal of concern and anxiety in their nearest and dearest as well. There are two main eating disorders, anorexia nervosa and bulimia nervosa, and each is closely related to the other to the extent that some people even believe they are part of the same basic disorder. The problem of obesity itself is so common that it can now be regarded as epidemic in Britain and other developed countries.

Michelle is a 15-year-old schoolgirl who started dieting because her friends were teasing her for being overweight. She weighed 65 kg (10st 3lb) and being only 1.6 m tall (5 ft 4 in) she felt very fat. She stopped eating carbohydrates and fats, and within 6 months was down to 49 kg (7st 9 lb) by which time her periods had stopped. Although to begin with her parents were pleased that she had lost weight, they became concerned when she continued to miss meals and exercised strenuously, and they suspected she was taking food up to her room only to flush it down the toilet when no one was looking. Even when her weight dropped to 38 kg (5 st 13 lb) she still believed she was fat, especially her hips and thighs. Rejecting all offers of medical help she was finally admitted to hospital weighing 29 kg (4 st 8 lb) when she was terribly skeletal and weak. Michelle has anorexia nervosa.

Anorexia Nervosa

Taken literally this means 'loss of appetite for nervous reasons'. This is misleading because people with this eating disorder lose weight but do not lose their appetite. Instead they suppress their desire to eat because of an intense fear of becoming fat. Even when the anorexic has lost considerable weight, they still regard themselves as being very fat, even when nobody else does. Doctors describe this as having a distorted body image. Most cases of anorexia are seen in females, with only 10 per cent coming from the male population. The usual age when it develops is the young teenage years up until the early twenties. Symptoms and signs of anorexia nervosa include weight loss leading to a body weight of at least 15 per cent below the normal or expected range for a person's height and age. The weight loss is deliberately obtained through the avoidance of a variety of foods. There is an overwhelming dread of becoming fat and a distorted body image based on a self-perception of being too fat. Finally there is a widespread hormonal disorder which in girls usually leads to abscence of periods and in boys to loss of sexual interest and potency.

Danielle is 24 and works as a nursery nurse. Her weight is fairly normal but she always tends to put on weight easily unless she is careful. Being a rather anxious person and not terribly happy in her job she often used to binge uncontrollably on everything and anything she fancied only to feel disgusted with herself afterwards and worry about getting fat. She began to take laxatives in an effort to counteract her excessive food intake and sometimes made herself sick deliberately after huge meals. She became moody and obsessed with the concept of reaching her ideal weight which she could only achieve by going on one diet after another. Danielle is suffering from bulimia nervosa.

BULIMIA NERVOSA

The main feature of this condition is binge eating. This is more than just the occasional blow-out or special feast. It means eating an unusually large quantity of food very frantically and is associated with the person eating feeling that they have become totally out of control. Like anorexics, bulimics have an exaggerated fear of fatness, but unlike anorexics their weight is often normal. In order to try to control the fattening effects of food, bulimics often make themselves sick, take laxatives to purge their intestines, undergo periods of relative starvation through crash dieting and may resort to drugs such as appetite suppressants or diuretics. There may also be a self-perception of being too fat even when their weight is relatively normal. Bulimia normally begins in the late teens and early twenties, is mostly seen in women and is considerably more common than anorexia. Some people, however, have features of both; indeed the umbrella term anorexia–bulimia has been described.

Obesity

Hal came to the surgery having failed a medical for a new job because of his excessive weight. He said that he had been overweight for some years, but that the problem had become worse since he had separated from his wife about 3 years earlier. He said that he used food to comfort himself after she left, preferring this to alcohol with which he had had problems before. He is now grossly obese and has pain in both knees from carrying the excess weight. His doctor remarked upon his high cholesterol level and his increasing risk of heart disease. Despite this he has been unable to stop eating huge meals, often 2 or 3 times as big as his colleagues would eat. Although he prefers pies, chips and fried foods, he admitted that he would eat just about anything. Hal is a compulsive overeater.

Compulsive overeating will always lead to obesity although there are often underlying issues, as in Hal's case, that need to be dealt with in psychotherapy. Perhaps some simple facts would be useful here. Basically, it is a simple mathematical problem. If you consume more calories than you burn, you will become obese. You need a lot of calories just to maintain your body at rest and to repair and renew cells. However, the leaner you are, the higher the proportion of your daily intake that is burned in this way. What you eat minus what you use in exercise and maintenance equals what you will store as fat. If you increase your energy output by exercise, then you will burn more calories and store less fat. The majority of excess calories that we eat come from fat, not sugar, although if something tastes sweet, better to eat it in moderation (that includes the artificial sweeteners). All the chemical reactions in your body require water. Drinking more water helps speed up those chemical reactions and therefore helps food to be metabolised and waste to be excreted. When you've made a decision to lose weight, set yourself reasonable goals and give yourself a pat on the back when you achieve them. If you constantly fail to meet your goals change them. Break them down into smaller steps which will give you a greater sense of success and being in control. A loss of 1 to 2 pounds or half to one kilogram a week is satisfactory and will allow your body to adjust without thinking there's a famine and that it must try to conserve every bit of fat in preparation!

Overweight children become overweight adults so it really is the responsibility of parents to watch their children's eating habits and help them learn how to have a healthy diet. Since obesity in childhood can lead to the risk in later life of heart disease, diabetes, breast cancer and cancer of the digestive tract, to say nothing of a shorter lifespan, not taking care of this problem in your children is a form of neglect.

Emotional and Spiritual Healing

Although eating disorders do occur in men, where they are often part of a greater addictive problem, they are much more likely to be the province of women. Over the last 40 years women have been subjected to pressure from the media, the fashion world, Barbie dolls, their men and the medical profession to be slimmer than our bodies were ever intended to be. It is natural for women's bodies to be curvy, to have breasts capable of feeding babies and hips that are round and soft. If we look at the icons of a few years ago, it's easy to see that the criteria for beauty have changed, but it is ridiculous to think that women should be able to change to accommodate such whims. Marilyn Monroe, perhaps one of the greatest beauties of this century, wore size 14 or 16 dresses. She had fat in all the places women are supposed to have fat. Just because designers then latched on to a thin waif-like look, were we supposed to suddenly change our whole metabolism? Thankfully the fashion is changing again, but the damage is done because most women follow an endless unwinnable battle to keep their bodies thinner than they are naturally supposed to be. Our bodies have an inner wisdom which tells us when we're just right despite what charts and tables decide. Tune in to your body and you will know whether you feel good in your skin or not. There are certainly benefits to being slim and in shape, but do not think that will-power is going to make you look like the pictures in magazines if in fact you are meant to be larger than what is now considered to be the norm. And please do not feel bad about yourself that you cannot make it happen or allow yourself to feel unhappy because you're less than perfect. You are perfectly you, and that's fine. What *is* important is that you're healthy.

Younger girls and women are much more likely to be affected by eating disorders these days. We are seeing some cases of established anorexia at the age of 8 or 9, although it is more usual for anorexia to appear in the early teens. Usually there is a history of previous disturbance often involving abuse of some kind. The typically perfectionist anorexic of 20 years ago – where the vast majority of girls suffering from eating disorders were from the families of professional parents, intelligent and diligent, often artistic and driven to succeed – has changed little. These young women are often very bright, intensely obsessional about their performance and their appearance and they set themselves very high goals. Their level of self-loathing is sad to behold as they punish themselves with a passion, having lost all insight about their real appearance, their body image being highly distorted. Although bulimia may be a separate disorder, often the anorexic person will become bulimic when she loses control of the ability to starve herself.

Amy presented at the surgery as a withdrawn 27-year-old woman of average weight. She appeared depressed and tearfully admitted that for the last 3 years she had been bingeing on carbohydrate snacks such as biscuits, chocolate, crisps, bread and cake, vomiting after each binge to keep her weight at the same level. She would take vast quantities of laxatives and was constantly in pain from abdominal cramps. Although ideally she would prefer to be slimmer, this is not as much of an issue as her lack of control over what she eats. She said that she had always been rather plump and had discovered that she could eat what she wanted and not get fat by vomiting after meals, although things had now got out of control. Her dentist has recently remarked on the decay of her teeth which is due to the stomach acid she vomits several times a day. There have been difficulties for some time in her relationship with her parents with whom she still lives having had several failed romantic attachments. Amy has bulimia nervosa.

In spiritual terms there has often been damage to the base chakra which develops usually before the age of 5. Women who have had some trauma before that age (such as separation from their mother, physical or sexual abuse, death of a parent, etc.) will have difficulty with their sense of self and with their identity as women. If there have been further difficulties through the years, especially in the 5 to 8 age group, then there can be problems with sexuality that may lead sufferers to try to remain emotionally and physically childlike. Healing therefore needs to be on all levels, physical (feeding slowly and gently while paying attention to any electrolyte disturbance etc.), emotional, to help heal the wounds of the past while gently coaxing the sufferer into adulthood, and spiritual, repairing damage to the chakras and to the aura, as well as rebuilding the spiritual strength necessary to cope with letting go of an illness which in its own way has been a comfort and protection, preventing the sufferer from having to live in the real world with all the responsibility that being an adult entails.

Sadie was 18 when she was brought along for treatment. She objected that she did not want to be seen and that her parents were fussing over nothing. She denied that she was starving herself and said that her mother was mistaken in her account of the tiny amount of food that Sadie ate and her tantrums if she was interrupted at mealtimes or the strict regime she had set was changed in any way. Weighing in at 39 kilograms and having lost over 25 per cent of her original weight, she still insisted that she was fat and said how disgusting she felt. She was fearful that she would put on weight and thought that she should lose at least another 5 kilos. She was compulsively exercising despite the fact that she was quite weak. Only much later did she confide that she had been sexually assaulted by a neighbour over a period of 8 months or so when she was about 5. Sadie has anorexia nervosa.

Often much of the work needs to be focused on the family who have usually also become embroiled in the illness and who may, with much love and the best possible intentions, have developed ways of communicating that are not really healthy or helpful. Sadie's treatment included individual, group and family psychotherapy. Supportive and spiritual therapy is ideal. However, there must be medical supervision in this potentially fatal illness where the metabolism has become so disturbed.

Women with eating disorders are making powerful statements about their womanhood which need to be heard. Although Amy eventually developed into a strong, proud, very competent woman, it took a long time and a lot of work for all those involved to help her take up her rightful place as an adult woman with responsibility for her own life. What was essential was that she was treated with love and compassion, tenderness and fairness, even though at times her therapist needed to be tough and to set limits with love.

Conventional Treatment

Whether professional treatment is obtained or not, there are three basic steps on the road to recovery from eating disorders which need to be achieved.

1. A sensible eating plan

The first step is to restore a healthy weight and a healthy pattern of eating. This means giving up the deliberate restraint from eating and the suppression of appetite, and allowing the weight to find a level where it can regulate itself naturally. The person needs to learn to trust the body's automatic pilot, as it were. This means eating normal meals with a normal calorific content, and hard though this may be for the sufferer, it is vitally important. It often means that someone will need to help the person with the eating disorder so that they remain feeling safe and secure in this new-found practice.

2. Separating body image from wider issues

The second step is to encourage the sufferer to disentangle their fears of fatness and their attitude to food from wider issues. This may mean exploding the myth that to be thin means to be happy and successful and that to be anything other than thin means low esteem and that one is a failure.

3. Confronting personal issues

Finally the third step is to confront special personal issues which are of immense significance and relevance to the individual sufferer and which will be crucial to their recovery. Achieving this means that the sufferer can start to get on with their life again and get it sorted out. It also means learning how to deal with new problems as they arise so that any triggers are avoided that might be capable of dragging the person back into their old eating habits and behaviour.

When broken up in this way, the steps to recovery may sound straightforward, but few people recover without professional help and a minority fail to recover despite extensive medical treatment. The problem is that although effective treatment exists for eating disorders, proactive contribution to the therapy has to be made by the sufferer because the treatment cannot be received in a passive way, as it might for example when recovering from a broken leg. Many eating disorder sufferers have very ambivalent feelings in that although they hate being as they are, they fear change because this could threaten their stability and sense of control. Professional treatment therefore needs to create confidence and a sense of safety to allow the sufferer to have the courage to move forward and to change.

Psychotherapy

For bulimia nervosa, short-term psychotherapy of the cognitive behavioural type is most successful, with the therapist working with the patient to get rid of undesirable behaviour such as bingeing and vomiting and to create healthy alternatives such as eating more regularly. A diary may be used to track relevant behaviours as well as feelings and thoughts. Eventually the ideas and beliefs that maintain the behaviour become more obvious and more open to change. Sometimes hospital admission is useful in the treatment of bulimia as are antidepressant drugs in certain cases.

The treatment of anorexia nervosa is usually more prolonged than that of bulimia and often takes months or even years. This is because a normal weight needs to be restored in the first place before learning to maintain that weight can be achieved. Also in fully developed anorexia, the entanglement of ideas of weight with wider personal issues is usually much more extreme. Despite this, most treatments for anorexia can occur on an outpatient basis with the core treatment involving some form of psychotherapy designed to make the patient feel comfortable enough to change.

In addition to the cognitive and behavioural techniques used for bulimia, dynamic psychotherapy may be used to detect and resolve underlying psychological conflicts that may be the root cause of any disturbed personal relationships and the unpleasant symptoms that commonly accompany them. Hospital treatment, however, is much more common in anorexia nervosa than in bulimia, and many hospitals have specialist units dedicated to the treatment of eating disorders. Self-help groups are also widely available throughout the country, providing useful information, advice and support for both the sufferers and their families. These complement professional help rather than act as a substitute for it, and many are organised by the Eating Disorders Association. Treatment for eating disorders will occasionally involve support for the family; in fact for anorexia, family therapy for young sufferers may be an essential part of the healing process.

Parents and other relatives must be sensitive in handling the situation that they feel so worried about as confrontation rarely gets anywhere with people who already have mixed and confused feelings. So choose the right time to bring up the subject if you suspect your son, daughter or partner has an eating disorder and, if necessary, pull back and try again another time. Avoid arguments and confrontations about their condition and about food rather than try to impose your own control over someone else's eating disorder. Seek professional help. It is hardly ever appropriate to force a person to accept treatment although professional advice may be essential. Finally bear in mind that most people with eating disorders make a full recovery eventually, and that although some sufferers may recover on their own, others can actually die from their condition if it becomes severe. A large number of people make an initial improvement from their disorder within months or years, but remain vulnerable to relapses in the future. The family GP is often the first port of call when help is needed (see Useful Addresses).

Nutritional Healing

Obviously eating disorders are superficially about eating, so getting the eating plan right is essential. It's a good idea to get away from calorie counting and to think instead of portions of food groups. The guidance of a good dietitian is invaluable here, and although there are other issues which are more important than food, refeeding not only your body but your brain is essential if you're to be able to deal with all the emotional baggage that got you into this state in the first place. A food diary is a good idea, in which you record accurately not only what you eat, but also the feelings that arise as you're faced with food. See the chart on p. 250 to help you get started. It would be useful to start this right away even if you haven't asked for help yet, and take it along with you to see either your psychiatrist or dietitian, or hopefully both. If either bulimia or overeating is your problem, then try to keep a diary of your trigger foods so that you can learn what to avoid, although if you follow the example of the food diary, you'll probably find that there are much more accurate pointers to what triggers your binge behaviour. Emotional factors such as insecurity, feelings of rejection or anger are probably underlying the more superficial aspects. Whatever, be gentle with yourself. Eating disorders are addictive disorders and whereas with other addictions such as alcohol or drugs, the sufferers never need face their substance of abuse again unless they wish to, for those with food addictions, the story is different. You have to have your addictive substance at least three times a day and confront your feelings about it and yourself every time. It's not easy.

Example of food diary

DATE	TIME	FOOD	FEELINGS
2.6.99	11.15 a.m.	2 biscuits Cup of coffee with milk	Feel guilty, as though I shouldn't have eaten anything. Angry that everyone else in the office just has a snack without even thinking about it. Why does it have to be such a big issue for me? I hate it.
2.6.99	1.45 p.m.	Tuna sandwich Yoghurt Apple Piece of cake	I'm so angry that I ate that piece of cake. I really tried not to. But then I'm so useless. Can't even say no to a piece of cake. Well I can't have anything else to eat today. I feel so fat. I'm really sick of this. I just want to disappear.
2.6.99	10.30 p.m.	Bowl of cereal with milk Packet of ginger snaps Mars bar	I can't even write down what I've eaten because I feel so ashamed of myself.

But more about nutritional healing. Drink plenty of water but not just before you're about to be weighed! Playing games like that will only prolong your agony and keep you sick.

If obesity is your problem, the same rules apply. You need good nutritious food in sufficient quantity to put your calorie intake in negative balance so the weight starts to come off *gradually*. High-fibre foods in grains, cereals, vegetables and fruits will increase the feeling of fullness, lower your insulin level which otherwise stimulates appetite, and oblige your body to use more calories during digestion and absorption. Wheat bran, whole grain cereals, brown rice, oats, corn, broccoli, asparagus, raspberries, dried apricots and pears are especially good. Get rid of any trigger foods you simply can't resist. Here are a few points of advice:

1. Keep a food diary. You can have whatever you want but you must justify it before you eat it.
2. Burn calories with aerobic exercise (see Basics, p. 7).
3. Check whether you have food allergies and intolerance (see box, p. 74) – sometimes these are the foods that we crave most.
4. Weigh yourself only once a week at the same time of day in similar clothes.
5. Could you have candidiasis? (See p. 330).
6. See your GP to check on the possibility of glandular disorders such as diabetes and hypothyroidism.
7. Spend some time smelling your food before you start to eat, then chew it slowly so that you thoroughly taste it. Your satiety centre starts to act at the mere smell of food and will have you feeling full much more quickly.

FOOD AND PHYSICAL WELLBEING

Since obesity is linked to higher rates of several cancers including breast and colon, be sensible and include in your diet fruit and vegetables which contain phytochemicals with anti-cancer properties. Fibre offers protection against colon, breast and prostate cancer. Limit your intake of alcohol, eat soya – tofu and soya milk – which lowers the risk of breast and prostate cancer, and ban saturated fat from your diet. Trans fats in margarine have also been linked to breast cancer.

WHAT IS A HEALTHY WEIGHT?

A good way to work out if your own weight is within healthy limits is to calculate your body mass index. See p. 253 and read off your own BMI from the chart.

Your Body Mass Index (BMI) is your weight in kilograms divided by your height in metres squared. For example, a man weighing 79 kilos and 1.78 metres tall would have a BMI of $79/1.78 \times 1.78 = 25$. This would represent a BMI within the normal healthy range for a man of 20–25. Now do the same exercise and calculate your own BMI.

Vitamins and Supplements

Whatever your eating disorder, a daily multivitamin and a multimineral supplement are a must. Often those with eating disorders have chromium deficiency and chromium picolinate can help reduce food cravings. Those with anorexia are often deficient in zinc which plays an important role in appetite and also in wound healing and tissue repair so add this to your daily regime also. L-carnitine and garcina extract have been said to help in weight reduction but the results of research are not convincing. There are lots of commercial weight loss products, but nothing succeeds as well as simple food balancing. The success of the Weight Watchers programme, which combines a good simple eating plan with simple group therapy and motivational talks, vouches for this approach.

Exercise and Lifestyle

Exercise not only promotes longevity and improves mood, it also helps regulate the biochemistry that affects your fat metabolism and ultimately your weight. It also tones and trims your shape and generally makes you feel better. However, those with eating

BODY MASS INDEX READY RECKONER

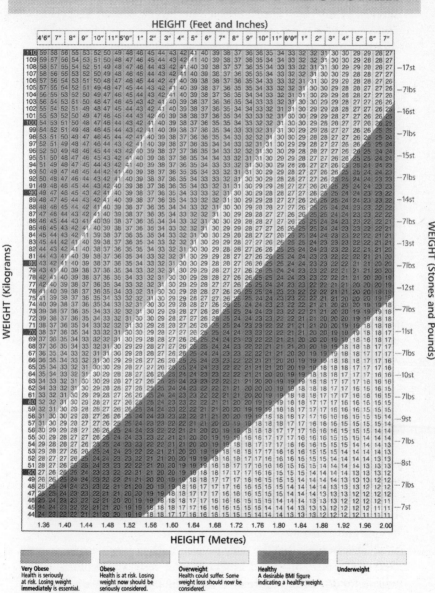

HEIGHT (Feet and Inches)

4'6" | 7" | 8" | 9" | 10" | 11" | 5'0" | 1" | 2" | 3" | 4" | 5" | 6" | 7" | 8" | 9" | 10" | 11" | 6'0" | 1" | 2" | 3" | 4" | 5" | 6" | 7"

WEIGHT (Kilograms)	1.36		1.40		1.44		1.48		1.52		1.56		1.60		1.64		1.68		1.72		1.76		1.80		1.84		1.88		1.92		1.96		2.00	WEIGHT (Stones and Pounds)
110	59	58	56	55	53	52	50	49	48	46	45	44	43	42	41	40	39	38	37	36	36	35	34	33	32	32	31	30	30	29	29	28	27	
109	59	57	56	54	53	51	50	48	47	46	45	44	43	42	41	40	39	38	37	36	35	34	34	33	32	32	31	30	30	29	28	28	27	
108	58	57	55	54	52	51	49	48	47	46	44	43	42	41	40	39	38	37	37	36	35	34	33	33	32	31	31	30	29	29	28	28	27	17st
107	58	56	55	53	52	50	49	48	46	45	44	43	42	41	40	39	38	37	36	35	35	34	33	32	32	31	30	30	29	28	28	27	27	
106	57	56	54	53	51	50	48	47	46	45	44	42	41	40	39	38	38	37	36	35	34	33	33	32	31	31	30	29	29	28	28	27	26	
105	57	55	54	52	51	49	48	47	45	44	43	42	41	40	39	38	37	36	35	35	34	33	32	32	31	30	30	29	28	28	27	27	26	7lbs
104	56	55	53	52	50	49	47	46	45	44	43	42	41	40	39	38	37	36	35	34	34	33	32	31	31	30	29	29	28	28	27	27	26	
103	56	54	53	51	50	48	47	46	45	43	42	41	40	39	38	37	36	36	35	34	33	33	32	31	30	30	29	29	28	27	27	26	26	
102	55	54	52	51	49	48	47	45	44	43	42	41	40	39	38	37	36	35	34	34	33	32	31	31	30	29	29	28	28	27	27	26	25	16st
101	55	53	52	50	49	47	46	45	44	43	42	40	39	38	38	37	36	35	34	33	33	32	31	30	30	29	29	28	27	27	26	26	25	
100	54	53	51	50	48	47	46	44	43	42	41	40	39	38	37	36	35	35	34	33	32	32	31	30	30	29	28	28	27	27	26	26	25	
99	54	52	51	49	48	46	45	44	43	42	41	40	39	38	37	36	35	34	33	33	32	31	31	30	29	29	28	27	27	26	26	25	25	
98	53	51	50	49	47	46	45	44	42	41	40	39	38	37	36	36	35	34	33	32	32	31	30	30	29	28	28	27	27	26	26	25	24	7lbs
97	52	51	49	48	47	46	44	43	42	41	40	39	38	37	36	35	34	34	33	32	31	31	30	29	29	28	27	27	26	26	25	25	24	
96	52	50	49	48	46	45	44	43	42	40	39	38	37	37	36	35	34	33	32	32	31	30	30	29	28	28	27	27	26	26	25	24	24	
95	51	50	48	47	46	45	43	42	41	40	39	38	37	36	35	34	34	33	32	31	31	30	29	29	28	27	27	26	26	25	25	24	24	15st
94	51	49	48	47	45	44	43	42	41	40	39	38	37	36	35	34	33	33	32	31	30	30	29	28	28	27	27	26	25	25	24	24	23	
93	50	49	47	46	45	44	42	41	40	39	38	37	36	35	35	34	33	32	31	31	30	29	29	28	27	27	26	26	25	25	24	24	23	
92	50	48	47	46	44	43	42	41	40	39	38	37	36	35	34	33	33	32	31	30	30	29	28	28	27	27	26	25	25	24	24	23	23	7lbs
91	49	48	46	45	44	43	42	40	39	38	37	36	36	35	34	33	32	31	31	30	29	29	28	27	27	26	26	25	25	24	24	23	23	
90	49	47	46	45	43	42	41	40	39	38	37	36	35	34	33	33	32	31	30	30	29	28	28	27	27	26	25	25	24	24	23	23	22	
89	48	47	45	44	43	42	41	40	39	38	37	36	35	34	33	32	32	31	30	29	29	28	27	27	26	26	25	25	24	24	23	23	22	14st
88	48	46	45	44	42	41	40	39	38	37	36	35	34	34	33	32	31	30	30	29	28	28	27	27	26	25	25	24	24	23	23	22	22	
87	47	46	44	43	42	41	40	39	38	37	36	35	34	33	32	32	31	30	29	29	28	27	27	26	26	25	25	24	24	23	23	22	22	
86	46	45	44	43	41	40	39	38	37	36	35	34	34	33	32	31	30	30	29	28	28	27	27	26	25	25	24	24	23	23	22	22	21	7lbs
85	46	45	43	42	41	40	39	38	37	36	35	34	33	32	32	31	30	29	29	28	27	27	26	26	25	25	24	24	23	23	22	22	21	
84	45	44	43	42	41	39	38	37	36	35	35	34	33	32	31	30	30	29	28	28	27	27	26	25	25	24	24	23	23	22	22	21	21	
83	45	44	42	41	40	39	38	37	36	35	34	33	32	32	31	30	29	29	28	27	27	26	26	25	25	24	23	23	23	22	22	21	21	13st
82	44	43	42	41	40	38	37	36	35	35	34	33	32	31	30	30	29	28	28	27	26	26	25	25	24	24	23	23	22	22	21	21	20	
81	44	43	41	40	39	38	37	36	35	34	33	32	32	31	30	29	29	28	27	27	26	26	25	24	24	23	23	22	22	22	21	21	20	
80	43	42	41	40	39	38	37	36	35	34	33	32	31	30	30	29	28	28	27	26	26	25	25	24	24	23	23	22	22	21	21	20	20	7lbs
79	43	41	40	39	38	37	36	35	34	33	32	32	31	30	29	29	28	27	27	26	26	25	24	24	23	23	22	22	21	21	21	20	20	
78	42	41	40	39	38	37	36	35	34	33	32	31	30	30	29	28	28	27	26	26	25	25	24	24	23	23	22	22	21	21	20	20	19	
77	42	40	39	38	37	36	35	34	33	32	32	31	30	29	29	28	27	27	26	25	25	24	24	23	23	22	22	21	21	20	20	20	19	
76	41	40	39	38	37	36	35	34	33	32	31	30	30	29	28	28	27	26	26	25	25	24	23	23	22	22	22	21	21	20	20	19	19	12st
75	41	39	38	37	36	35	34	33	32	32	31	30	29	29	28	27	27	26	25	25	24	24	23	23	22	22	21	21	20	20	20	19	19	
74	40	39	38	37	36	35	34	33	32	31	30	30	29	28	28	27	26	26	25	24	24	23	23	22	22	21	21	20	20	20	19	19	18	
73	39	38	37	36	35	34	33	32	32	31	30	29	29	28	27	26	26	25	25	24	24	23	23	22	22	21	21	20	20	19	19	19	18	7lbs
72	39	38	37	36	35	34	33	32	31	30	30	29	28	27	27	26	26	25	24	24	23	23	22	22	21	21	20	20	20	19	19	18	18	
71	38	37	36	35	34	33	32	32	31	30	29	28	28	27	26	26	25	25	24	23	23	22	22	21	21	21	20	20	19	19	18	18	18	
70	38	37	36	35	34	33	32	31	30	30	29	28	27	27	26	25	25	24	24	23	23	22	22	21	21	20	20	19	19	19	18	18	17	11st
69	37	36	35	34	33	32	32	31	30	29	28	28	27	26	26	25	24	24	23	23	22	22	21	21	20	20	20	19	19	18	18	18	17	
68	37	36	35	34	33	32	31	30	29	29	28	27	27	26	25	25	24	24	23	22	22	21	21	21	20	20	19	19	18	18	18	17	17	
67	36	35	34	33	32	31	31	30	29	28	28	27	26	26	25	24	24	23	23	22	22	21	21	20	20	19	19	19	18	18	17	17	17	7lbs
66	36	35	34	33	32	31	30	29	29	28	27	26	26	25	25	24	23	23	22	22	21	21	20	20	19	19	19	18	18	18	17	17	16	
65	35	34	33	32	31	30	30	29	28	27	27	26	26	25	24	24	23	22	22	21	21	21	20	20	19	19	18	18	18	17	17	17	16	
64	35	34	33	32	31	30	29	28	28	27	26	26	25	24	24	23	23	22	22	21	21	20	20	19	19	18	18	18	17	17	17	16	16	10st
63	34	33	32	31	30	30	29	28	27	27	26	25	25	24	23	23	22	22	21	21	20	20	19	19	19	18	18	17	17	17	16	16	16	
62	34	33	32	31	30	29	28	28	27	26	25	25	24	24	23	22	22	21	21	20	20	20	19	19	18	18	18	17	17	16	16	16	15	
61	33	32	31	30	29	29	28	27	26	26	25	24	24	23	23	22	22	21	21	20	20	19	19	18	18	18	17	17	17	16	16	16	15	7lbs
60	32	32	31	30	29	28	27	27	26	25	25	24	23	23	22	22	21	21	20	20	19	19	19	18	18	17	17	17	16	16	16	15	15	
59	32	31	30	29	28	28	27	26	26	25	24	24	23	22	22	21	21	20	20	19	19	19	18	18	17	17	17	16	16	16	15	15	15	
58	31	30	30	29	28	27	26	26	25	24	24	23	23	22	22	21	21	20	20	19	19	18	18	18	17	17	16	16	16	15	15	15	14	9st
57	31	30	29	28	27	27	26	25	25	24	23	23	22	22	21	21	20	20	19	19	18	18	18	17	17	16	16	16	15	15	15	15	14	
56	30	29	29	28	27	26	26	25	24	24	23	22	22	21	21	20	20	19	19	18	18	18	17	17	17	16	16	16	15	15	15	14	14	
55	30	29	28	27	27	26	25	24	24	23	23	22	21	21	20	20	19	19	19	18	18	17	17	17	16	16	16	15	15	15	14	14	14	
54	29	28	28	27	26	25	25	24	23	23	22	22	21	21	20	20	19	19	18	18	17	17	17	16	16	16	15	15	15	14	14	14	13	7lbs
53	29	28	27	26	26	25	24	24	23	22	22	21	21	20	20	19	19	18	18	18	17	17	16	16	16	15	15	15	14	14	14	14	13	
52	28	27	27	26	25	24	24	23	23	22	21	21	20	20	19	19	18	18	18	17	17	16	16	16	15	15	15	14	14	14	14	13	13	
51	28	27	26	25	25	24	23	23	22	22	21	20	20	19	19	19	18	18	17	17	16	16	16	15	15	15	14	14	14	14	13	13	13	8st
50	27	26	26	25	24	23	23	22	22	21	21	20	20	19	19	18	18	17	17	17	16	16	15	15	15	14	14	14	14	13	13	13	12	
49	26	26	25	24	24	23	22	22	21	21	20	20	19	19	18	18	17	17	17	16	16	15	15	15	14	14	14	14	13	13	13	12	12	
48	26	25	24	24	23	23	22	21	21	20	20	19	19	18	18	17	17	17	16	16	15	15	15	14	14	14	14	13	13	13	12	12	12	7lbs
47	25	25	24	23	23	22	21	21	20	20	19	19	18	18	17	17	17	16	16	16	15	15	15	14	14	14	13	13	13	12	12	12	12	
46	25	24	23	23	22	22	21	20	20	19	19	18	18	18	17	17	16	16	16	15	15	15	14	14	14	13	13	13	12	12	12	12	11	
45	24	24	23	22	22	21	21	20	19	19	18	18	18	17	17	16	16	16	15	15	15	14	14	14	13	13	13	12	12	12	12	11	11	7st
44	24	23	22	22	21	21	20	20	19	18	18	18	17	17	16	16	16	15	15	15	14	14	14	13	13	13	12	12	12	12	11	11	11	

HEIGHT (Metres)

Very Obese
Health is seriously at risk. Losing weight **immediately** is essential.

Obese
Health is at risk. Losing weight **now** should be seriously considered.

Overweight
Health could suffer. Some weight loss should now be considered.

Healthy
A desirable BMI figure indicating a healthy weight.

Underweight

disorders will often abuse exercise and therefore it needs to be taken in moderation the same as anything else. Those who have already lost considerable amounts of weight perhaps still need to have some toning exercise, but beware the dangers of exercise when your body has become frail and all your muscles including your heart are fragile. Cardiomyopathy, a condition where the walls of the heart have become dangerously weak, can lead to heart attack on exertion during exercise, so if you have anorexia, then check with a physician about the amount of exercise that would be safe for you. Those with bulimia also put great stress on their hearts by vomiting and upsetting the delicate electrolyte balance of the heart muscle which, unlike any other, can never stop for a rest. Here again, toning is fine, but beware putting sudden strain upon your heart by rushing into strenuous exercise. Before, during and after exercise drink plenty of water.

All this healthy living will leave you less time to watch TV which is a good thing. You'll have less temptation from food commercials! If you have a television in the bedroom, move it. If you continue to watch it, take a note of not only how long you watch but of what you eat while you watch. You'll be shocked! And lastly, get enough sleep. Appetite increases when we're sleep deprived.

Complementary Therapies

If obesity is the problem try some creative visualisation, seeing yourself at your ideal weight dressed in your favourite clothes, looking good. And just before you go to the loo, imagine fat cells being flushed down the toilet. It may sound crazy but it works! Positive thinking can work wonders and 'thinking thin' can bring about benefits not only in feeling more confident but in helping your mind to create what you are already accepting as a reality.

Hypnotherapy may be very helpful with eating disorders, but first of all you really need to want to get well. The problem with the major disorders, anorexia and bulimia, is that there is often at best ambivalence and at worst no desire to be well at all. Self-hypnosis and meditation will have numerous benefits (see p. 10).

Herb teas such as burdock, ginseng and Oregon grape will help if you're overweight. Kava tea will help calm you if you have anorexia or bulimia and – in case you're worried – it contains no calories! Two or three cups a day maximum. Green tea will also help since it's full of antioxidants and again is calorie-free. Many people with eating disorders have caffeine addictions as they drink lots of black coffee to keep them going when they would otherwise be fainting from hunger. Do try to cut this down, although you're bound to have a headache for a few days to begin with. Try in the first place to substitute some green tea. It still contains caffeine, although a bit less, and it will be less constipating and put less strain on your heart.

Integrated approach

1. Eating disorders and obesity are common so nobody should feel they are misunderstood or that they must deal with their problems alone.
2. Solutions may be difficult and complex but in time treatment outcomes can be excellent.
3. Emotional and spiritual aspects of treatment can help disentangle eating behaviour from deeper, personal issues.
4. Nutritional adjustments, vitamin supplements, exercise and complementary therapies are all beneficial.
5. For bulimia nervosa, cognitive and behavioural psychotherapy is successful, either on an individual or group basis, especially if a food diary is strictly kept.
6. Anorexia nervosa is the most serious eating disorder of all and needs to be recognised and treated as early as possible. In severe cases admission to hospital is needed and can save lives, but individual group and family psychotherapy may all be required.
7. Local self-help groups and the Eating Disorders Association can offer excellent practical help and support.

Eczema

There are about 5 million sufferers of eczema in total throughout Britain, so clearly the condition is very common. The usual type leads to severe itching with reddened, dry and scaly skin which, if the ailment has been present for some time, becomes thickened, cracked and sometimes infected. There are many different kinds of eczema, however, and because of this it is easy to become confused about the causes and the treatment.

Kirsty, aged 2, continuously scratches the red, flaky, angry-looking areas of skin on her wrists, fingers, elbows, knees and feet. She even does it in her sleep at night and now the patches are oozing a yellowy straw-coloured fluid and staining her clothes. She also suffers a little with asthma. Kirsty has atopic eczema.

Atopic eczema, otherwise known as infantile eczema, affects around 12 per cent of all children and the good news is that 90 per cent will have grown out of it by the age of 8. The two other common types of eczema are seborrhoeic eczema and contact eczema. Seborrhoeic eczema tends to be seen in teenagers and adults and produces a thick yellow crust over the skin particularly where there are areas of lots of sebaceous or oil-producing glands. Contact eczema occurs where chemical irritants produce a reaction in the skin, characterised by redness, itching and blistering, and common examples include washing powders, certain plants and the various metals used in jewellery.

Self-Help

Since childhood eczema has a very strong genetic component which cannot be altered, the next best policy to aim for is to avoid as many exacerbating environmental factors as possible. If a mother decides to breastfeed her child, then it is to the child's advantage that this is continued for as long as possible. It is advisable that cow's milk, eggs, orange juice and wheat in the diet should be deferred until the age of one. Exposure to these common causes of allergy make the development of eczema all the more likely. Remember to check the labels on baby foods to confirm that these products are not among the listed ingredients. When weaning your child, it is best to wean them onto vegetables, fruit, gluten-free cereals and a form of baby rice which is milk-free. Remember also that some children seem to react badly to additives and colourings in food so again check the E-numbers and ingredients on all food labels. Cut down on exposure to house dust mites by ensuring adequate ventilation, by keeping the house cool, by hot-washing bedclothes and by putting cuddly toys in the deep-freeze for 12 hours every couple of weeks to kill the mites. Regular vacuuming of all soft furnishings and the use of some of the newer mattress and pillow covers to cut down on the number of house mites to which the child is exposed are helpful measures. Woollen clothing should be avoided and household pets, if responsible for allergy, should sadly go. There are also an enormous number of irritants capable of inflaming eczematous skin including biological washing powders, fabric softeners, scented or perfumed soaps, bubble baths and shampoos. For most of these, more natural substances may be substituted.

Conventional Treatment

It is distressing not only for the child to suffer from eczema, but also for the parents too. It is always helpful therefore if a doctor can tell parents that it is very likely that the child will grow out of the condition in time, and that modern treatment is highly effective provided it is used in an appropriate way. Advice can be given about the avoidance of trigger factors and sometimes specific help with elimination diets may be required. These are designed to identify factors in the diet that trigger the eczema and cow's milk alternatives such as soya milk can be provided on prescription. If the eczema is weeping or oozing, the doctor may prescribe antibiotics to eradicate any bacterial infection that is likely to be present since until this is treated the eczema will certainly not improve. When severe itching is a problem antihistamines may be given which these days may be entirely non-sedating. Sedating antihistamines are still sometimes used, however, especially at bedtime so that sleep is not disturbed by severe itching but is actually promoted. The active treatment of eczema generally consists of a combination of emollients and steroids.

An emollient is a mixture of oil, fat and water. It comes in the form of ointments, creams and lotions or in liquid form in order that it can be added to bathwater. Emollients are designed to be used every day to keep the skin moist and soft and may be purchased directly over the counter at the chemist or obtained on NHS prescription. Avoid excessive drying of the skin which in itself will cause itching. Regular application of emollients means that any steroid use can be kept to a minimum which is a real benefit in cases of severe eczema where absorption of steroids through the skin with resulting side effects is always a possibility. Hands should be washed before applying creams to the skin to avoid the transmission of any possible chemical and the emollient should be massaged well into the skin. Sometimes the child's skin can be wet-wrapped at night which keeps the skin even more moist and concentrates the active treatment in the affected site. It also prevents any staining of the bedclothes with certain preparations. Emollient bath liquids are very useful for children who bath in water alone, especially in hard water areas. Commercial soaps and shampoos should be avoided as these merely remove any natural oils from the child's skin. Alternatives to soap are aqueous cream or emulsifying ointment which are totally inert but effective.

STEROIDS

The conventional treatment of eczema involves the use of steroid creams. Their effectiveness depends on the strength of the preparation, and as a general rule the mildest strength that controls the symptoms should be used. More potent steroid creams should be kept to a minimum or hopefully avoided altogether as they may be absorbed through the skin into the bloodstream leading to possible side effects such as abnormal skeletal growth and a moon-shaped face. However, 1 per cent hydrocortisone cream or ointment is almost entirely safe, even with long-term use. Sometimes wrapping the skin with cling film or polythene can improve and accelerate results. Very occasionally in severe cases low-dose oral steroids such as prednisolone are used under close medical supervision.

OTHER TREATMENTS

Antihistamines to prevent itching are best taken in oral form. Some medical studies have suggested that oil of evening primrose may, in a proportion of eczema sufferers, result in significant improvement. It should not, however, be used in children under the age of one, nor in epileptics because of possible side effects. It is available on prescription in the form of Epogam (gamolenic acid) where it is taken in the dose of 1–2 capsules twice a day.

Chinese herbal medicine has also been proved to be of definite benefit in trials at Great Ormond Street Hospital for Sick Children, and this is well worth considering. The active ingredient of the many different herbs that are used to produce these Chinese herbal preparations has not yet been identified, however, and the herbal tea is still only available privately. Its disadvantage is that it can taste vile and it does not work for everyone. The initial fears about its side effects on the liver have come to very little and this appears to be a useful complementary therapy to use alongside the conventional approach.

Nutritional Healing, Vitamins and Supplements

Often eczema has an allergic basis and it is worth looking at the nutritional recommendations in the section on allergies. Infants will often respond to the replacing of cow's milk and dairy products with goat's milk. Try eliminating dairy produce for at least a month and then reintroducing it very carefully, keeping a diary of what happens. Eggs and peanuts may be the culprits in childhood eczema. Keep up the child's intake of cold water fish and flax seed (linseed) oil which provide essential fatty acids. Liquorice will help, either taken internally or in lotions to apply externally. Vitamins C and E are essential for skin care, and zinc and flavinoids will help the healing process. Green tea, with its complement of antioxidants, and gingko biloba will also help. Beetroot and carrot juice will help detoxify. Copper and chromium supplements are useful since sometimes these are found to be low. See the section on skin disorders for other nutritional recommendations.

Exercise and Lifestyle

Wearing soft, natural fibres as much as possible will help skin breathe and reduce irritation. Clothes should be washed in good non-biological soap and rinsed thoroughly. Using an extra rinse cycle on your washing machine may help. Cotton gloves worn at night will help prevent excoriation of the skin during sleep and will aid the absorption of creams and other products into the lesions on the hands. Yoga, T'ai chi and Chi gong are excellent exercises since all of them not only stretch and exercise the physical body but promote relaxation of the mind and stimulation of the spirit also. Try having regular baths with a handful of baking soda (bicarbonate of soda) in the water, dabbing gently with a soft towel to dry yourself before applying creams with calendula, chamomile or witch hazel (check there is no alcohol in the product since it can cause irritation and excessive drying).

Complementary Therapies

As well as Traditional Chinese Medicine, calendula either as a soothing cream or as a tincture is useful, while creams or lotions made from aromatherapy oils such as roman chamomile, neroli, lavender, tea tree or bergamot will soothe and promote healing. Aloe vera as a cream has been used with good effect. The classic homeopathic remedy to try is Pulsatilla, although Proicum, Calc Carb and Graphites may be useful too. Acupressure, acupuncture and reflexology can help as can magnetic therapy.

Emotional and Spiritual Healing

There is undoubtedly an emotional component in the development of eczema and stressful issues can usually be pinpointed that are associated with the flare-up of the condition. Therefore it will always help to deal with whatever stresses there are. In children do look not only at what is going on at home but also at school and in the playground. Sometimes bullying and other forms of abuse are first suspected because of eczema that fails to respond and gets worse, for instance, during term-time, subsiding in the holidays. If this is so, then check with teachers about how your child is doing at school so that a special eye can be kept on what is happening. To have constantly painful itching skin is of course wearing and can lead to anxiety and depression which may need treatment in their own right. Psychotherapy can often help adults come to terms with painful events of the past and also with recurrent worries that may be causing the illness to surface.

INTEGRATED APPROACH

1. Identify all trigger factors and avoid them wherever possible.
2. Substitute alternatives for any allergic components in the diet. The advice and help of a qualified dietitian would be helpful.
3. Choose clothing and bedding from materials less likely to irritate.
4. Experiment with nutritional and vitamin supplementation including oil of evening primrose or Chinese herbal medicine.
5. Use emollients liberally at all times to soften the skin and avoid perfumed soaps and detergents.
6. Use antihistamines when necessary to suppress itching.
7. Do not be afraid of using carefully selected dilute steriod creams or ointments under medical supervision if eczema is severe.
8. Antibiotic creams are required where infection complicates eczema.

Epilepsy

At 33 Jack has had epilepsy since he was a child. He had a traumatic birth with a forceps delivery and began having convulsions when only a few days old. Despite taking prescribed medication regularly all his life, he still occasionally has a fit during which he wets himself, goes blue and awakes feeling confused and with a headache. He often knows a few hours in advance that the fit is coming and has noticed that sometimes, when he has been very depressed beforehand, his mood clears a little once the after-effects of the fit have gone. Often he is moody and depressed and feels awkward with his work colleagues because he thinks they are frightened of the fact that he may have a fit at work. He's angry that he isn't allowed to learn to drive and that his life is somewhat restricted because of his illness. Jack has grand mal epilepsy.

Many people believe that epilepsy is merely a tendency to have recurrent convulsions or seizures, but there are many forms of epilepsy and not all of them involve such dramatic symptoms. A seizure in fact is a temporary abnormality of the nervous system where unusual electrical activity occurs in the brain. Normally all emotions, ideas, thoughts and movements are organised by the orderly excitation of nerve cells but during a seizure the electrical discharge becomes chaotic and disorganised.

About 1 in 200 people suffer from epilepsy in one form or another, and it usually starts in childhood or adolescence, although a few develop epilepsy in later life.

Causes

In many cases there is a recognised cause such as previous head injury, trauma at birth or damage to part of the brain due to infection such as after meningitis or encephalitis. Brain tumours, strokes and the effects of drugs including excess alcohol may also be responsible. For the majority of people with epilepsy, however, there is no identifiable cause and it is likely that they have an inherited tendency to the condition as a result of a lowered threshold at which the seizures are triggered by a variety of internal and external factors.

Symptoms

There are two main types of epileptic seizure, generalised and partial. Which type the patient suffers from depends on the part of the brain affected and how widespread the electrical discharge becomes. Partial seizures are due to just a limited area of the brain being affected. In a generalised seizure the whole or a large part of the brain is affected, and loss of consciousness always occurs. This is the most dramatic form of epilepsy and the one which carries most stigma in our society. Along with the loss of consciousness the body stiffens and then twitches and jerks uncontrollably. Breathing is irregular or even absent during the seizure and biting of the tongue, frothing at the mouth and incontinence may occur. Afterwards the person is confused and disorientated, may have a headache and want to sleep. This can last for several hours. First-aid treatment of a seizure of this kind is summarised below.

FIRST-AID TREATMENT FOR AN EPILEPTIC SEIZURE

1. Loosen tight clothing, especially around the neck.
2. Do not restrain the victim or attempt to put anything in the mouth.
3. Do not try to move the person unless they are in danger of hurting themselves further by their surroundings.
4. When the attack has finished, place the person in the recovery position, where they are lying on their side with their head tilted back and the airway unobstructed, and allow them to come round in their own good time.

In children, there is a form of seizure that is a lot less dramatic and that sometimes goes completely unnoticed. It can happen for example in the classroom at school where it involves just a momentary loss of consciousness without any abnormal movements and the child concerned remains sitting or standing while exhibiting a totally blank expression. During this time, however, the child is unaware of anything untoward but as this type of seizure (petit mal) can occur many hundreds of times every day, it can gradually impair educational performance and learning. There are many other types of partial epilepsy where twitching of just one part of the body occurs without loss of consciousness or where there are hallucinations of vision, smell or taste.

Daisy is 7. She has not been doing very well at school, where her teachers have complained that she doesn't pay attention and she has sometimes been witnessed sitting daydreaming as though she were in a trance. Sometimes she will be talking and suddenly stop mid-sentence, then start again a few seconds later. She has never fallen down in a fit and seems unaware that anything untoward has happened. Daisy has petit mal epilepsy.

Diagnosis

Many people experience a single seizure throughout their life at some stage, but cannot be considered as having epilepsy, which by definition is recurrent. It is also easy to confuse some seizures with a faint or a period of dizziness, so a proper history of the seizure-like event is essential in pinpointing the diagnosis. Often a witness to any epileptic 'attack' is the most reliable source of the history. A full examination and a brain-wave test called an EEG or electroencephalogram is carried out, and sometimes CT scanning of the brain and blood tests are also required.

Prevention and Treatment

The first-aid treatment of an epileptic seizure itself is described on p. 263 and it is something that everybody can master. The way to deal with recurrent seizures, however, is a lot more complex. Since 1 in 20 people will have a convulsion at some stage in their lives, doctors generally take the view not to investigate and treat until a second episode occurs. When this happens a full investigation is carried out, and if necessary anticonvulsant drugs are used to prevent further attacks. Patients are given advice about how to avoid any trigger factors that may cause their seizures such as stress, too much alcohol, sleep deprivation, fevers and flashing lights (photosensitivity). After that, the most effective anticonvulsant drugs that control the symptoms but also keep the side effects to a minimum are selected and the patient remains on them until they have been seizure-free for at least 2 years. The aim is to introduce the medication cautiously and to increase the dose in gradual steps. The final dose will be determined by the balance between control of seizures and side effects. Any possible interactions with other drugs such as aspirin, antidepressants and antacids need to be explained to the patient. It is also important that the recipient of the medication keeps a careful record of their seizures in a diary which will help the doctor adjust the correct dosage of the drug against the symptoms. Sometimes blood tests are taken to see if the blood level of the drug is therapeutically correct.

Another form of treatment for epilepsy is surgery and important steps have been made in the last few years using 'stereotactic' surgical techniques for the treatment of epilepsy. So much so that it has been estimated that up to 12,500 people in the UK could benefit from this method of treatment. In this procedure, MRI scanning enables the precise location of the source of the seizures to be identified so that that tiny part of the brain can be surgically removed or destroyed. This is, however, not without risk and tends to be restricted for use with drug-resistant, 'refractory' or 'pharmaco-resistant' patients, as they are called. Before contemplating such an invasive method of treatment there are three main criteria that have to be fulfilled:

1. The seizures themselves have to be one of the main causes of the patient's disability.
2. Both the doctor and the patient need to feel that stopping the seizures would result in significant improvement to the patient's quality of life.

3. The patient must be able to understand the possible risks and benefits of the epilepsy surgery.

The results of the surgery depend on the part of the brain involved and the type of the operation but about 70 per cent of people with an identifiable defect in the temporal lobe of the brain will become seizure-free and another 20 per cent will experience some improvement. It must be borne in mind, however, that 1 in 10 will appreciate no improvement, or may even be made worse. With modern advanced imaging and surgical techniques the outcome of this kind of surgery continues to improve.

Established drugs used commonly in the treatment of epilepsy include: carbamazepine, clonazepam, ethosuximide, phenobarbitone, phenytoin, primidone and sodium valproate. Newer drugs include gabapentin, lamotrigine, topiramate, vigabatrin and at the current time a dozen new compounds are being developed which look very promising. However, there are no cure-all anticonvulsants that are free of side effects and the search to find an epileptic panacea continues. It is good to recognise that although newer drugs may have fewer side effects than some of the more established ones, the long-term side effects are not yet fully known as they have not yet been exposed in clinical use to a large population.

The Social Implications

Derek was injured in a car crash at the age of 27. He was unconscious for several days following the accident and on recovery had headaches and some difficulties in remembering things. About six months later he suddenly felt very frightened, could smell a familiar smell that he couldn't quite name at the time and had a strange feeling in his tummy. He reported that this feeling arose in his chest and then he had what he could only describe as a religious experience. He could see things in wonderful colour and felt that he had been transported to another place. His wife said that he started to put on his clothes as if he was going to work and she was unable to reach him even though he appeared to be wide awake. The whole thing lasted about half an hour during which time she noticed that he had a twitch in his right hand that eventually spread to his face. When it was over he reported feeling frightened and said that he would hate to have a similar experience again. Derek has temporal lobe epilepsy (TLE).

A great deal of worry and concern revolves around the effect of a person's epilepsy on their social welfare. Parents become frantic with anxiety when their young child has a febrile convulsion, but they must remember that very few of these children go on to develop epilepsy itself. In pregnancy the risk of anti-epileptic drugs to the baby are very small and certainly much smaller than having uncontrolled seizures. It is also generally safe for women to breastfeed their baby while taking anticonvulsants. All people who have a driving licence need to tell the DVLA if they develop epileptic seizures and must refrain from driving. However, they can reapply for a licence if they have had no epileptic attacks during the previous year while they were awake and provided that any epileptic attacks they have had only occurred during their sleep. If this pattern of seizures has been present for at least 3 years their licence will be renewed. It is helpful if employers are informed that an employee has epilepsy and high-risk occupations involving strenuous or dangerous activity should be avoided. Most sports can still be enjoyed as long as there is adequate supervision. No parent should overprotect an epileptic child, as this can lead to social isolation. It is important that adults who have difficulty in forming relationships regard themselves as normal people with epilepsy, rather than as epileptics. In other words, they must take care to control their condition rather than let their condition control them.

The Outlook

Epilepsy resolves in most people with about 80 per cent of patients on anti-epileptic medication becoming seizure-free. It is generally advised that a patient waits to be seizure-free for about 2 years before they think of stopping medication. Some 60 per cent of patients who have been seizure-free for 2 years then successfully come off their drugs.

Emotional and Spiritual Healing

The emotional concomitants of epilepsy, whatever form it takes, will usually respond to healing even if the actual illness does not. Often those with such a long-term illness suffer from the accumulated side effects of quite potent medication, are angry, sometimes feel aggressive and tend toward depression. Suicidal thoughts are not uncommon and of course these need to be checked out by a psychiatrist. Although epilepsy is nowadays seen as the province of the neurologist, there was a time when the psychiatrist alone treated it, and many neurologists and psychiatrists still work hand in hand to give the patient the best possible care. There is almost always a place for psychotherapy. Jack's lack of self-esteem and his worries about his colleagues' opinion of him and his illness would respond well to this approach. Often the partner of someone like Jack also needs some care. There is often a great deal of concern from the partner and codependent relationships tend to occur, one person mothering the other and then feeling resentful and angry about their own needs not being met. Partnership issues are best dealt with early by a compassionate therapist who understands not only the illness, but the pitfalls for both individuals separately and the relationship as a whole.

As far as spiritual healing is concerned, some people with temporal lobe epilepsy do have an almost spiritual experience, feeling that they have left their bodies and communed with God. On the other hand some find it a terrifying experience of which they are ever fearful. Healing can usually help settle some of the fears which in turn may have a pacifying effect on the brain. Healing is certainly worth trying but do be patient and don't expect overnight success. Why not keep a seizure diary, or if you're the parent of a child with epilepsy, keep it for them, scoring the fit from 1 to 10, 1 being very mild and 10 being severe. You may find that there is a general trend towards health and, in the end, a time when medication can be reduced, in negotiation with your physician.

Exercise and Lifestyle

Sadly, as Jack found, the life of someone with epilepsy can be quite restricted leading to anxiety and depression and loss of self-esteem. There are some sports which, because of their potentially dangerous nature, are not open to you and driving can be potentially hazardous. People with epilepsy do sometimes drive, however, hiding their illness from the authorities. If this applies to you, perhaps you could ask yourself how you would feel if someone you knew was using a potentially lethal weapon around your children and on this basis make the decision about whether such behaviour is fair to yourself, your family and others. Why not talk it over with someone you can trust and then make a decision.

Exercise is important and you may find that something like T'ai chi or yoga would be ideal, bearing in mind its relaxing and spiritual qualities. Relaxation would help with the anxiety often associated with epilepsy, particularly in Derek's case. Any anxiety or tension is counter-productive, leading to stress which is not good for the already irritable brain. It's a good idea to think of your brain as being irritable and to avoid those things that will irritate it further. Noxious fumes, sitting for hours at the computer, being in noisy surroundings or where there are flashing lights are just some of the situations you should avoid. Both caffeine and alcohol will interact with your medication, so be careful about both. We have known several people with epilepsy who have been very angry at having to continue to take medication. We understand this, but nevertheless would suggest that you make no changes without consulting your doctor.

Nutritional Healing

As always, good nutrition is essential and the basic recommendations on p. 5 will help considerably. Take those foods rich in antioxidants to minimise damage as much as possible and give you all the nutrients necessary for cell growth and repair.

Vitamins and Supplements

Since the role of antioxidants is to repair cell damage, they are as relevant here as anywhere else. Often there is damage to brain tissue following periods of cerebral anoxia and Vitamins A, C and E, flax seed (linseed) oil and green tea would be useful. Gingko biloba can help to open the circulation in the brain, but do check with your physician before adding anything to your regime. Some of the orthodox medications necessary to treat epilepsy may interact with anything else you may take and since your medication will be finely balanced for your needs, it's important not to do anything that will disturb it.

Complementary Therapies

There are therapies that will help, sometimes to the point that seizures no longer occur and the brain has healed. We have certainly had patients who have been able to cease their medication and who have no further difficulties through using complementary therapies, but do be cautious. There is no guarantee that this will be so. Spiritual healing with a well-trained and registered healer is certainly worth a try and if nothing else, you will find that you can become much more peaceful and accepting of your condition, sometimes working out why this should have happened to you and what positive gifts it has brought to your life. The anger, anxiety and depression sometimes accompanying it can certainly be ameliorated and your whole being, including your brain, can become more tranquil. If you want to try aromatherapy, see a good therapist since some oils may be contraindicated. Homeopathy may help, but again, have a full consultation and try not to dabble with the remedies you can buy over the counter. One complementary therapy to avoid is autogenic training and any attempt at hypnotherapy should be approached with extreme caution.

INTEGRATED APPROACH

1. A single seizure does not constitute a diagnosis of epilepsy.
2. There are many different forms and symptoms of epilepsy.

3. Full medical investigation of recurrent seizures is essential.
4. Avoidance of recognised trigger factors can reduce the frequency of seizures.
5. Lifestyle adjustments bear significant dividends.
6. Emotional and social repercussions of epilepsy need to be addressed.
7. Complementary therapies can help but some can harm, so always consult your doctor first.
8. Anticonvulsant medication means that 80 per cent of patients with epilepsy become seizure-free.
9. Stereotactic surgery is well worth considering for people with drug-resistant epilepsy.

Fainting

Harry will always remember his wedding day. While his bride-to-be repeated her marriage vows, he simply wilted and fell to the floor where he remained for a few moments, twitching and jerking his limbs. The emotion of the occasion had induced a simple faint and a temporary reduction in blood flow through his brain had caused a very minor and short-lived convulsion. Once his legs were raised by a first aider as he lay on the floor he quickly recovered and the ceremony was able to continue.

Fainting is a common symptom but may often be confused with giddiness or dizziness. In medical terms, fainting is a temporary loss of consciousness which occurs when the blood flow to the brain is reduced, resulting in an insufficient supply of oxygen. Dizziness, on the other hand, refers to a spinning sensation so that the sufferer feels that the room is rotating or the ground falling away from them. So when you tell your doctor that you feel 'faint', it is well worth making sure you are describing your symptoms correctly. Your doctor will double-check anyway.

People often experience warning signs that they are going to faint. Sweating, feeling sick, weakness, seeing stars and ringing in the ears can all precede a faint, and as the blood pressure drops resulting in loss of consciousness, the person falls to the floor in a heap. The most dangerous aspect of fainting, however, is the risk of head injury on the way down. Most people soon regain consciousness within a few minutes, as their new-found horizontal position on the floor quickly raises the blood pressure once more, re-establishing an adequate supply of oxygen to the brain. This explains the cardinal rule of first-aid treatment for someone who has fainted – never sit them up or hold them erect. Leave them flat on the floor with their head down and their legs and feet raised. This is the quickest and most effective way to speed recovery.

Causes

Many factors can trigger faints including shocks, emotion, pain and fear. Any kind of physical straining involving an increase in abdominal pressure can also bring it on, such as coughing, urinating, being constipated or even blowing a trumpet! Standing still in warm weather can allow blood to pool in the legs and reduce the blood flow to the brain, as can pregnancy, and jumping up quickly from a hot bath. Certain medication like pills for high blood pressure and anti-angina drugs can also reduce blood pressure and produce episodes of fainting. Two causes of particular clinical importance, however, include vertebro-basilar insufficiency and cardiac arrhythmias. In the former, there is a partial obstruction to blood flow in the arteries that pass upwards through the vertebrae in the neck to the brain, and in the latter an abnormal heart rhythm results in a temporary drop in blood pressure. Both conditions are potentially serious and require full investigation and treatment.

Mary, 68, is a widow who likes to lead as independent a life as possible. While standing on a stool to rehang her curtains, she suddenly became extremely faint and fell from her stool. The warden who took care of the elderly folk found her with a broken wrist and a laceration to her head. She quickly recovered from her temporary loss of consciousness which had been induced by looking vertically upwards, thereby blocking off the blood supply to the brain from the neck area. Mary has vertebro-basilar insufficiency, a circulatory disorder caused by arthritis in the neck.

Prevention and Treatment

When you experience the warning signs of a faint, sitting down and putting your head between your knees can often result in symptoms abating. A more effective alternative is to actually lie down flat on your back with your legs raised on a chair or pillow. Some individuals seem particularly prone to fainting, especially those who have naturally low blood pressure or who may have become anaemic for any reason. Both conditions can be excluded in a simple medical check-up. Other vulnerable people seem to have rather sluggish reflexes in the blood pressure-sensing organs located in the larger blood vessels at the root of the neck. Lack of exercise and leading a particularly sedentary lifestyle will predispose to this.

In Europe, doctors often prescribe medication to raise blood pressure in people in whom it is considered to be lower than normal, although in Britain naturally low blood pressure in the absence of disease is not a condition that is recognised or considered worthy of treatment.

Conventional Treatment

The conventional method of treating recurrent episodes of fainting would be first to ascertain how frequently the attacks are occurring and which trigger factors contribute. Tests to measure the blood pressure in a sitting, standing and lying position may then be taken on different occasions and at different times of the day. This is to monitor the normal fluctuation that occurs from hour to hour in response to daily activities. Sometimes a 24-hour ambulatory blood pressure machine is supplied to the patient which is worn for a full 24-hour period while normal daily activities continue. With older people, it is especially important to rule out any heart rhythm abnormality or blood vessel obstruction, and electrocardiograph (ECG), ultrasound and echo cardiograph tests may be required. These conditions would be treated appropriately if detected. Any evidence of osteoarthritis in the neck such as stiffness, restriction of movement or light-headedness, especially when looking up towards the ceiling, can also indicate pressure on blood vessels in this area, in which case a neck collar and postural correction would be warranted. Most cases of fainting are simple and benign, especially in younger people. In the older age groups, however, the symptom of fainting should never be dismissed, and a proper examination, investigation and diagnosis is essential. This is particularly true if other symptoms occur in association with the fainting such as chest pain, blurred vision or slurred speech, any of which could indicate abnormal nervous system function due to a more sinister cause.

Nutritional Healing

If you are prone to fainting, make sure you plenty of iron in your diet. Iron deficiency is the commonest nutritional deficiency in Britain and it leads to anaemia, which can bring about fainting. Lean red meat, eggs, nuts, cereals and green leafy vegetables like spinach are ideal sources of dietary iron (see also p. 544). Since fainting in often due simply to low blood pressure, drinking plenty of fluids is important as even mild dehydration inevitably leads to a fall in the circulatory blood volume and lowers blood pressure. Water is the essential element but an isotonic sports drink or some form of fruit juice or squash is even better as the minerals in them help to retain water within the circulation for longer. Sodium chloride, otherwise known as common salt, is the mineral with the most powerful action when it comes to raising blood pressure, so by adding a fraction more salt to your cooking or to the food on your plate, you may often be able to counteract any regular feelings of faintness. Too much salt in the diet, on the other hand, can elevate the blood pressure above normal levels and this can have serious health consequences too.

Eating smaller but more frequent meals is advisable, as the blood sugar level is then likely to remain more evenly controlled and you avoid the reduction in blood pressure brought about by large, indigestible meals that divert a large amount of blood to the intestine and reduce the circulatory blood volume elsewhere.

Food sensitivities and allergies may also lead to faintness as these cause circulatory changes within the gut and other organs. Keep a mental note of the frequency and timing of any symptoms and see if they generally occur after eating certain foodstuffs. If so, a food sensitivity is a distinct possibility.

Vitamins and Supplements

Iron supplements are especially useful for vegetarians and vegans who, unless they are extremely careful to eat a well-balanced diet, may not get enough absorbable iron from their usual diet. If iron supplements are taken together with

Vitamin C in either natural or synthetic form, the absorption and assimilation into the body is more efficient.

Gingko biloba is useful in that it stimulates the cerebral circulation and counteracts poor blood flow through hardened arteries. It is especially worth trying in elderly people with postural hypotension – the feeling of faintness they get when they suddenly stand up quickly from a sitting or lying position. Ginseng, Chinese angelica and Don quai are herbal treatments used for low blood pressure but the latter should not be taken in pregnancy. Rutin tablets along with ginger and cinnamon tea and buckwheat infusions are useful too. All of these are gentle and readily available solutions to faintness that are safe. There can be little harm in trying them.

Exercise and Lifestyle

The body's ability to keep the blood pressure within a normal physiological range depends on highly developed reflex sensors located in the walls of some of the major arteries. Without regular exercise, they can become sluggish and react only slowly to environmental change such as temperature differences, vigorous exercise or emotion. The best way to tone them so that our blood pressure can instantaneously react to these changes is regular aerobic-style exercises. Swimming, cycling, jogging or keep-fit are all ideal. Taking a proper Swedish-type sauna interspersed with 2 or 3 dips in a cold bath or shower is another great way of toning up those reflex blood pressure sensors, as the circulatory changes in the skin that this induces start to happen faster than in normal circumstances.

Keeping cool generally is another vital tip as the warmer you are, the more likely you are to faint. Why do soldiers out on parade in the height of summer regularly keel over? Why do you feel faint when you suddenly jump out of a hot bath? The reason is that so much blood has been shunted into the blood vessels in your skin in an effort to lose heat from the surface of your body, the blood pressure in your heart and brain drops as a result. By keeping cool at all times, fainting can be avoided. So wear loose-fitting clothes without restricting items such as tight neckwear, corsets or belts. Even splashing a little cold water on the face can reverse the early symptoms of low blood pressure.

For people with postural hypotension, making a habit of rising slowly from a chair or bed – taking the movement in 2 or 3 gradual stages and keeping your head well down to begin with – will pay dividends.

Even mental exercises can help to overcome postural hypotension. So practise an isometric handgrip exercise or count backwards from 100 in chunks of 7 at a time – this alone can ward off a full-blown faint when you feel one coming on.

Complementary Therapies

While conventional doctors may still use ammonia-based smelling salts to 'bring round' a victim of fainting, two complementary alternatives include camphor or rosemary oil. The face can be wiped with distilled extract of witch hazel and the body sponged down with a 1 in 20 mixture of cider vinegar in water.

Acupressure is another technique you can practise on yourself if you feel faint, or use on someone else to revive them. Press firmly between the base of the nose and upper lip, applying pressure for about a minute. Rub your fists against someone's lower back for 1 minute and rub the groove between the big toe and the second toe for 30 seconds. Stimulating these three acupressure points can help the body rebalance and rejuvenate its energy fields, and nip any falls in blood pressure in the bud.

Homeopathy offers lots of additional help. If faintness is due to emotional upset or grief and is accompanied by sighing, take Ignatia. If it is from fright or apprehension and you feel shaky, trembly and are having to go to the toilet frequently, take Gelsemium. Aconite is best if symptoms are due to shock or great agitation, but if your faintness is due to pain, try Hepar sulph. Pulsatilla is recommended when the temperature is very hot and Carbo veg if you desperately need more air but at the same time feel cold.

The Bach Flower combination Rescue Remedy is well

regarded, either taken in tea (3–4 drops in water first), applied under the tongue or rubbed directly into the temples or navel.

You could also consider seeing a reflexologist. Stimulation of the appropriate zones on the soles of the feet is thought to influence the electrochemical energy within that part of your nervous system responsible for the regulation of blood pressure. Finally, relaxation and biofeedback techniques can be learned, enabling you to gain better mental control over your feelings and emotions. In just the same way as embarrassment can lead to socially disabling blushing, emotional fears and concerns can paralyse the involuntary nervous system and lead to fainting. This can be overcome with a little patient practice.

INTEGRATED APPROACH

1. Lean forward and put your head down between your knees if you feel faint, or better still, lie down flat.
2. Raise your legs whenever possible if you regularly suffer from faintness. Take regular aerobic exercise and have saunas to sharpen your circulatory reflexes.
3. Drink plenty of water and try taking a little extra salt.
4. Avoid too many layers of tight clothing and get out of a chair or hot bath slowly. Keep cool.
5. Eat little and often.
6. Ensure plenty of iron in your diet and consider iron and herbal supplements.
7. Learn some of the complementary therapies such as acupressure and biofeedback, and try homeopathic or Bach Flower Remedies and reflexology.
8. Remember that older patients who faint or feel faint should *always* be fully investigated to rule out a serious cause.

Headaches

Diana had a heavy cold 3 weeks previously but could not shake it off. She still suffered from nasal congestion, but she had a heavy feeling in her head, a permanent headache that got worse if she coughed, sneezed or bent forward, and she had a feeling of complete detachment from her surroundings as well as a faint sensation of giddiness when she moved around. The paracetamol and aspirin mixture she got from the chemist did not relieve her symptoms, and eventually her doctor diagnosed chronic sinusitis on the strength of X-rays which revealed fluid in the air cavities within her facial bones.

Headaches can represent something fleeting and quite trivial, or be the first sign of some serious underlying disorder. But it is relatively rare for a headache to be caused by something sinister, while the common migrainous or tension-type headache is experienced by a large proportion of the general population. Simple short-lived headaches are usually easily explained. Many of us can expect a headache when we are tired, stressed, hungry, worried, anxious or dehydrated. Anyone who has driven a long distance especially at night, or has sat in front of a VDU for too long will know the headache of eye strain. Pain from the teeth and gums, a strenuous workout in the gym or too many drinks the night before are also trigger factors. When we can readily explain our symptoms most of us do not worry, and broadly speaking headaches by themselves represent a very small percentage of all reasons for visiting a GP.

However, when the symptoms become particularly annoying, recurrent or chronic, that is when we take the problem to the doctor. A very common worry is that a frequent headache may be the first sign of a brain tumour, but in reality less than 1 per cent of all severe or persistent headaches are caused by major disease processes, and even these by no means defy definitive treatment.

Phil has had a very stressful time recently as he is covering the work of two other colleagues, and the second of his 3 children is in hospital with a glandular fever-type infection. He suddenly developed flashing lights on the right side of his field of vision followed by blindness in the same area. He soon felt nauseated and sick, which was swiftly followed by a splitting headache on the right side of his head, just behind his eye. The doctor was able to reassure him that he was not going blind nor did he have a brain tumour, he had simply had a classic migraine attack.

Characteristics of Different Types of Headache

Tension headaches are the most common type of headache, particularly in people suffering from stress or anxiety. The pain is usually felt at the back of the head or neck, and unlike some headaches, is usually on both sides. This type of headache does not generally interfere with sleep, and may well be improved by a good night's rest. It is described by the patient as crushing, pressing or like having a tight band around the head.

Headaches accompanied by visual disturbances and nausea and which are one-sided suggest migraine.

Short-lived and very frequent headaches may represent cluster headaches, a type of migraine found more commonly in men, and which are so called because they can occur as frequently as several times a day for some weeks.

High temperatures can cause headaches usually because of dehydration, but also because the toxins produced by the micro-organisms that caused the fever in the first place are capable of dilating the blood vessels both inside and on the outside of the skull. This results in a throbbing headache similar to a hangover.

In fact the causes of headache are legion and include depression or anxiety, sinusitis, glaucoma, cervical spondylosis (wear and tear arthritis in the neck), ear problems, throat infections, inflammation of the temporal arteries (temporal arteritis), head injury, meningitis, side effects of medication, and rarely, high blood pressure and benign or malignant brain tumours.

The Conventional Approach

Faced with so many possibilities as to the precise diagnosis of the cause of a headache, the conventional doctor seeks to identify the problem by exclusion. He or she takes a full and thorough medical history from the patient and then examines them. These two fundamental procedures are sufficient to come up with the correct answer in the vast majority of cases. Occasionally the clinical picture remains confusing, in which case further investigations including blood tests, X-rays, scans and a number of other tests may be required.

Linda, a happily married 35-year-old, works in a busy office as PA to the head of marketing. She is conscientious about her work and worries if she cannot completely clear her desk every evening which sometimes causes her to work late and have less time to unwind at home in the evenings. Her workload has grown over the last year as her company has become increasingly successful and she admits that although she loves her job, there is certainly more strain than there used to be. Though her husband is supportive, they both agree that Linda does more of the household tasks than he does. Lately she has had headaches several days a week which present as a tight band around her head making her feel irritable and tired. Linda has stress-related tension headache.

When Might a Headache Be Serious?

Headaches can very occasionally be the first sign of a serious illness, so any unexplained persistent headache should be brought to the attention of the doctor, especially in certain circumstances. Most headaches are improved by a good night's sleep, but when a headache is sufficient to actually produce sleep disturbance, vomiting or is present first thing in the morning it is ominous. Also if the headache is paroxysmal, coming and going in violent ways, it suggests something out of the ordinary. If the headache is made worse by coughing, sneezing or movements of the head, or if the headache is in the temple area and is accompanied by visual disturbances in the eye on the same side, it warrants urgent attention. Finally anyone suffering from a migraine headache for the very first time after the age of 40 should at least let their doctor know so that if it should happen again, secondary causes of the migraine such as increased pressure of fluid within the skull can be eliminated.

Conventional Treatment

Most people self-medicate in the first instance with simple analgesics such as paracetamol, aspirin or codeine. It is only when these self-help measures fail to work or when the headaches are persistent that the doctor is usually consulted. Tension headaches tend to be treated with advice regarding lifestyle changes with rest, relaxation, massage, physiotherapy and osteopathy. Migraines respond to some of the more modern anti-migraine drugs that are available in tablet or injectable form, and recurrent migraines can be efficiently prevented using drugs such as beta blockers or pizotifen. When infections are responsible for headaches, antibiotics may be appropriate. Where headache is due to hangover replacing fluid in the body as quickly as possible is important. Fruit juice will help as will having a meal to boost sugar and mineral levels in the bloodstream.

Depression and anxiety may be relieved by counselling, psychotherapy and medication. The headache of sinusitis may respond to antibiotics, antihistamines, decongestants and, if chronic, surgery to drain the sinuses. Pain originating in the eye in glaucoma may respond to eyedrops and possibly surgery. When neuralgia or muscle tension emanates from wear and tear arthritis in the neck, physiotherapy, osteopathy, wearing a neck collar, anti-inflammatory medications and very occasionally surgery may all be appropriate. Problems within the teeth and gums can be solved by proper dental treatment, and ear and throat inflammation will require anti-inflammatory or antibiotic treatment. Where temporal arteritis is suspected (a condition resulting from inflammation of the temporal artery at the front and side of the skull), steriod treatment is urgently required in order to reduce the possibility of sudden loss of vision due to obstruction of the artery supplying oxygen to the back of the eye.

Head injuries resulting in persistent headache will need medical or surgical therapy, and if meningitis is ever suspected, urgent admission of the patient to hospital is mandatory to confirm the diagnosis and start treatment immediately with antibiotics. GPs seeing patients with suspected meningitis at home should give benzylpenicillin immediately as time is of the essence and this simple measure can be life-saving. It should be remembered that any other medication that the patient has been prescribed could be the possible cause of headache, in which case discontinuation of the drug or a reduction in the dosage is the obvious answer. In the very rare instances where high blood pressure is the cause, medical treatment can alleviate the symptoms, and in the equally rare cases where a brain tumour proves to be the underlying cause, radiotherapy with or without surgery will follow. Doctors should always help patients to discover the true underlying cause of their headache and wherever possible use non-pharmaceutical means to overcome it. There is no doubt that far too many people abuse painkillers and that a proportion of such abusers actually induce the headache itself as a side effect of the analgesic. Often a simple change in lifestyle and a more relaxed approach to life is the answer.

Terry has had increasingly painful headaches over the last few months. The pain now wakes him in the night. A few days ago he had a brief loss of vision accompanied by some dizziness and nausea. He has also had brief episodes of numbness in his hand. Today he had a convulsion. Terry needs urgent assessment to rule out the possibility of a brain tumour.

Nutritional Healing

Food allergies (see p. 74) are worth looking at, and keeping a food and headache diary to see if there is any correlation between the two can often pinpoint the triggers. You could use the model on p. 250. While you're at it why not chart just how much coffee, tea, caffeinated drinks and chocolate you consume, since caffeine can also be a cause. However, if you already have a headache, sometimes a single cup of coffee can help. If you've been drinking a lot of coffee and are trying to give up, then expect a headache for a few days, as you would if you were trying to come off dairy produce. Other fairly common foods that precipitate headache are alcohol (especially red wine and beer), cheese and artificial sweeteners such as aspartame, found in diet drinks. Dehydration may precipitate headache so look at how much water you drink and adjust it to 8 glasses a day at least. Eating regularly will also help. Try to get into a proper routine and keep to it. Small, light, regular meals are better than a fast followed by a feast. Be sensible with your fruit and vegetable quota and watch your salt intake (although if you're in a hot climate, exercise a lot or perspire excessively, you may need extra salt or even a salt tablet). The monosodium glutamate (MSG) in prepared foods, especially Chinese, can cause headache in some. Don't skip your intake of cold-water fish (salmon, mackerel, tuna and others) since omega-3 fatty acids can also help bring relief to the chronic headache sufferer.

Margaret complained of throbbing pain involving the left side of her head accompanied by feeling nauseous. She said that she knew when an attack was coming and that she usually had to lie down and draw the curtains because she couldn't bear the light. Noise affected her badly too and she would feel depressed. She is always afraid of the next attack which could go on for several hours or a couple of days. The headaches began in her teens and were always more likely around ovulation or at the time of her period. Her doctor said that they were most common in women and were in some way linked to falling levels of oestrogen. Now that she is menopausal they have increased in frequency. She says that her grandmother had the same 'sick headaches'. Margaret suffers from migraine.

Vitamins and Supplements

The B vitamins, especially riboflavin (Vitamin B_2) and B_6, are known to be helpful. Migraine sufferers who take riboflavin have been found to reduce their frequency of attacks by about a third according to a Belgian study, although the severity was not reduced. The effects seem to begin only after a month of taking the supplement regularly and give maximum benefit after 3 months of regular use. Of course riboflavin has numerous other benefits too. If you're vegetarian and do not eat fish, take flax seed (linseed) oil or another supplement containing omega-3 fatty acids. Gingko biloba can help by improving the circulation in your brain, and guarana and melatonin may be useful for cluster headache. A magnesium supplement may also help.

Self-Help Methods for Avoiding Stress and Headaches

* Fit a diffuser to your computer screen and ration the time you spend at it.
* Replace all fluorescent lights in your home and office if possible since often the almost imperceptible flicker may be triggering your headache.
* Ensure that you get enough sleep and that it's truly restful. You won't benefit if your neck is at an odd angle because of a poor pillow, or your shoulders and back are not supported by a good mattress.
* Enjoy a jacuzzi or massage for your neck, shoulders and back.
* Check your posture. Have a look at your desk chair; check it is at the right height, and confirm that your neck posture is correct as you work. You should also check how you hold the phone etc. Neck exercises and stretching will help.
* Get enough sleep. Too much sleep is just as likely to precipitate headache as too little, and if you wake feeling fuzzy, grumpy and with a headache, try getting up a little earlier.
* Avoid very hot sun and wear good sunglasses to reduce glare.
* Exercise. Hot, stuffy, smokey atmospheres are bound to leave most people with headaches, whereas taking plenty of exercise, outdoors if possible, will stimulate your circulation and the release of your own antidepressant analgesics, the endorphins.

* Use the stress reduction techniques on p. 482. And if you do have a day when you can't avoid the pressure and come home with a headache like Linda's, then take some time for yourself, listen to some relaxing music or simply go somewhere quiet, put your feet up, close your eyes and allow your body and mind to stop racing. Or go for a walk in the fresh air and while there do some breathing exercises (see breathing techniques, p. 114). Your headache may well respond quite quickly.
* Rest even if you're not sleepy – half an hour with a good book or in a hot bath with an ice pack on your head can work wonders.
* Make sure that if you're reading, you have adequate light and that if you wear glasses, they are the right prescription for you.
* Ask your partner if you grind your teeth in the night, and check whether you could have a tempero-mandibular joint (TMJ) problem. Chewing gum can exacerbate this and contribute to developing a headache. If so, reduce stress and see your dentist.
* Come off contraceptive pills or HRT for a while and see if it helps, but if you do, remember that you need to find an alternative contraceptive that is as reliable as possible.
* Try changing your perfume and see what happens. Sometimes powerful scents can trigger headaches.
* Smile. Although the very last thing you may feel like doing when you have a headache is smiling, this will actually help. The simple act of working the facial muscles you use to form a smile releases endorphins that not only improve your mood but are nature's pain relievers.

Complementary Therapies

Depending upon the cause of your headache, there are a myriad of complementary possibilities. Meditation, yoga, relaxation and massage, all of which are comforting, improve circulation and reduce tension, and can be accompanied by visualisation, in which you first imagine the shape, location and colour of the pain and with the power of your mind change these. If, for instance, your headache feels like a red, jagged pain, try smoothing it into a round shape, changing the colour to a cool pale blue and letting the size of it reduce and reduce until it's only the size of a pinhead, then simply let it go. Osteopathy and chiropractic are both helpful, especially if headache is due to sinus problems or to an old neck injury such as a whiplash. Alexander Technique will improve posture and reduce strain which causes tension headache. Acupressure, massaging the web of skin between your thumb and first finger while applying pressure in the direction of the first finger, will help, as will applying pressure at the base of your skull, above your eyebrows, over your temples and under your cheekbones. Acupuncture, autogenic training, biofeedback and craniosacral therapy can also help.

Why not consult a homeopath and have them prescribe for you? Some common remedies for headache include: Apis, for when the headache is throbbing at the left side of the head usually from above or behind the left ear to the temple, improves with pressure and worsens with motion. Bryonia is good for left-sided headaches starting at the back of the head and moving into the left eye, being worse in the morning and improved by closing your eyes. Coffea may help if your headache is associated with emotional issues or coffee withdrawal, is worsened by noise or music and feels as though a nail is being driven through your head. Lycopodium, Pulsatilla and Silicea may also be useful, but your homeopath will prescribe only after looking at the whole picture, of which your headache is just a part.

Migraine is so dreadful for its sufferers, yet sometimes orthodox medicine does little except to briefly and incompletely ameliorate the situation. Homeopathy may also help here and among the remedies you may be prescribed are Natrum mur, Lac canium, Lac defloratum and Sanguinaria. For cluster headaches Aconite, Belladonna or Lachesis might help. Aromatherapy offers chamomile which relaxes and relieves stress, peppermint, sweet orange, sandalwood and ylang-ylang. If the quality of the air is poor either in your home or office, try using juniper berry, tea tree, lavender or lemon in a vaporiser, or rub the diluted oil over your temples. A herb you may find useful is feverfew which helps reduce both the frequency and severity of migraine attacks in 6 to 8 weeks, although it tastes awful. It can't be used in pregnancy since it may trigger uterine contractions and it may cause a reaction if you're allergic to daisies. White willow could also help. Try Australian Bush or Bach Flower Essences.

Reflexology could be useful and if you want to try to do it yourself before you can manage a consultation, then concentrate on your big toe which corresponds to your head, the other toes which also correspond to the head and the sinuses, and the ridge under the toes which will relieve your neck and shoulders. Have a consultation with a chiropractor to see if either your facial sinuses or your TMJ need manipulation. A TENS (transcutaneous electrical nerve stimulation) machine may help in migraine and tension headaches, and acupuncture may be very effective. Have plenty of plants around, since not only do they keep the air oxygenated, but they can also remove undesirable substances that are potentially hazardous and may be causing your headaches. Peace lilies will absorb the radiation from electronic equipment, spider plants can absorb formaldehyde from new carpets and upholstery, and chrysanthemums absorb fumes from sprays such as hair lacquer, glue and varnish. If you still get attacks, take yourself off to a cool, quiet, dark place to rest, perhaps with an amethyst crystal and some lavender or peppermint oil if you have some, and take plenty of water with you to keep well hydrated. Wearing a headband might help by reducing the blood flow to the scalp. If all else fails, try to keep your hands warm, diverting some of the blood supply away from your head, and relax.

Emotional and Spiritual Healing

Whether you have migraine or cluster headache, suffer from tension, eye strain or the side effects of medication, or if your headache is a complication of premenstrual syndrome, food allergies or physical pain elsewhere, perhaps involving emotional upset or trauma or some other cause, obviously the primary basis needs to be addressed if possible. However, sometimes it's difficult to find the root cause and we find ourselves searching for the reason. It's at times such as these that we need to return to basics and look at where we are in our lives, what seems to be out of sync with who we really are and what we believe, to see if getting back in line with our true path and our integrity affects our physical state. Often we can be amazed at the difference it makes. If our bodies are signalling that there is something wrong, the cause can usually be traced through the emotional messages we're not heeding and even further to the spiritual ones.

So if you have persistent headache, let's have a look at where it might be coming from on a higher level. Are there any outstanding emotional issues you need to address? Is there something you feel angry about that you're not dealing with? Is there something you know you have to deal with, have to say, have to confront that you're avoiding? Are you staying in some relationship or situation which you know isn't good for you, isn't what you really want, that causes you pain? What is it that is making you so tense and anxious? What moves do you need to make in your life? We usually know deep down even if we're afraid to bring the answers into our consciousness. If you're sleeping badly, waking in the night and getting up with that hung-over feeling and a headache all morning, what is it that's disturbing you so? Why not write these questions on separate pieces of paper and spend a little quiet time alone trying to answer them really honestly. Doing so doesn't mean that you have to commit yourself to changing things right now, so don't be afraid that if you discover your marriage is really causing you to feel tense and angry, you have to leave it. What will happen, however, is that you'll become aware of where the problems are and in doing so, already you will feel less confused and can begin the process of starting to sort them out. When you realise, for instance, that the headache you've been nursing for so long is really because you haven't forgiven your best friend for something she did, or that the irritability you now displace onto your children and that you blame on your headache is actually because you haven't spoken your mind on another issue, it all starts to make sense and the pain can subside. You will have to do something about the things you discover at some point, and maybe you will want to start right now. Or maybe you'll need some help in the form of counselling to help you mobilise the courage you need to confront them, but whatever, you will start to be back in control and your body will no longer need to be signalling distress by giving you physical pain in order to get your attention. Why not start the process now and get the help you need by asking the wisest person you know for the answers – and that's yourself.

INTEGRATED APPROACH

1. Be determined to seek a precise diagnosis for your headaches wherever possible.
2. Look at spiritual and emotional aspects where diagnosis proves elusive.
3. Bear in mind the signs and symptoms of headaches of sinister cause.
4. Rule out lifestyle and environmental trigger factors.
5. Adjust exercise levels and nutritional dietary content.
6. Remember that chronic abuse of painkillers in itself may be the cause of headaches and that other medication too may be responsible.
7. Experiment with relaxation and various other complementary therapies.
8. Where migraine is frequent and severe, ask your doctor about more effective acute and preventative treatments.

Heart Disease/Heart Attack

John, aged 54, is the finance director of a national mobile telephone network. His work is largely office-based but he does travel several times a year to Europe and the United States. He is slightly overweight and smokes about 20 cigarettes a day. The only exercise he gets is a gentle cycle ride with the children at weekends and a spot of gardening. While digging the vegetable patch the other day he experienced a pain in the centre of his chest which felt like a tight band of pressure preventing him breathing properly. It stopped after a minute or two, but came back again whenever he resumed heavy digging. He has angina.

Heart disease can manifest itself in many ways. Among other things it can cause pain in the chest, breathlessness, intolerance of exercise, blueness of the lips and tongue, swelling of the ankles and feet, and palpitations. Most of us will have known someone who has had a heart attack and most of us are aware that heart disease is the second commonest cause of death overall in Britain. It kills somewhere in the region of 300,000 people every year and the disability and devastation it causes even when it is not fatal, for patients and families alike, is enormous.

Next to the human brain, our hearts are the most important organ in the body and when the heart does not function well, it affects us not only physically but psychologically and emotionally too. This is something that orthodox doctors, trained as they are in anatomy, biochemistry and physiology, would do well to remember when talking to patients with heart disease.

Congenital Defects

About 800 babies in every 100,000 are born with a congenital heart defect of some kind or another where there is a structural abnormality of the heart resulting from a problem in fetal development. Not all are serious and many require no intervention whatsoever, but common ones include septal defects, otherwise known as holes in the heart, and certain kinds of abnormal heart valves. Occasionally the large blood vessels leading to and from the heart are interposed, and these provide the greatest of all surgical challenges to treatment.

Zak is only 3 weeks old. He was dusky blue when born and fairly unresponsive at first to stimulation by the obstetrics team, so he was nursed on the Special Care Baby Unit. This 'blueness' continued despite oxygen treatment. He fought for breath and did not satisfactorily gain weight. It soon became evident he had a hole in his heart – a congenital abnormality resulting in the mixing of oxygenated with deoxygenated blood so that his body became chronically starved of oxygen.

INFECTIONS

The lining of the heart, the endocardium, can become infected, either as a result of infectious diseases such as rheumatic fever, or through the introduction of bacteria into the bloodstream as might occur when drug addicts inject drugs without using an aseptic technique. Where there is any abnormality of the heart valves themselves, infections can even arise from procedures as trivial as dental work. Scaling of the teeth, for example, can introduce what would otherwise be fairly harmless bacteria into the bloodstream which then lodge on the abnormal valves and produce growths that may be dispersed into the bloodstream, leading to ministrokes.

Even very fit young athletes can develop infections in and around the heart as a secondary result of a simple viral infection. This is why athletes competing in events sometimes collapse if they vigorously exercise under the influence of a cold.

Dorothy suffered from rheumatic fever as a child and has been told several times by different doctors over the years that she has a heart murmur. All she really knows is that this has something to do with the valves of her heart being a little scarred. She is now 68, however, and feels that this cannot have done her much harm. On the other hand, she has certainly begun to feel somewhat breathless and weary of late and her son is eager for her to explore the possibility of cardiac surgery to 'get her going again'. Dorothy has mitral incompetence – a leaky heart valve – resulting in the onset of heart failure.

CARDIOMYOPATHY

In these muscle disorders of the heart, the heart muscle becomes inflamed or enlarged, leading to obstruction of the outflow of blood from the heart. This can result in sudden death in young people who have up to that moment shown no evidence of any problem with their health. In these cases the problem is often inherited but in other situations it can be acquired, for example through vitamin deficiency or alcohol poisoning.

RHYTHM DISTURBANCES

Known as cardiac arrhythmias, abnormal heart rhythms can cause anything from simple palpitations to fainting, blackouts and even sudden death. Many arrhythmias are due to the stimulant effect of caffeine, found in tea, coffee, cola drinks and certain foodstuffs, but others may represent an anatomical aberration or the toxic effect of medications such as asthma treatments or antidepressents.

POOR BLOOD SUPPLY

Otherwise known as ischaemic heart disease, this is the commonest cause of heart disease in developed countries, and is responsible for angina and heart attacks. The heart is a muscle like any other in the body and it can only function properly when supplied with sufficient oxygen. This comes by way of the circulation, and if the circulation is impaired or interrupted in any way, the heart muscle will be starved of oxygen and produce pain. Just as a leg muscle goes into cramp in the latter stages of a sprint race when oxygen levels are low, so the heart muscle will cause a cramp-like pain in the chest. In the heart, however, this will affect its ability to pump blood around the body, and the greatest risk of all is an interruption to the nervous impulses that enable the heart to contract rhythmically in the first place.

Risk factors for ischaemic heart factors

smoking
lack of physical exercise
high blood pressure
high cholesterol and triglycerate (blood fat) levels
high homocysteine level
obesity
family history of heart disease
stress
diet high in saturated fat
diabetes

Diagnosis

People are much more aware of heart disease at the end of this century than they were at the beginning. Because people are not dying at a younger age from other diseases, because we take less exercise, and because we can enjoy a rich and plentiful diet, heart disease has become the epidemic of our time. Consequently, for every person who has a real physical basis to their symptoms there is another who is unduly anxious about the state of their heart. However, by listening carefully to most patients it is possible for doctors to gauge a reasonable idea of the proportion of their symptoms that are real and those that are imagined. Symptoms can tell us a lot, but there is much overlap, and making the distinction for example between indigestion and angina can sometimes be impossible based on the patient's history alone, even for the super-specialist. All chest pain should be taken seriously by doctors, therefore, and every case should be investigated and explained before it can be dismissed as 'non-cardiac' in origin. No patient should feel awkward or reserved about asking medical advice when they suffer from chest pain, and no recurrent twinge, however slight, should ever be neglected. Far too many middle-aged men have died prematurely as a result of this nonchalant attitude on behalf of their doctor.

After the doctor has taken a full and thorough history, including an appraisal of lifestyle and dietary habits in particular, the physical examination can throw further light on the symptoms. The physical appraisal starts with the general appearance of the patient. Any undue breathlessness, pallor, blueness around the lips or even change in weight may be important. The rate and regularity of the pulse provide important information, and so does listening to heart valves and heart rhythm using a stethoscope. Sometimes a murmur may be heard, which is the rushing noise as blood is pumped through narrow blood vessels or valves and which is very reminiscent of the rushing sound heard when water runs through a hose with a kink in it. Murmurs are not always abnormal, however, as some are heard in young fit athletes who simply have a powerful flow of blood around the body. Further evidence of poor heart function can be gleaned from the presence of any fluid in the feet, ankles and lower legs, and can even be indicated by tenderness in the liver resulting from congestion occurring in the venous system of blood vessels. Sometimes fluid can accumulate in the bases of the lungs leading to breathlessness especially when the patient lies flat in bed at night and the presence of this fluid can often be heard by a doctor by means of the stethoscope.

In recent years many technological milestones have been passed with the development of investigative and diagnostic machines that have made the diagnosis of heart disease much more precise. The electrocardiogram (ECG) is a major asset in the detection of heart arrhythmias, and the echocardiogram using ultrasonic sound waves has helped enormously in the identification of heart valve and heart muscle abnormalities. The ECG also gives the earliest evidence of a recent heart attack in the majority of patients where this has happened. It is a portable machine, often combined with a defibrillator, and is carried by many GPs in their cars on home visits should a patient's heart ever need restarting in the emergency situation of cardiac arrest. Chest X-rays provide the simplest and most widely used method of providing an image of the heart, and from it doctors can determine the size and shape of the heart and whether the lungs are congested as a result of venous congestion and fluid build-up. These findings would indicate a degree of heart failure. Angiography is another imaging technique where X-rays are taken after a contrast medium has been injected into the circulation. It can show any obstruction to the coronary blood vessels that supply the heart, as well as the size of the heart chambers and the function of the muscular walls of the ventricles of the heart. More recently radio nuclide scanning, CT scanning and MRI techniques have made it possible to further assess heart function and to scrutinise the results of coronary artery bypass surgery.

Conventional Treatment

The duty of any family doctor is to try to prevent as much heart disease in their patients as is humanly possible by encouraging the patients themselves to learn about the risk factors and to live as healthy a life as they can. Nobody can change who their parents are, so nobody can alter any genetic predisposition to heart disease they may have. But there is much you can do to reduce their risk of dying prematurely from heart disease. For example, you can:

- stop smoking
- reduce your intake of saturated fat in your diet
- take regular aerobic-type exercise for at least 20 minutes at a time, for a minimum of 3 times a week
- make sure your blood pressure is under control
- make sure that any diabetes is treated

* make sure that your cholesterol level is checked and kept under control
* learn to deal with excess stress in your life

Tara, 31, is an interior designer and combines the job with looking after her two children aged 4 and 6. She has had a number of yellowy-cream flecks and spots around her eyes for as long as she can remember, but lately, people have commented that they have become more noticeable. Both her parents died before they were 45 of heart disease and Tara is beginning to wonder whether she should still be on the oral contraceptive pill and whether these spots are anything to worry about. Unknown to her, she has hypercholesterolaemia, a condition she has inherited from her parents which results in a dangerous elevation of the cholesterol level in her blood. This puts her at much greater risk of heart disease.

In the area of heart disease perhaps more than any other, prevention is so much more important than treatment. By the time treatment becomes necessary, the patient can never ever return to a satisfactory state of health; they can merely prevent the problem from becoming worse. That said, so much is possible now with modern treatment. Coronary bypass surgery has become a commonplace operation with a successful outcome and low mortality. Heart valve surgery, even in the relatively elderly, to correct or replace narrowed or leaky heart valves, can transform a breathless, exhausted, weak individual into a person of strength and good stamina, and valves made from metal or plastic, or even fashioned from human or bovine tissue, may be used. On top of this, heart and lung transplants are now proceeding apace. The outcome, once the immediate post-operative period is complete, is good with some 80 per cent of patients surviving the first year in many hospitals, with a death rate of only about 5 per cent per year after that.

Modern medicines have made all this possible through the use of immuno-suppressant drugs such as prednisolone, cyclophosphamide and cyclosporin. Anticoagulants also play an important role in reducing any tendency of the blood to clot too easily, leading to obstructions of the coronary arteries. Antibiotics prevent life-threatening infections relating to heart disease. Another important group of drugs control abnormal heart rhythms and heart failure, and includes diuretics or water tablets to prevent excess build-up of fluid. Antianginal medicines to ease chest pain are important, as are drugs that lower blood pressure and again reduce the risk of heart attacks and strokes. Even those who have recently suffered an acute heart attack can be significantly helped through treatment with anti-thrombotics or fibrinolytics as these can, in that vital time between the heart attack occurring and the patient being transferred to hospital, dissolve a potentially fatal obstructive blood clot. We also now have at our disposal very effective hypolipidaemic (lipid-lowering) agents to effectively reduce blood fats and cholesterol, as well as a variety of pharmaceutical products that can correct anaemia or inflammation of the blood vessels themselves.

On the face of it, the investigations and treatments that modern doctors have at their disposal to assess and treat heart disease appear complex and bewildering. It can be perplexing and frightening for a patient to have to put their lives in the hands of doctors who may take a lot of this for granted. But by asking relevant and appropriate questions and doggedly insisting on answers, the patient can still feel in control of their destiny. Most of these procedures are relatively straightforward these days and have an excellent safety profile. But tests and therapies are always more likely to be successful if the patient is involved with the decision-making process with the doctor, and fully understands what is going on. No doctor should underestimate the degree of anxiety that accompanies heart disease.

The post-operative treatment is just as important as the pre-operative and operative treatment, and patients and their families should avail themselves of any information about how they should lead the rest of their lives. No person – be it an infant with congenital heart disease, a middle-aged person with ischaemic heart disease or an older person with valvular disease should ever be allowed to become a cardiac cripple. Organisations such as the Family Heart Association can supplement the advice and information provided by conventional doctors.

Exercise and Lifestyle

An active lifestyle is still the most important factor in the reduction of heart disease. That includes being generally active as well as taking formal exercise. Exercise can greatly reduce the risks to your heart by strengthening the whole cardiovascular system. But not only that, it makes you feel better! Walking remains the best exercise for those with heart disease but yoga is gentle and not only does it keep you supple and fit, but it also helps with stress and anxiety and prompts you to slow down. T'ai chi is another form of exercise which, like yoga, involves the emotional and spiritual and will add a new dimension to your life. Research has shown that having 6 weeks of T'ai chi (30 minutes 4 times a week) can significantly reduce the blood pressure of older people while improving flexibility and balance.

If you're a high-powered executive type, please try to slow down and take some time for yourself. It would be very sad if you joined the ranks of those who have strived all their lives to build up a nest egg to enjoy later, only to have a heart attack or stroke intervene.

Although most women think of breast cancer as being the major scourge, post-menopausal women succumb to heart disease 8 times more often than they do to breast cancer. So take care of yourself.

Smoking is a major risk factor in the development of heart disease. Giving up smoking is the single most important self-help measure you can take to maintain a healthy heart. Both smoking yourself and inhaling smoke from other smokers causes the aorta to lose its elasticity with resultant extra strain on heart muscle to pump blood around. The *Journal of the American College of Cardiology* found that of 336 adults admitted to hospital after suffering a heart attack, 43 per cent lived with someone who was a smoker. According to this research, non-smoking husbands of smoking wives increase their chance of heart attack by 92 per cent whereas non-smoking wives of smoking husbands increase their risk of heart attack by 50 per cent. Non-smokers who live with a partner who smokes 20 or more cigarettes a day have increased their risk of heart attack by 400 per cent! (This greatly raised figure is due to the fact that the risk to those who don't smoke would generally be very low.) We have found no figures for the increased risk for children, but it must be high. It's worth pondering on whether smoking in a house where there are children, especially if they have a heart or chest problem, could amount to child abuse.

Nutritional Healing

Look at the basic eating plan on p. 5 and see what you need to change (gently and gradually) to help you achieve optimum nutrition. The incidence of heart disease decreases as the intake of fruit and vegetables increases, so make sure that you have your full quota of 5 to 8 servings daily and include at least one serving of dark leafy vegetables. Fruit and vegetables are the main sources of antioxidants and fibre, which not only benefit your heart but are also effective in the management of cancer (see p. 154). Have a fibre-rich cereal at some time in the day. If not at breakfast, could you have cereal as a bedtime snack? Although a low-fat diet is recommended, the total amount of fat you consume is less important than the type of fat. Olive oil contains monounsaturated fats which have not been shown to be harmful in any way. But when oils are partially hydrogenated to make them semi-solid as in margarine, the fats are converted to trans fats which have been linked to major diseases such as heart disease and cancer. Cakes and biscuits, etc. are major sources of trans fats and it is for this reason, as well as their being high in calories, that they should be avoided. Oily fish (salmon, sardines, mackerel) eaten at least twice a week which will give you omega-3 essential fatty acids (EFAs) although these can also be obtained from flax seed (linseed) oil and to a lesser degree canola and walnut oil. As their name implies, they are essential to your health so don't skip on them.

Reduce your alcohol intake to between 7 and 14 units spread over the week – less if your heart is already compromised. And do cut down on caffeine-containing drinks such as coffee and cola. Remember chocolate also contains caffeine. Tea contains antioxidants and, drunk in moderation, is fine. Green tea is especially beneficial.

Oranges, broccoli, fortified cereal, lettuce, eggs and spinach are particularly good sources of folic acid (sometimes called folate). A huge study at Harvard Medical School strongly suggests that higher folate intake is cardio-protective. Not only does Vitamin B_6 reduce the risk of heart disease but it's necessary for energy and for the health of the immune and central nervous system. Deficiency causes nervousness, dermatitis, hair loss, acne, depression, anaemia, arthritis and weak muscles as well as heart problems. Natural sources of Vitamin B_6 include meat, milk, peas and beans, whole brown rice and brewer's yeast. Spinach is a natural source of alpha lipoic acid, a newly isolated antioxidant which protects cardiovascular muscle as well as reducing the damage to both heart and brain when there's stroke or heart attack. (It can also be purchased as a supplement.) Flavinoids are compounds found in tea, onions and apples and are the pigments that give wine its colour. They can help cardiac function and reduce risk of stroke. There is also a substance in grape seeds that can help protect the heart as well as showing great promise in both the prevention and treatment of cancer (see p. 154).

A study in Germany found that people who took garlic supplements had greater flexibility in their blood vessels than those who didn't, while another in China showed that blood pressure was quite dramatically controlled by taking garlic oil. The active constituents of garlic can lower both your blood pressure and your cholesterol. You can eat it raw (if you do, chew some parsley afterwards to be less antisocial), cooked or as a deodorised supplement. One of the active ingredients, allicin, is released when garlic is either crushed or cut but starts to degrade almost immediately, so use it very fresh. If you're taking tablets, check the sell-by date.

Ginger reduces the tendency of blood platelets to stick together and therefore reduces the risk of clotting and thrombosis. Hot foods such as chillis and peppers act similarly. Both are available as supplements, but as always, it's preferable to get what we need naturally from food if we can. Do discuss it with your GP first if you're already taking the anticoagulant warfarin.

Vitamins and Supplements

The B vitamins play several important roles in the prevention of heart disease. Vitamin B_6 and folic acid (folate) are essential for the breakdown of homocysteine, high levels of which have been recognised for over 30 years as a predictor for heart disease. More recently, the health of 80,000 women was followed for 14 years by researchers at Harvard and a report in the *Journal of the American Medical Association* confirmed that women who add B vitamins (particularly folate and Vitamin B_6) to their diet can lower their risk of heart disease by about 45 per cent. Although vitamins are obviously found in our food, this study looked at the place for supplements. Generally we need a folate supplement to boost levels and provide protection. Besides its effect on coronary heart disease, it helps prevent neural tube defects in the fetus and is necessary for growth (see Pregnancy, p. 404). Diuretics (drugs which help treat or prevent water retention), oral contraceptives and steroids can reduce the absorption of Vitamin B. A strong Vitamin B complex tablet and a healthy diet should give you sufficient B vitamins.

Vitamin C may prevent fatty deposits in arteries from rupturing and causing heart attack. Researchers in Boston who measured blood levels of Vitamin C found that those with lower levels were likely to have more severe heart disease and angina.

Vitamin C, Vitamin E and other antioxidants lower the risk of heart problems but need to be taken in higher than the usual daily recommended dose to achieve this aim. We would usually recommend about 2000 to 3000 mg of Vitamin C and 800 to 1200 IU of Vitamin E daily. Vitamin E taken at this dose can reduce the risk of heart disease by 70 per cent. If you're taking any medication to prevent clotting (for example, warfarin), then please talk to your medical practitioner before taking Vitamin E since it has the effect of thinning the blood a little.

It has been said that everyone who is in a high-risk group for heart disease should be taking CoEnzyme Q10, a vitamin-like substance that releases energy from cells and is necessary for the metabolism of virtually every cell in the body, particularly the muscle of the heart which of course can never rest. We produce less as we get older and some people with heart disease just don't have enough. Some cases of even quite serious cardiac illness can respond dramatically to a supplement of CoQ10. It can help relieve angina and in some cases will improve the function of the heart when there's congestive cardiac failure. It's also useful in the treatment of cardiomyopathy where there is abnormal enlargement of the heart muscle.

Magnesium deficiency increases the risk of hypertension (raised blood pressure), artery constriction and blockage, arrhythmias and heart attack, yet this is an element whose level is rarely checked. A good way to take magnesium if you do need some is to have a combined calcium and magnesium supplement. Alpha lipoic acid, mentioned earlier, is even more useful when used in combination with Vitamin E.

Emotional and Spiritual Healing

So many people with the so-called Type A personality, dashing through their lives busily allowing their brain to be in charge, miss the joy of a happy heart. Have you noticed how some people are always trying to control everything, from those around them to the universe in general? Are you one of these? Beware! Your heart is at risk. Then there are those who appear unable to see the world as a benign place and instead are constantly on guard for the next event that's going to come along and get them. Not only do they repeatedly feel to be the victim of some slight or another, but they are usually in the process of blaming someone or something for whatever befalls them. Again, your heart is suffering. It's time to take responsibility for you and only you, unless you have small children in which case your responsibility extends to them also. You don't need to be responsible for anyone else, their behaviour or their difficulties. We're all responsible for ourselves. We do, however, have responsibilities *towards* other people, but if you take responsibility for them, not only are you wearing yourself out and expending energy unnecessarily, you're giving others the message that they can't take care of themselves and rendering them helpless into the bargain. Time to back off and take responsibility for your own health and wellbeing and this will allow others to do the same. You don't have to be a victim or a martyr.

Adopting a softer, more loving and caring attitude towards yourself and others not only relaxes you, but makes you nicer to be around, allows you to accept yourself and others in a totally different, non-competitive and tolerant way, and releases energy that has previously been squandered on the futile attempt to change those around you. Once you do that, you'll find that everything seems to change quite miraculously, the world is a happier place than you thought and the stress upon you and your heart is reduced.

How about learning to meditate? Meditation has amazing effects on stress, blood pressure and a variety of illnesses including angina and heart disease in general. It would also be worth working through the HEART questionnaire in Paul Pearsall's book *The Heart's Code: Tapping the Wisdom and Power of Our Heart Energy* (Broadway Books, 1998) to see what message you're putting out to the world.

In spiritual terms, love is the energy of the heart centre. Read the chapter on the heart in *The Rainbow Journey* (Dr Brenda Davies, Hodder & Stoughton, 1998). The more we can open our hearts to love ourselves and others, generally the more healthy our physical hearts will be also. However, beware being so open in your heart that you allow your whole life to be taken over by other people's needs and pain until you have little time or energy left for yourself. Those who work in the caring professions need to be very wary of this phenomenon, which is called burn-out. Loving also has a barbed edge of course, in that when we lose the object of our love, we suffer grief. Those who are grieving have a higher risk of all kinds of illness and even increased risk of dying. Those who are lonely, isolated and depressed have five times the risk of premature death from any cause. A broken heart is not only something we hear about in songs. The pain of loss can actually weaken us physically as well as emotionally and spiritually. Dealing with anger is also essential to reduce the stress upon your heart. Some good therapy would help you here and some spiritual healing would soothe your aching soul.

Please don't let the fear of loss stop you having relationships that are intimate and fulfilling. People who have such relationships, characterised by good communication, caring, commitment, touch and compassion (even with a pet), are much less likely to have heart attacks or strokes, and if they do, they recover from them more easily. Those who have a sense of commitment and community have not only longer survival times but greater quality of life. No drug can do this for us. Being with those we love isn't a luxury, it's essential to our survival. If you feel alone, then look into joining some club or support group or do some voluntary work. Your GP may possibly be able to help you, or you could have a word with your local librarian. They can often be an amazing source of information.

Complementary Therapies

Heart conditions need to be thoroughly investigated and treated by an orthodox practitioner, although there are methods that can complement the help you are receiving. There are several herbs you may find useful but see a qualified herbalist and check the situation with a sympathetic doctor. Hawthorn helps dilate blood vessels and lower blood pressure, reduces shortness of breath and improves heart function. It also helps with peripheral circulation, especially in hands and feet. Cayenne can reduce both the level of triglycerides in the blood and the risk of clot formation. Gingko biloba has a marked effect on the blood vessels to the heart and brain as well as to your limbs, but talk to your GP about using it if you're taking warfarin.

To reduce stress and prevent heart disease, oils such as lavender and ylang-ylang are useful (see Stress, p. 481). There are several homeopathic remedies that will help angina, Cactus perhaps being the classic. Arnica, useful wherever there is shock, can be helpful when there is heart pain, also Apis and Lachesis. Please see a good practitioner if you wish to use homeopathy – that is, someone well trained, registered and who will be willing to work hand in hand with your allopathic doctor. Massage will help relax you and the power of human touch shouldn't be underestimated as a healing technique.

Integrated approach

1. Identifying risk factors for heart disease and adopting strategies to minimise them could save countless lives.
2. Prevention of heart disease, the biggest killer of all in Britain, is perfectly possible.
3. Increased levels of regular exercise, stopping smoking and a low-fat diet are among the most important lifestyle changes you can make.
4. Accept offers of medical screening on a regular basis. In particular, cholesterol, blood sugar and blood pressure levels should be monitored.
5. All episodes of chest pain should be taken seriously and reported to a doctor.
6. Modern diagnostic techniques are less invasive and more accurate than previously, and the success rates for coronary artery surgery and other cardiac operations are very good and improving all the time.
7. Most symptoms relating to heart disease can be vastly improved with the help of pharmaceutical intervention.
8. Adopt a more gentle, loving attitude to yourself and those around you.
9 Have a committed loving relationship even if with a pet.

High Blood Pressure (Hypertension)

Robert was watching television at home when he suddenly noticed weakness in his right arm and leg. Both limbs felt heavy and clumsy. When he tried to tell his wife, his speech was slurred and he dribbled from one corner of his mouth. Robert has had a stroke as a result of undiagnosed and untreated high blood pressure.

Abnormally high blood pressure affects 10–20 per cent of adults in Britain, and is said to exist when a person's resting blood pressure is persistently elevated. When doctors measure the blood pressure it is expressed by two values, for example 160/90, the higher value representing the systolic pressure and the lower value the diastolic. The systolic pressure is the maximum pressure within the artery which occurs when the heart actually beats, forcing a pulse wave of blood into the major arteries. The diastolic pressure is that between the beats of the heart and represents the resting blood pressure within the arteries. The actual figures measured merely refer to the height of a column of mercury which in millimetres is capable of exerting the same pressure as that of the blood in the arteries.

Assessing your blood pressure

'Normal' blood pressure varies with age but is generally defined as lying between certain parameters.

Borderline high blood pressure: from 120/90 up to 160/94.
Mild: from 140/95 up to 160/104.
Moderate: from 140/105 up to 160/115.
Severe: 180/115 or over.

Hypertension hardly ever causes symptoms but despite this, it is a serious disorder. If neglected it increases the risk of stroke and heart disease. It leads to enlargement of the muscle chambers of the heart, the 'ventricles', contributes to poor circulation in the lower limbs, may bring on angina and heart attack, can damage the kidneys and lead to the warning signs of a stroke (transient ischaemic attacks) or to strokes themselves. This is why doctors take the condition seriously and why patients should undergo frequent health checks (at least every 2 years), especially over the age of 35, to detect hypertension which occurs without symptoms. Obviously checks should be more frequent if there are any symptoms.

Causes

The vast majority of those with hypertension, some 90 per cent, have no identifiable cause for their raised blood pressure. This is known as 'essential' hypertension. What we do know, however, is that high blood pressure is more common in men than in women and that it seems to be more common with increasing age. Other aggravating factors include smoking, obesity, excessive alcohol intake, lack of regular exercise, a high degree of occupational and social stress, and a family history of high blood pressure. In less than 10 per cent of cases there may be an underlying medical condition such as narrowing of the arteries to the kidneys, narrowing of the major artery exiting from the heart, kidney disease, adrenal gland abnormality or a side effect of certain medications and drugs. The combined oral contraceptive pill also seems to increase the risk of high blood pressure.

Dan, aged 72, looks and acts young for his age, and has always lived by the motto 'work hard and play hard'. Unfortunately his playing hard involved heavy drinking, and when he experienced two near blackouts close together, he was diagnosed as having extremely high blood pressure. He was shocked, as his previous medical records were almost non-existent, but the doctor was able to identify arterial damage at the back of his eyes, and an enlarged heart on his electrocardiogram. Initially reluctant to take drugs every day when he felt quite well, he was persuaded by the doctor and the practice nurse that this was in his own best interests. This was confirmed by a specialist and, once settled on medication and free of side effects, he complied fully with the treatment prescribed by his doctors.

Diagnosis

Normal blood pressure fluctuates all the time. It tends to rise when people are emotional or stressed, or take exercise, and it decreases during sleep. However, only a persistently elevated and abnormally high blood pressure can be considered as representing hypertension. For this reason, nobody should be diagnosed as having high blood pressure on a single reading, and several readings on different occasions should be taken in the sitting, lying and standing positions.

Conventional Treatment

When blood pressure is mildly raised, it should be monitored on a frequent basis, and lifestyle measures should be instigated. These include those measures listed below.

Self-help measures to reduce blood pressure

1. Reduce weight if obese.
2. Reduce stress levels.
3. Reduce salt intake.
4. Stop smoking.
5. Reduce dietary fat.
6. Take more exercise.
7. Cut back on alcohol.

When these lifestyle changes have been made and the hypertension persists, usually with a diastolic value above 100 mm of mercury, drug therapy is usually recommended. This includes the use of various groups of medications including diuretics, beta blockers, ACE inhibitors, calcium antagonists, alpha-1 antagonists and angiotensin-2 antagonists. All work in different ways to lower the blood pressure, and all have different advantages and disadvantages. The conservative medical approach to drug treatment for hypertension would be to choose the right drug or combination of drugs to suit the individual patient and their needs. Since diabetes and coexistent blood fat abnormalities may be present in association with high blood pressure, the patient may require adequate diabetic management and use of lipid-lowering agents. Thereafter people with high blood pressure should have their blood pressure frequently measured so that adjustments can be made to their therapy according to how their condition progresses. It is quite possible for some patients to stop taking their medication, particularly if they succeed in losing weight and stopping smoking, but the majority may need to continue with treatment for life in order to minimise the attendant risks.

Check-ups

Because high blood pressure is a silent and often asymptomatic disorder, it can be present for many years causing damage to many organs in the body unless it is recognised and treated. For this reason, all those over the age of 35 should have their blood pressure checked frequently. Although people feel completely fit and healthy with high blood pressure, they are well advised to accept treatment as it will significantly reduce the risk of a future heart attack, stroke and the development of kidney and other disorders. With today's modern drugs, side effects may be kept to a minimum if experienced at all, and there are perfectly palatable substitutes for sodium (salt) that can be used in cooking (sodium can have the effect of raising blood pressure).

Sue made an appointment with her family doctor for a check-up prior to applying for a repeat prescription for the oral contraceptive pill. The doctor was as surprised as she was when her blood pressure was found to be significantly elevated. It had been normal when she first started the pill, but was now at a level necessitating its withdrawal. Within 3 weeks her blood pressure had settled back to normal, and a substitute prescription for the minipill, containing only progestogen and no oestrogen, gave her the contraception she needed without any elevation in her blood pressure.

Nutritional Healing

This is yet another of those illnesses where the first advice needs to be to trim excess body fat, or in more simple terms, lose weight. The good news is that even a few pounds can make a difference. Following a healthy eating plan (see p. 5) will help, although if you need to shed more than a few pounds have a look at p. 242. Vegetarians generally have lower blood pressure than those who eat meat, so perhaps you could make some changes there. The essential fatty acids in cold-water fish (salmon, tuna, mackerel and sardines, for example) can be beneficial, although you can derive the same benefit from taking flax seed (linseed) oil as a supplement. We have already said that you need to limit your salt intake too. Beware of fast foods, processed and pre-prepared foods which are often have a high salt content. Melons, bananas and green leafy vegetables, which are rich in calcium and magnesium, are helpful, although perhaps the most beneficial food is celery. Not only is it a natural diuretic, but it can lower blood pressure quite significantly. Eating more broccoli and citrus fruits will boost your intake of Vitamin C. On your healthy eating plan you will reduce your intake of saturated fats, refined sugar, alcohol and caffeine, and increase the amount of fibre you eat. Much has been said about the amazing qualities of garlic, and its active ingredient allicin lowers blood pressure while also having a beneficial action on your cholesterol level. Onions have a similar action. If you're over 65 and don't respond very well to orthodox medication to control your blood pressure, or if you're prescribed diuretics by your GP, you may benefit considerably by increasing your intake of potassium (bananas are a good source). However, ask your GP to keep an eye on your serum potassium since its level is crucial to good health.

Vitamins and Supplements

As always, it's best to get what you need from your diet if possible. Calcium, magnesium and potassium can be taken as supplements but please only take the latter under the supervision of your doctor. Vitamins C, E and B_6 are useful and CoEnzyme Q10 has been reported to have good results although these may only become evident if you have taken it regularly for several weeks. Flax seed (linseed) oil is a good source of omega-3 fatty acids. Hawthorn berry may have an effect on mild hypertension

Emotional and Spiritual Healing

Are you the kind of person who gets angry and upset, can't let go of grudges and feels that injuries need to be avenged? Do you find yourself in the middle of disputes in shops, in relationships, at work? Are you determined to fight your corner and have the last word no matter what? If so, if you haven't got high blood pressure now, you may soon have. Not only is life too short to be holding onto anger and being unwilling to let things drop, but generally, the person who's being hurt most in such situations is yourself. Could you try just letting go and rising above it? Let go of negativity and try the positive thought that things may just go well if you let them. Holding onto old grudges and pursuing the possibility of revenge waste your precious time, force you to carry yesterday into today and spoil the joy you could be having now if you were willing to open your eyes and your heart to the new gifts that abound every day. The power of positive thinking to change not only your outlook but your life has been written about for decades, as Norman Vincent Peale's book of that title testifies. We're not suggesting that you should always be submissive and give up on your rights, but if you can learn to walk away and take a few deep breaths, coming back to discuss things when you can do so rationally, then you'll spare not only your blood pressure but your dignity too. And in the final analysis, as long as you know what you know, does it really matter what the other person thinks or who has the last word? Just let it go.

People often ask how to do this and it's difficult to describe. But a lovely exercise you might like to try is to repeatedly visualise walking through a doorway into the next moment, firmly closing the door behind you and leaving the past where it belongs. If you could do this every morning, or better still each night before you go to sleep, you can always be ready to start with a new beginning unhampered by the past. That is not to say that we should close the door on our responsibilities, but we can on things that no amount of worrying or anger will change. Open yourself to a fresh new beginning every moment and you will always be in the present, and your blood pressure will benefit. You may like to do some work on your sacral chakra. This is the one that develops between the ages of 5 and 8 (see p. 539) and among other things controls the fluid systems of your body. If you had any trauma between those ages, then do see a healer to work through that and rebalance and cleanse your chakras.

Exercise and Lifestyle

A healthy active lifestyle will benefit you, but do choose as exercise something you enjoy so that you will stick to it. Gentle dancing and swaying to soft music or yoga will do a great deal for you by keeping you supple and lowering your blood pressure, and aerobic exercise would also be good, whereas lifting weights is not a good idea since it may cause a brief but rapid rise in blood pressure. Walking, swimming or cycling may suit you. Why not have a talk with your GP about how to monitor your own blood pressure at home and during exercise. Breathing exercises are good for you especially if you can do them in front of an open window or better still outdoors, although not if you live in the middle of a polluted city. You already know that cutting out alcohol is a good idea and stress reduction (see p. 481) is a must. If you have a mobile phone you might like to consider getting shot of it. They increase the blood pressure not only of those using them, who are constantly prepared to be interrupted wherever they are, but of those who have to suffer others using them in restaurants, on trains, etc., not to mention the divided concentration of those still trying to drive while having a phone conversation. The emanations from cellular phones may also cause measurable rises in blood pressure. Managing high blood pressure is a lifetime commitment. Don't stop the good work because you feel better. You're feeling better because of all you're doing, so keep it up.

Complementary Therapies

Anything that will reduce stress is useful here (see p. 481). Aromatherapy, reflexology and meditation will help, as will simple breathing exercises. Try relaxing to your favourite piece of gentle music, perhaps in a warm, not hot, lavender-scented bath. Add some blue chamomile oil for a particularly relaxing soak that will reduce your blood pressure and leave you feeling wonderful. If you add to that some soft lights, preferably from candles (but do be careful with them) and follow it by a massage with lavender massage oil, you'll find it very therapeutic. Autogenic training, biofeedback and hypnosis can all give you control over this physiological state which we generally think is automatic and beyond our control. Shiatsu massage has been reported to be useful.

Try to have at least a short period of quiet solitude each day, whether you choose to simply sit alone, mediate, listen to music or pray, since communication, even cordial conversations, can increase your blood pressure. And lastly, have you thought of having a pet? A well-behaved animal that you can stroke and pat can work wonders for you on many levels, not only improving your blood pressure control but boosting your self-esteem as well by feeling loved and loving.

INTEGRATED APPROACH

1. Exercise, dietary and other lifestyle changes can prevent as well as significantly reduce elevated blood pressure.
2. Regular checks of blood pressure after the age of 35 are highly recommended especially if there is a family history of hypertension.
3. Stress management and relaxation exercises can dramatically reduce hypertension if practised regularly.

4. Basic medical investigation of the cause of high blood pressure, once diagnosed, is important and should include blood tests, cholesterol and blood lipid measurement, urine tests, ECG and chest X-ray.
5. Modern medication to lower raised blood pressure can be very effective and is acceptably free of side effects.
6. It is vital to take any prescribed medication on an uninterrupted daily basis, exactly as the doctor has advised, to maintain adequate control of the problem.
7. Make changes to your diet and use complementary techniques to help you live in a more relaxed fashion.

Hypochondriasis

Monica is forever at the doctor's surgery with one minor ailment or another. Nothing serious or even worthy of treatment has even been found and after several years, all of the six doctors at the practice are now thoroughly fed up with having to continually reassure her. She has been referred to a number of different specialists over the years, including psychiatrists, but it has made no difference to the way she feels. Her whole social life revolves around talking about her non-specific symptoms such as headache, backache and abdominal gripes and she still nurses a nagging conviction that the doctors are missing something terrible or that she might have cancer. Monica is an undoubted hypochondriac.

Despite this condition remaining the butt of much medical humour, suffering from hypochondriasis is no fun. The hypochondriac has an unrealistic expectation or obsession that they have a serious condition and, even when it is shown not to be true, despite investigation and medical reassurance, this belief endures. People affected by hypochondiasis worry about their health and bodily functions all the time, and regard any symptom, however trivial, as proof of some life-threatening or serious disorder. Consequently, such people are always making appointments at the doctor's surgery and receiving a battery of tests, investigations and unnecessary treatments as a result. The very fact that they receive such medical attention reinforces in their mind that something really is wrong, yet when they are reassured that nothing has been found, they merely convince themselves that the doctor has either missed something or knows too much and is holding something back. Not surprisingly, hypochondriacs remain anxious and depressed, do not function well socially and cannot get on successfully in their everyday lives. Nevertheless it is in itself a psychological complaint which warrants treatment.

Causes

Sometimes hypochondriacal thoughts may be associated with obsessive–compulsive behaviour or form part of another condition such as depression, anxiety, schizophrenia, dementia or phobias. Other people who have none of these have been brought up by parents who over-relied on medical reassurance or who at a young and formative age were constantly exposed to family members affected by serious disease.

Conventional Treatment

Looking after hypochondriacs is a challenge to the conventional medical fraternity as ignoring them makes them worse, and over-investigating them and being too sympathetic encourages them. A friendly but firm approach is required, involving educating them at every opportunity and teaching them to cope with minor complaints and symptoms as best they can prior to seeking professional help. Sometimes referral to psychologists can be advantageous, and there are specialist clinics in some British hospital psychiatry units where all hypochondriacs are warmly received and given individual and group psychotherapy to good effect. Where an underlying associated condition is found, such as depression or obsessive–compulsive disorder, it is treated appropriately.

Exercise and Lifestyle

It is important to normalise your life as much as possible, following all the basics for good living (see p. 4) as far as you can. Taking regular exercise will reduce the stress associated with this painful illness.

Complementary Therapies

Relaxation techniques will help you take the focus off your physical body and enable you to get things in perspective. Any technique that will help you align mind, body and spirit will help, such as yoga, T'ai chi or Chi gong, all of which will also give you good exercise. Several homeopathic remedies could be helpful. Actaea is indicated if there is also a feeling of depression, as though there is a black cloud hanging over you or a sense of impending doom. If the symptoms are worse at night and with a large anxiety component, then Arsenicum is worth a try. Sometimes those who have hypochondriacal fears feel that they are going crazy, especially since what they perceive is very real to them, but apparently to no one else. Try Calc carb here. If there is a tendency to become hysterical, Ignatia is useful, and Natrum mur will help if there is melancholy with a feeling of being tired of life and just wanting to be left alone with your misery. Sometimes those with hypochondriasis are so positive that there is something wrong which their medical advisers are missing, they can become hostile and argumentative, alienating those around them who are trying to be sympathetic and helpful. Nux vomica may be useful in such cases. The herb valerian can be calming and help with anxiety where there is a fluctuating mood. Aromatherapy oils which may help will be found in the sections on anxiety and depression.

Emotional and Spiritual Healing

To be constantly feeling that there is something wrong with us, to worry that we are going to be ill, or that we are ill and indeed may not survive what we perceive ails us, is a frightening and painful state to be in. Unfortunately the attitude of those around the sufferer often makes matters worse since eventually they cease to even take notice of complaints and ignore the person, which only serves to increase their anxiety even further, and sometimes precipitates hostility and a sense of abandonment. Reassurance works up to a point, but in the end what is needed is a strong but kind approach asking the hypochondriac to look at living with the fear that something is actually wrong. Some psychologists are very adept at such techniques and a referral by the GP would be in order.

It is also useful to find someone whom you respect and know will always be honest with you and make a vow that you will always listen to their counsel and know that they are telling you the truth with your ultimate good in mind. There is an old saying that just because you are paranoid, it does not mean that people are not out to get you. And similarly, just because you're hypochondriacal, it does not mean you cannot get ill. This is why you need to have someone who will listen to you and filter out what is real from what is your hypochondriasis talking, and point you in the right direction when necessary. Sadly sometimes the hypochondriac has cried wolf so many times that no one listens anymore.

Finally have some healing. Although there may not be any physical complaint that is causing your problem, you do have a problem! You are obviously lacking peace and inner calm for you to be in this state, so having a healer to help you align can only be beneficial. In particular, have a look at some grounding exercises to help you be firm and stable and more self-confident with better self-esteem.

If you are the partner or friend of a hypochondriac, try to encourage them to focus on their anxiety itself rather than on any imagined symptoms. By acknowledging the hypochondriasis itself and gaining insight into it, a gradual management programme can be set up involving some desensitisation to trivial symptoms and breaking the dependence on professional reassurance.

Integrated approach

1. All other genuine physical and psychological disorders must first be excluded through thorough examinations and investigations.
2. A firm but sympathetic medical approach is required.
3. Once a diagnosis of hypochondriasis has been made, referral to a specialist clinical psychology unit is appropriate.
4. Exercises to build confidence and self-esteem are important.
5. Find at least one person you trust absolutely and listen to their counsel.

Hysterectomy

Overall, hysterectomy is one of the most common operations performed in Britain, and up to 1 in 5 of all women may undergo this procedure. Hysterectomy is an operation to remove the womb and sometimes the fallopian tubes and ovaries as well. It is an operation many women fear and try to avoid at all costs, although when it is used appropriately it can dramatically improve the quality of life, or even prove life-saving. It need not, as it did too often in the past, change the way a woman feels about herself in terms of her sexuality and femininity. The loss of the organs of reproduction need not induce depression; in fact with adequate counselling women can feel younger, more energetic and revitalised – sexually and otherwise.

Types of Hysterectomy

Total Hysterectomy

A total hysterectomy removes all of the womb including the neck of the womb (the cervix). The ovaries and fallopian tubes are left alone and this type of hysterectomy is the most common type of operation performed.

Hysterectomy with Bi-lateral (Two-Sided) Salpingo-Oophorectomy

This operation removes both the tubes and the ovaries, as well as the uterus. Because removal of the ovaries means that production of female hormones will stop, some surgeons may leave one ovary and one tube, but if not, hormone replacement therapy (HRT) can prevent the consequences of absent female hormones.

Werthheim's or Radical Hysterectomy

Here not only are the uterus, tubes and ovaries removed, but nearby lymph glands and some fatty tissue are excised at the same time. Although this is surgically extensive, it would only be needed for the treatment of a cancer that was in danger of spreading. It would probably be combined with radiotherapy, with or without chemotherapy, and this operation may well be life-saving.

Stella was tired and felt constantly drained. She no longer had any zest for life and at 43 she felt that she could no longer keep up with her husband and take pleasure from the hobbies they had usually enjoyed together. She had been having very heavy periods for a long time and her doctor recommended a hysterectomy some months ago. She thought that she would feel strange about having her womb removed and that she would no longer feel like a woman. However, she finally made the decision to go ahead and was amazed to find that within 3 months of the operation she felt younger, more healthy and more energetic, and her husband commented that she was like her old self.

Why Might it be Needed?

REASONS FOR HAVING A HYSTERECTOMY

fibroids
endometriosis
prolapse
pelvic inflammatory disease
cancer
heavy periods

Mavis is 36 and has had gynaecological problems since puberty. Her periods started late and she was found to have polycystic ovaries when she was investigated for infertility. Over the years she has complained of painful periods with dragging backache and pain during ovulation. Finally she had a laparoscopy which showed that she had endometriosis, with cells from her uterus implanted on her fallopian tubes, ovaries and bowel. After initially trying medication to suppress her periods to see if that helped, her consultant finally recommended a hysterectomy with a bilateral salpingo-oophorectomy, followed by hormone replacement therapy. Mavis had counselling to deal with her sadness that she would be unable to have children and she agreed to the procedure which released her from the monthly pain she had experienced for decades.

FIBROIDS

These are solid, round growths of muscular tissue in the wall of the uterus. They may be single or multiple and up to 20 per cent of women over the age of 30 will have them. They are almost always benign, but as they grow they can interfere with fertility, with periods and with a woman's love life. For some women who have completed their family, who have very frequent and heavy vaginal bleeding, and whose fibroids are growing fast, a hysterectomy is the best possible solution.

ENDOMETRIOSIS

This is a condition where the cells that normally line the cavity of the uterus become established in other parts of the abdominal cavity causing pain and bleeding. Where symptoms are severe, a hysterectomy offers considerable relief.

PROLAPSE

If at all possible, a prolapse of the womb will be surgically repaired vaginally, but in some cases a hysterectomy to remove an enlarged womb and to tighten up slack tissues within the vagina will offer a better result.

PELVIC INFLAMMATORY DISEASE

Where infection has caused scarring of the fallopian tubes and ovaries, infertility, irregular heavy periods and pain may result. Again a hysterectomy can resolve these symptoms.

HEAVY PERIODS

For some women, often around the menopause time, their periods become unpredictable, frequent, painful and extremely heavy. Sometimes this responds to hormone treatments, but these are not normally sufficient nor are they ideal in view of their side effects. Because women can become anaemic, worn out and inconvenienced by their symptoms, a hysterectomy can offer them a much better quality of life. There are alternatives to hysterectomy, however, such as a TCRE (trans-cervical resection of endometrium) which is like a D&C (dilatation and curettage) operation but merely removes a proportion of the lining of the womb that bleeds at period time, resulting in much lighter periods. This is something that can be discussed with the gynaecologist.

Cancer

Hysterectomy is required in the presence of cancer of the cervix, the womb itself or the ovaries. If there is any sign that the cancer may have spread beyond these organs, a Wertheim's or radical hysterectomy would be the operation of choice.

Is Your Hysterectomy Necessary?

It is vital that you are fully informed and counselled before contemplating having a hysterectomy. Any concerns regarding your sexuality and femininity need to be addressed and it is essential that you are included in the decision about whether or not to undergo hysterectomy thus prompting a more satisfactory outcome. You're much less likely to become depressed or resentful about the operation if you make a fully informed choice. It is also less likely that complications will occur. You should be made aware of all the possible alternatives to the operation, and whether or not you will require hormone replacement therapy afterwards.

There are a number of alternative choices to hysterectomy in the conditions listed above, but whereas some can be helpful and avoid the need for surgery, many others will not be sufficient to cope with the symptoms and will merely postpone the inevitable procedure that will ultimately help. It is important to explode any myths, such as that you will have an empty space inside you, that you will become fat, that you will age prematurely or lose your figure. None of these are true if good medical care is obtained. Many gynaecology departments now employ a nurse who specialises in counselling women both prior to and following hysterectomy, and there is no doubt that their role is enormously important in achieving the best result for everyone concerned.

What You Need to Know

Part of the job of the counsellor is to encourage you to talk about your feelings and to tell you about the surgery itself. Hysterectomies can be carried out vaginally in cases of prolapse of the womb, the advantages being that there is no visible scar, that the slack tissue of the vagina can be tightened and that the prolapsing womb is removed. Usually, however, the operation is carried out abdominally resulting in a vertical or horizontal scar about 6–8 inches (15–20cm) long. An advantage of this method is that a surgeon has easy access to the organs concerned and can check other abdominal organs for any problems while the procedure is being carried out.

A counsellor can help you to predict what will happen immediately after the operation and can give you special exercises to practise that will tone up the muscles, prevent thrombosis (blood clots) and get you moving again. You will need advice about hormone replacement therapy, whether it is necessary and if so what type to use. Be assured that your sex life after a hysterectomy can be as good as it was before the operation, if not even better in view of the fact that the reasons for the hysterectomy and for a troubled love life have now disappeared.

A lot depends on your age and health as to how long full recovery takes, but most women are ready to return to normal work after 3 months, and sex may usually be resumed after 4 weeks. It may sound obvious, but you must clearly be aware that you will not be able to have children, that you will have no periods and that you will not need any contraception after the operation.

Emotional and Spiritual Healing

So much needs to be said about hysterectomy that a whole book could be dedicated to it. This is a time when you would be wise to ask for a second opinion and to weigh all the pros and cons. It may be that hysterectomy is the only way forward and if so, then you need to take time to prepare yourself well. The most sensitive and beautiful thoughts on hysterectomy that we have ever come across are in Christianne Northrup's wonderful book, *Women's Bodies, Women's Wisdom* (Piatkus, 1995) which we would recommend that you read. It deals with the emotional and spiritual preparation for the loss of a part of yourself that has been a major aspect of your womanhood, whether or not you have borne children, whether or not you are now at the point that it is giving you problems and you have to make the decision to let it go. It would be a good idea to spend some time with someone you can trust to allow you to put into words your feelings about your womb and what it has meant to you. As a nest for your babies, a place which along with your ovaries has guaranteed your femininity, it has been one of the essentials of being a woman. Should you have had difficulties gynaecologically, or if you have been abused in some way, you may have very different feelings. You may have felt angry with your womanhood and those feelings may surface now, often with some relief that you can rid yourself of that part of you at last. Whatever your feelings, now is the time to allow yourself to feel them, to acknowledge them in your life and finally to heal them and let them go.

Before your surgery spend some time sending healing to the whole of your pelvic region, visualise light there (orange light would be good), cleansing, healing and balancing your womb, tubes and ovaries, and ensuring that there will be healing and health after the surgery has taken place (see the sacral chakra, p. 539). Be aware that there may be feelings of grief afterwards, and that this is perfectly normal. But the more work you can do beforehand the less likely there are to be emotional consequences. Try to have someone with you, both immediately before and immediately after your surgery, who is in tune with your feelings and if you feel that you would like a ceremony focusing on the loss of your womb, then she can validate that with you. Don't let anyone rush you and ensure that you have both emotional and practical support afterwards. To have someone who cares for you, to make a cup of tea, a bowl of soup, wrap you in a blanket and put an arm around you is so healing in itself. When all is over, there's no reason why you shouldn't be able to give thanks for renewed vigour and move into a new phase of your life happily and healthily.

So let's have a look at what else you can do both before and after the operation.

Nutritional Healing

If fibroids are the problem, then a high protein diet may help reduce their size, especially if the protein comes from vegetable sources such as peas and beans. Soya will help in any form, as will increased fibre in your diet. Citrus fruits and berries containing high levels of Vitamin C are also helpful. Try to avoid meat, diet drinks, refined sugar and fat. If there has been excessive bleeding, your doctor will probably prescribe iron, and dark green leafy vegetables will be good for you. Also try some extra ginger and garlic in your cooking. If there is no choice but surgery, then prepare yourself well (see Surgery, p. 29).

Vitamins and Supplements

Vitamins C and E are indicated here along with the other supplements mentioned for menstrual problems on p. 379 and for surgery p. 29. Ensure that through this period you adhere to all of the recommendations on p. 4 (Basics for Good Living).

Exercise and Lifestyle

Whatever you do keep as active as you can! Walking daily will strengthen all your muscles including those of your pelvic floor which will help in your recovery and your ability to enjoy sex afterwards. See p. 518 for Kegel exercises which would be particularly useful pre-surgery. Pelvic tilts will also prepare your muscles and help you in the post-operative phase. If surgery can't be avoided, get back to some gentle exercise as soon as your surgeon gives the OK.

But do be sensible, take plenty of rest with your feet up and a good book and gradually return to whatever activity you enjoy. You may well find that if you've been dragged down by heavy periods and pain, you have a new lease of life. Why not take this opportunity of getting yourself really physically fit now that you have a head start? One close friend who had a hysterectomy in her late forties over 30 years ago began dancing as soon as she felt well enough to do so after her surgery. In her seventies she is happy, healthy and still dances 3 or 4 times a week, has no sign of osteoporosis and loves her life. She feels that her hysterectomy, which at last freed her from the pain and excessive bleeding that had restricted her in so many ways, was one of the best things that ever happened to her.

Complementary Therapies

Don quai has a beneficial effect on the whole female reproductive system. Other herbs you may find useful are red raspberry leaf, ladies' mantle, yarrow and motherwort. Shepherd's purse may help control bleeding whereas white ash can reduce the size of fibroids. The homeopathic remedy that is most useful in reducing the size of fibroids is Aurum muriatium. Acupuncture may also help. On p. 29 you'll find recommendations for preparing for surgery and for afterwards. They are all relevant here.

INTEGRATED APPROACH

1. Take time to get a second opinion if you wish and look at all the pros and cons of having surgery.
2. In the meantime use acupuncture, herbs, and other remedies to try to curb the problem.
3. When a decision to have surgery has been made, prepare yourself well with diet, supplements and exercise.
4. Spend some time preparing yourself emotionally and spiritually for your hysterectomy, either alone or preferably with someone who understands you and your feelings.

5. Have someone with you pre- and post-surgery who can validate your feelings and support you emotionally and practically.
6. Return to a healthy lifestyle as soon as possible.
7. Give thanks for your survival and renewed fitness.

Infections

Most of the infections that trouble the British population these days are of a fairly mild nature. We are all subjected to the common cold, sinusitis, tonsillitis, thrush and boils at some time or another. Yet it was not so very long ago that infections were of a much more serious nature, at a time, for example, when pneumonia, diphtheria, scarlet fever and osteomyelitis (infection of the bone) were so rife that they were a major cause of illness and death. In fact in the third world, infections that we regard here as treatable and preventable are responsible for millions of deaths each year.

Nevertheless, in Britain we must still be aware of the sometimes dreadful consequences of serious illnesses such as meningitis, encephalitis (inflammation of the brain), pelvic inflammatory disease, tuberculosis and AIDS, for example. All of us are potentially subject to any of these infections so it behoves every one of us to try to keep our health in tip-top condition if we are to avoid contact with the micro-organisms responsible. To give ourselves every possible chance of fighting infections should we come across them, we must keep our immune system in as healthy a condition as possible (see p. 535).

Types of Organisms Responsible

Most infections are caused by bacteria, viruses or fungi. But there are other less common germs such as rickettsia (responsible for infections such as typhus), micaplasma (infections such as TB) and chlamydia (infections such as pelvic inflammatory disease in women). There are also other types of micro-organisms, such as single-celled protazoa, worms and flukes, that can invade our bodies.

Susie was aware that she had hurt her foot when playing in the sea while on holiday. She looked at the cut briefly and put an adhesive dressing on it. On the flight back she became conscious of a throbbing in her foot and was aghast to find when she got home that the area was swollen and inflamed. Her doctor needed to incise the abscess to remove pus and also put her on antibiotics. He reminded her to take some peroxide with her on holiday next time and to be careful to cleanse all wounds very carefully before dressing them.

Brad gave a party a few days ago and encouraged his girlfriend to come along even though she complained of having a sore throat. This morning he awoke with pain in his throat especially on swallowing, swellings in the glands in his neck and a temperature. His doctor diagnosed a throat infection caused by streptococcus and recommended salt gargles and penicillin.

Infections may be transmitted through water, food, air, blood, skin contact, by insects, by sexual transmission and by transmission across the placenta from mother to baby. Once within the body, the micro-organisms either damage the body's cells directly or cause inflammation as a result of the toxins that they produce. Our bodies then mount a resistance using our immune system, and it is the battle between our immune system and the infection which is responsible for many of the signs and symptoms of that particular disease. If you want to know more about your immune system, see Appendix 1.

Candida (thrush)

An unhealthy diet, stress or antibiotic treatment can result in an eradication of the useful bacteria in the gut and an overgrowth of the natural yeast cells that inhabit the vagina and surrounding areas as well as the intestinal tract. This can result in candida, either locally in and around the genital organs or more widely spread throughout the gut. Symptoms include diarrhoea, constipation, lethargy, weight gain, food cravings (especially for sweet things), as well as itching around the vagina and anus and a vaginal discharge that resembles cottage cheese.

Although the vaginal infection can be cleared very quickly (see p. 320), the systemic infection needs special care.

* Herb teas to soothe vaginal irritation: ginger root, horsetail, Oregon grape, uva ursi.
* Stop sugar in any form and have no fruit for 3 weeks.
* Avoid all dairy products (except butter), gluten, wheat, oats, yeast (in all forms, including bread), alcohol, commercially prepared foods, Marmite, roasted nuts, vinegar, soya, ginger beer, tamari, miso soup, vitamin and mineral supplements containing yeast, spices and dried foods, deep-fried foods.

Vaginal Yeast Infections

* These are associated with reduced acidity in the vagina and excess sugar in that area. After sex, always cleanse the whole area carefully.
* Use natural antifungals such as garlic taken internally, grapefruit seed extract or artemisia, or ask your doctor for a pack which usually contains one pessary and some cream.
* Pro-biotics such as lactobacillus and bifidus help restore natural flora.
* Take capryllic acid which is available as capsules or pessaries.
* Have garlic, eaten raw, cooked or taken as a tablet.
* Thyme and oregano oils can be diluted and used as a wipe, or put them in your bath and soak. Add them to your cooking, fresh if possible.

Symptoms

Initially, during the incubation period (that is, the time between your exposure to germs and the time when symptoms start), although you're capable of transmitting the infection to someone else, you won't feel ill. Later, if the infection becomes generalised throughout the body, or 'systemic' as doctors call it, there will be a fever, aching joints, muscular weakness, headache and malaise. If the infection remains localised to one organ, system or part of the body, there will be pain, redness, swelling, fever and possible abscess formation. There may also be restriction of the function of the part of the body affected, although much depends on the exact location.

Diagnosis

Clinically your doctor can obtain a great deal of information both by listening to you and through his initial examination. If you've been abroad to a tropical country or have been exposed to suspicious food or contaminated water, this is of course relevant. If you've been to a malaria-affected country and didn't take an antimalaria preparation, then the search for the cause becomes more complex. Specimens of infected tissues or body fluids can be examined in a laboratory and it may also be necessary to take samples of serum to measure antibodies to various infections. If the cause of an infection remains undetermined by simple means, further tests such as X-rays and scans may be necessary.

Prevention of Infection

Few people die in Britain from infection these days because with better sanitation, pest control, housing, water purification and personal hygiene; generally we have learned to avoid contact with infectious micro-organisms in the first place. Antibiotics, which only became available during the Second World War, have saved millions of lives, as has vaccination against some of the world's greatest killers. Diseases such as smallpox have even been eradicated worldwide through the process of immunisation. Combined with better general health and nutrition, these factors have made death today from infection a relatively rare thing. However, we must not be complacent. Resistance to antibiotics is increasing, resulting in much more virulent and fulminating infections; there are many micro-organisms which cannot be vaccinated against, such as some types of meningitis, and in some parts of the world, resistance to malaria preventatives and treatments for tuberculosis has resulted in increasing levels of disease. Furthermore, if we are to curtail the death rate from the massive spread of some infections such as AIDS which require an alteration in human behaviour, we need mass educational campaigns.

All of us must remember the basics of good hygiene:

* Washing hands after going to the toilet is essential.
* Cuts and grazes must be cleansed aseptically.
* Regular dental appointments prevent transmission of germs from the mouth into the bloodstream.
* Immunisation is extremely safe and confers protection against many disabling or fatal diseases.
* Food should be stored and prepared in clean conditions.
* Water purification must be of the highest order.
* Contact with animals and their secretions must be made with caution.
* When travelling abroad do take your antimalarial treatment, protect yourself from insect bites and have whatever inoculations you need to protect you from infections that are more prevalent in hot countries.
* The use of condoms is a simple, cheap and effective way to protect against sexually transmitted diseases.

Wound Healing

If we're in good health, then we have all that we need within ourselves to heal most wounds, although large wounds or those of a crushing nature usually need expert care. The basics are to keep the wound clean (hydrogen peroxide cleans wounds admirably), to have the cut surfaces brought together as much as possible and to have good circulation to the wound to help the growth of new tissue.

It has been said that aloe vera accelerates wound healing faster than anything else on the market. It can be applied locally, to scars to help them fade, or taken internally. It can even reduce the inflammation caused by radiation therapy and will increase circulation in those with peripheral vascular disease when taken internally.

Tea tree oil diluted with a carrier oil and applied direct to cuts and scrapes is a good natural disinfectant which is both antibacterial and antifungal. It is able to fight staphylococcal infections that are antibiotic-resistant, yet without affecting the normal skin flora (healthy bacteria that are found on the skin). It may sting a little as you apply it. A drop of lavender oil applied directly to a clean wound will also promote healing and of course there is the old standby, Dr Bach's Rescue Cream. Echinacea as an oil, tincture or tea is another disinfectant which simultaneously stimulates the immune system and can be applied directly to cuts and other lesions. Calendula has anti-inflammatory properties as well as hastening wound healing. It can be applied as a cream, oil or tincture. Vitamins A, D and E are also good when applied as dressings or creams while Vitamin C is better taken internally in high doses (1000 mg every 3 hours or so for severe wounds and burns). Organic honey applied to small wounds will help keep them clean and promote healing. Similarly sugar applied to a clean dressing and changed twice daily will clean a wound or minor infection.

Ozone therapy is popular in some areas of the world and can be used in different ways. As a local application the therapy includes placing a bag containing ozone over the wound so that it can be absorbed. It accelerates wound healing and is an antiviral and antibacterial agent. However, it can also be used as an intravenous therapy where a little of the patient's blood is removed, is mixed with a small amount of ozone and then reintroduced into the patient. It has been found effective not only in promoting wound healing but in cleansing the wound by carrying extra oxygen to the site, fighting infection and improving circulation. It is said to be effective in the treatment of cancer. Ozone can also be given rectally.

Although most wounds are sustained accidentally, we are lucky to be have the opportunity to prepare ourselves if the wound is to be inflicted because of surgery. If this is the case, see p. 29, Surgery.

Nutritional Healing, Vitamins and Supplements

It would be wise to pay particular attention to your nutrition since your requirements will be different when you have tissues to repair. Increase your intake of protein and add natural sources of zinc where possible (see p. 545). Also take extra garlic. Fruit and vegetable juices will give you concentrated vitamins, chlorophyll, antioxidants and other goodies. Try mixing fruits such as kiwi, strawberries, bilberry and orange; and vegetables such as carrot, celery and beetroot. Soup made from natural antivirals such as garlic, onions, ginger, broccoli, carrots, cabbage, mushrooms and beetroot, will be soothing and healing. This is one of those times when you will probably need extra supplements, so add Vitamins A, B, C and E for starters along with extra zinc if necessary and magnesium. Zinc lozenges can ease coughs and shorten the duration of sore throats and the common cold. Try to get time-release Vitamin C with bioflavinoids. Echinacea will bolster your immune system and help wound healing if applied topically, but avoid in autoimmune disorders such as lupus or MS.

Exercise and Lifestyle

A positive mental attitude, good food, supplements, adequate rest and antibiotics if you really need them should soon have you over your difficulty. Take exercise, reducing the intensity somewhat until you feel stronger. Keep your stress down as much as possible since stress can significantly affect the immune system and delay healing. If you're going to be outside, cover scars with sunblock since they may burn easily and are also prone to develop skin cancer more easily than the rest of your skin.

Complementary Therapies

Traditional medicine generally aims to kill the organism that has infected you, whereas complementary medicine tries to help you kill it yourself. It also protects against further infection by facilitating your natural healing processes and boosting your immune system. If you have a fever, have lots of juices and try herb teas including elderflower, thyme, chamomile or linden. Suck ice to bring your temperature down and if necessary use tepid sponging. Homeopathic remedies to try include Ferrum phos, Aconite, Belladonna and Bryonia. Reflexology may also help. For the prevention of colds and flu, try a mixture of antiviral herbs such as astralgus, boldo leaf, jalapeno, cayenne and rose hips made into a tea.

INTEGRATED APPROACH

1. Prevent infection wherever possible by using good hygiene.
2. Discuss preventative measures such as immunisation and prophylaxis with your doctor.
3. Clean any wounds with care and protect with clean dressings.
4. If you have an infection, look after yourself. That means eating a healthy diet, drinking lots of fluids and resting.
5. Have a proper diagnosis made by your doctor.
6. If you have a cold or flu stay away from areas such as the work environment where you may spread the infection.
7. Keep your immune system healthy.

Infertility

Most couples consider trying for a baby and a woman may get pregnant relatively easily. However, for some it can take quite a while, often between 6 months and 2 years. In fact, 1 in 6 couples in Britain have trouble conceiving, and many of them require help and treatment in order to do so. Women over 35 who have tried to start a family without success for more than 6 months should therefore consult a doctor to see what the problem might be. Often an infertility problem is compounded by the fact that friends of roughly the same age are starting families without difficulty. However, help is at hand. Perhaps the first step is to ensure that both the man and the woman are in peak condition, and there is much they can do themselves to achieve this.

Preparation for Pregnancy

Women should have a blood test to ensure they are immune to rubella (German measles). Many women are uncertain whether they have been made immune by natural infection in the past, and if there is any doubt a blood test will clarify this. If you have no antibodies to rubella, you should definitely have a vaccination which protects against rubella since contracting this during pregnancy can damage the baby. You should then take contraceptive precautions for 3 months after the vaccination to prevent any possible damage to a baby conceived straight afterwards. Also, women should take 400 mcg of folic acid (folate) every day from the time contraception is stopped, up until the 12th week of pregnancy, as this reduces significantly the risk of the baby having neural tube defects such as spina bifida.

Valerie is 36 and has been married for 7 years, during the last 5 of which she and her husband have been trying to have a baby. She complains that her periods have been regular but difficult since her mid-twenties. They are usually accompanied by quite severe abdominal pain, dragging backache, nausea and cramps. She feels bloated and bleeding is heavier than it used to be. Although she has been having intercourse regularly, she admits that it is no longer pleasurable because of pain while making love. After a laparoscopy, her diagnosis is confirmed. Valerie has endometriosis which is the cause of her infertility.

Women who may have been exposed to a sexually transmitted infection, either recently or in the past, should have a check-up at a genito-urinary medicine clinic (GUMC) since sometimes this may reveal asymptomatic chlamydial infection which may be causing inflammation of the fallopian tubes and preventing the passage of the egg from the ovaries to the womb. Attendance at a GUMC can be anonymous if you wish.

The most fertile time for love-making

Women release an egg from the ovary some 12–16 days before the next expected period. The egg survives for roughly a day, although sperm can live for up to 7 days. Knowledge of the menstrual cycle is therefore helpful in that you can work out the most fertile time to make love. The menstrual cycle starts on the first day of a period, and ends the day before the next period starts. So count back 12–16 days from when the next period is due to start as this is the most fertile time. Fluid from the vagina (cervical mucus) becomes thinner at this time, more slippery and wetter, and this provides a further clue. You can buy ovulation predictor tests from chemists which will test ovulation from a urine sample, but they are of limited value if your periods are irregular or if your menstrual cycle is very short or very long.

According to Oriental medicine it's best to avoid sexual intercourse during menstruation and adopting the missionary position (man on top) gives you the best chance of impregnation. It has been said that using egg white as a lubricant has a beneficial effect on sperm motility (active movement) and survival.

Causes for Concern

If after carrying out all the above checks you don't conceive, you may wish to see your doctor, or even earlier if you have any particular reasons to worry. If you have irregular periods or very short or long cycles or find love-making painful, you would do well to be medically advised.

Shelley, now 28, had a severe pelvic infection in her mid-teens. Now she and her boyfriend are having difficulty in conceiving the child they both desperately want. Having tried for almost 2 years they have embarked upon investigation, which has found that her boyfriend has a good sperm count with good motility. However, a hystero-salpingogram shows that Shelley's fallopian tubes are blocked (a hystero-salpingogram is a special X-ray which shows the outline of the fallopian tubes and uterus).

Previous pelvic infection, abdominal surgery, sexually transmitted disease or being very under- or over-weight can reduce fertility. If Shelley was over the age of 35, her fertility would also be waning naturally. Men who have had testicular problems such as cancer or an undescended testicle may like to seek reassurance, as should men who are very overweight, who have had mumps with testicular swelling after puberty or who have had sexually transmitted infections. Doctors can advise on all these issues and either reassure you or commence investigations.

Tests or Investigations

Tests on the woman include:

* Blood and urine tests, to measure hormone levels and the presence or absence of ovulation. Cervical mucus tests and temperature charts can also indicate ovulation but are less reliable.
* Ultrasound scans, to determine whether eggs are being released from follicles in the ovary.

* Post-coital tests, to ascertain whether a woman's cervical mucus is allowing her partner's sperm to penetrate into the womb.

* Endometrial biopsy, which takes a sample of womb lining to ensure the absence of infection and that ovulation is occurring.

* A salpingogram, which involves the passage of a dye (which shows up on X-ray) into the uterus and along the fallopian tubes to see whether the tubes are patent (accessible) and allowing the eggs to move along the central canal. A hystero-salpingogram examines the uterus at the same time.

* A laparoscopy under general anaesthetic, which involves passing a narrow telescope-like instrument through a small incision below the navel so that the reproductive organs can be viewed directly by the surgeon to identify possible problems. These may include: scar tissue, fibroids, abnormalities in the overall position of the womb, ovaries or fallopian tubes, and endometriosis, a condition where the cells that normally line the uterus spill out, covering the ovaries and tubes and causing inflammation and scarring.

The simpler tests can be organised by your family doctor and the more invasive and more complicated tests are available at the local NHS gynaecology or infertility clinic.

Being Realistic

Neither infertility treatment which results in natural conception nor assisted conception techniques are miracle cures and the results depend largely on the age of the woman and the reasons for which she is seeking treatment. The overall success rate in the various infertility clinics is somewhere in the region of 15–30 per cent. Couples may find infertility treatment particularly stressful. Counselling is essential to find out what the treatment involves, how you feel about it and how much support exists. Organisations such as Child and Issue are tremendously helpful in this regard.

Find out before you start fertility treatment what kind of tests are involved, what treatments are available, what restrictions might be imposed, how long the waiting lists are and how often the clinic will need to be attended and at what times of the day. Find out about the costs and what they include. Find out what is involved in the treatment and if there are any risks involved. Ask about the second stage of treatment should the first be unsuccessful, and get help from patient support groups, which can advise where you can obtain counselling. Finally, obtain an accurate idea of the success rate for the different treatments and, if necessary, for the assisted conception treatments mentioned below. Remember that private clinics have different success rates and it is useful to compare these before deciding where to go for treatment. Always write down a list of questions you wish to ask the specialist as it may be some time before your next appointment.

Assisted Conception

Sometimes there is a limit to the amount of treatment you can receive on the NHS. About 80 per cent of *in vitro* fertilisation (IVF) treatment is carried out privately. Your GP, practice nurse or local Community Health Council can advise you as to your eligibility. A more direct approach would be to contact the Human Fertilisation and Embryology Authority (HSEA), which can supply a copy of its patients' guide to the National Infertility Awareness Campaign (see Useful Addresses). This has very good information for couples who have no option but to go privately but who have problems with funding.

Assisted conception is required when a couple fail to be helped to have a child naturally.

In vitro fertilisation (IVF) is the best-known of these techniques, involving removal of eggs from the woman and their fertilisation in the laboratory using her husband's sperm. The fertilised egg or embryo is replaced into her womb where hopefully implantation will occur.

Donor insemination (DI) uses sperm from an anonymous donor and this is carried out where the partner's sperm is not of sufficient quantity or quality.

Gamete intrafallopian transfer (GIFT) uses the couple's own sperm and eggs or those of donors which are mixed together and then placed in the woman's fallopian tubes where fertilisation hopefully occurs.

Introcytoplasmic sperm injection (ICSI) involves the injection of a single sperm into the woman's egg which is later transferred to the womb after fertilisation.

Nutrition

Good nutrition is essential. Although there are specific considerations for men and women, both would be wise to eat as many natural, whole, unprocessed foods as possible with no additives and completely free of pesticides and herbicides. Clean, purified water is essential, especially for men, since even tap water is polluted with oestrogens following the advent of the oral contraceptive. Large amounts of oestrogen now find their way into our water systems. Add to this the fact that livestock are fed oestrogens to fatten them and it's no wonder that the sperm counts of men throughout the world, and of many animals too, have declined over the last 30 years. Fruit and vegetables high in antioxidants and bioflavinoids (such as broccoli, cauliflower, green peppers, parsley and citrus fruits) are of course essential, but even more so for men (see below). Both men and women with fertility problems should cut down on caffeine intake. If either are of you are overweight this would be a good time to trim down a bit.

Men need to eat more whole grains and fibre. We've all heard about oysters being an aphrodisiac, but whether that's so or not, they do contain a lot of zinc which will help increase sperm count and motility. Other zinc-containing foods include lean red meat and crab. Reishi mushrooms are good for sperm health.

Vitamins and Supplements

Both of you need a good multivitamin and multimineral supplement. Gingko biloba will improve circulation to the reproductive organs as well as everywhere else. Men should, add an antioxidant or Vitamin C up to 3000 mg daily and 800 mg of Vitamin E daily which will improve sperm motility and count. Since sperm are made almost entirely of DNA, free radical damage can be particularly harmful to their production and development. Vitamin D, folic acid (folate) and Vitamin B_{12} would be useful as well as selenium and beta carotene. A zinc supplement will help especially if testosterone levels are low. Carnitine also increases sperm count and motility. Ginseng and pygeum africanum will improve general vitality. For women, Vitamins C, B_6, B_{12} and folic acid (folate) are essential, with an iron supplement only if your GP has found your iron to be low. Colloidal silver will cleanse the whole reproductive system and especially clear chlamydia, an infection that often gives no symptoms to warn you of its presence. A simple urine test annually will screen you for the presence of chlamydia infection, a very common sexually transmitted disease (see p. 447).

Exercise and Lifestyle

Both of you would be wise to reduce stress to a minimum and get enough restful sleep. You should both cut down on alcohol intake, stop smoking and also stop the use of any recreational drugs such as marijuana or cocaine. Should either of you have any chronic infection, have it treated.

SMOKING AND ITS EFFECTS ON FERTILITY AND CHILDBIRTH

If you have any doubt about stopping smoking and need a bit of a push, the following information may help. Smoking decreases sperm quality and motility. Women who smoke may pass on genetic mutations to their offspring, putting their babies at risk of cancer later in life. Women who smoke during pregnancy also run a higher risk of miscarriage, giving birth prematurely or having a stillborn infant. Babies born to mothers who smoke are smaller than average and run a higher risk of dying from Sudden Infant Death Syndrome (SIDS), also known as Cot Death. Also check your prescription drugs for their side effects.

Dave is a weight trainer and he exercises every day. He enjoys competition and takes anabolic steroids to help his muscle development. He and Susan have been trying to have a baby for about 3 years. Susan underwent a variety of investigations and was found to be healthy. Dave's sperm count was found to be low. He was advised to discontinue his use of anabolic steroids for a few months, to train only 3 times a week, to wear looser-fitting underwear and jeans and to have cold showers regularly. His sperm count increased in a few months to the point that they were able to conceive.

As Dave found, men would benefit from keeping their scrotal temperature down by wearing loose underwear and keeping cool. If you work in the garden with pesticides or herbicides or use solvents at work, wear a mask and be careful to wash very carefully afterwards. Viral illnesses especially if associated with a fever can depress sperm production for 3 months or more, so if you've had such an illness, be patient and take care of yourself. Sperm production should recover. Anabolic steroids can reduce sperm count as can pollution with heavy metals. If you're an exercise fanatic, try to cut back a bit since excessive exercise can elevate prolactin levels to the point that they depress ovulation. Incorporating some exercise such as T'ai Chi, yoga or Chi gong into your daily routine will have a marked effect on your whole wellbeing.

Complementary Therapies

Acupuncture will help clear blocks that may be interfering with your ability to conceive, while anything that will help destress you (see p. 481) will be beneficial. There are several herbs that may help, including red raspberry leaf, which acts as a tonic for whole reproductive system, fennel and anise which increase fertility, and don quai which increases female vitality. Homeopathy offers among other things Sabina, Sepia and Lycopodium. Bach Flower Remedies and Australian Bush Essences could help, in particular pomegranate which balances the female reproductive system. Reflexology and Traditional Chinese Medicine may also be of value. Sitz baths are an old remedy which help detoxify the pelvic organs and although they are rather laborious, you may like to try them. You need a bath of hot water in which you can sit with your arms and legs out of the water, and close by a smaller bath in which you put cold water enough to simply sit your bottom in, the water coming up just to your lower abdomen. You need to alternate between the two, having a few minutes in each for about 15 minutes in all, 3 or 4 times a day. Don't expect results quickly. It may take several months during which time you shouldn't have unprotected intercourse since you'll be releasing all sorts of toxins from your uterus, fallopian tubes, etc. You might find that you develop a discharge as old products of infection, scar tissue or retained products from menstruation start to be released. This is a good sign although it might not be very pleasant. Before we had modern surgical techniques or antibiotics, this was one of the few remedies open to women whose tubes were blocked and it often worked.

Emotional and Spiritual Healing

Being beset with the natural desire to have a child and being unable to conceive is not only painful but frustrating, and leaves many women leapfrogging from one month to the next, their whole lives revolving around their period and whether or not it will appear this month. So much of the joy of the present and of the other blessings in life are lost including the joy of making love because it feels good, using sex as a healing crowning of the love they have for their partner, and gaining from it comfort and closeness. In some couples sexual intercourse becomes a researched, planned, timed and charted scientific experiment devoid of emotion, being evaluated only by the result (or not) of conception. If this is where you find yourself, it's time to stand back and have a good look at what you really want and what has happened to the feelings that brought the two of you together in the first place. It's time for some counselling, some professional support and perhaps some group therapy to help you get it in perspective and take the tension out of it. It's time to relax! Some therapy will also help you deal with the anger and resentment that arises and the tendency to blame each other for the deficiency which results in your not being able to have a child . . . yet. There is more chance of that happening when you start to live a more balanced, fulfilled and creative life.

One of the questions that needs to be answered is whether or not you really want a child.

Roy and Andrea have been talking about having a family ever since they came together 5 years ago. Roy is 10 years older than Andrea and has two adolescent children from his first marriage. Andrea, also previously married, has never had children. Tests showed that both were fit and healthy and that there was no physical reason for Andrea not to conceive. A joint counselling session revealed that Roy was somewhat ambivalent about starting a new family despite the fact that he loves Andrea and wants to please her. After some therapy, Roy fully committed himself to the relationship and Andrea became pregnant within a few months.

As Roy and Andrea found, ambivalence can often be sorted out, but it is better to do so now and to face the facts if one of you doesn't really want a family.

Sometimes there is unspoken fear about being a parent and coping with the extra responsibility especially if you've had some trauma which has left you feeling needy and sometimes like a child yourself. Low self-esteem can often make us think we are unworthy to be a parent, and any history of sexual abuse can result in a subconscious fear that we ourselves may similarly abuse a child. Bearing in mind that body, mind and spirit are so intimately involved, our minds and spirits can profoundly affect the functioning of our bodies. If there are any unresolved issues from your own childhood, these may be causing you to subconsciously block your ability to conceive.

There are many wonderful healers who combine psychotherapy and spiritual healing and this may be the time to find one of them. Try to get your partner to come along too, at least at first, so that you have support and so that your therapist can meet and assess your partner as well. We have known healing alone to result in pregnancy shortly thereafter, although whether this is due to general healing and relaxation or some divine intervention, it's not for us to say. You have nothing to lose and potentially much to gain!

There comes a time for many couples when they have to come to terms with the fact that despite full investigation and treatment, with or without vast expense, they have to accept that it may fail. Once fertility treatment has ended, adoption may be a possibility and the local Social Services department and the British Agencies for Adoption and Fostering can then advise on your eligibility and the procedures that have to be followed (see Useful Addresses). You may be surprised at how utterly and completely you can love a child who is not biologically yours so do consider this if all else fails. Another possibility is fostering, enabling you to look after children when their own parents temporarily cannot be there to care for them. As for the couple themselves, acceptance of their infertility can involve a devastating grief-like reaction that can seriously affect their quality of life. Organisations such as Issue can be very helpful to them in this situation, getting them to come to terms with everything, and encouraging them to enjoy life without children of their own in the future.

INTEGRATED APPROACH

1. Take care of yourself pre-pregnancy and have tests etc. that may highlight any problems.
2. Have a well-balanced diet, vitamins and supplements where necessary and clean water.
3. Avoid pesticides, herbicides and pollution as much as possible.

4. Avoid excessive exercise and the use of anabolic steroids.
5. Use complementary therapies to improve your general health and vitality as well as your potency.
6. Have counselling or psychotherapy to sort out any underlying psychological issues.
7. Have proper investigations and explore methods of assisting you to conceive.
8. If all else fails, don't forget that there are many children who are available for adoption and longing for loving parents.

❧ ME

ME is short for myalgic encephalomyelitis which translated into layman's terms means muscle pain with inflammation of the brain and nerves. This is in fact a total misnomer as there is no detectable inflammation of the brain and nerves, so doctors now tend to use alternative terminology. It is more likely that doctors will refer to ME as chronic fatigue syndrome (CFS), post-viral fatigue syndrome (PVFS) or persistent viral disease (PVD).

Symptoms

The diagnosis is based on certain key findings. There is severe fatigue which is always brought about by exercise and this includes muscle weakness and pain, with or without twitching of the muscles, which starts up to 72 hours after activity and lasts for at least 24 hours. There are also at least two of the following symptoms: impaired concentration, short-term memory loss, disturbed sleep, feelings of detachment from one's surroundings and unpredictable mood swings. Furthermore, these symptoms will fluctuate at different times during the day. When the above symptomatology has persisted for at least 3 months and other recognisable causes have been excluded, it is reasonable to assume that the patient is suffering from ME.

Reyna complained of feeling unwell for about 8 months. She had a recurrent sore throat with painful swollen glands in her neck, a feeling of generalised weakness and pain in her muscles which disappeared from time to time only to return. She also had painful joints, although her main complaint was of tiredness. She found that if she exerted herself at all she would feel so fatigued that the following day she would be unable to do her housework and would have to spend much of the day in bed. She felt listless and depressed and felt that her family were starting to ridicule the fact that she would be too tired in the evening to wash up and no longer wanted to join her husband in taking the children to the park at the weekends. She was feeling ashamed of the state of her home and the fact that she could never catch up on the endless pile of ironing.

Reyna demonstrates the fact that there may be an extraordinary array of symptoms in this illness, and indeed they also vary enormously in different individuals. If you have overwhelming fatigue and weariness, flu-like symptoms, including mild fever, headaches, sore throat, aching muscles and enlarged tender glands, insomnia, short-term memory loss, poor concentration and mood swings, then it may be that you are suffering from ME. Depression is a major feature in many sufferers. All these symptoms tend to be more apparent after exercise, either physical or mental, and most cases of ME can be linked with a recent viral infection such as glandular fever, sickness and diarrhoea or flu. In many ways it is a puzzling disorder but many researchers believe that ME arises as an abnormal reaction to a viral infection and may have something to do with an inappropriate response of the immune system.

Diagnosis

One of the problems of diagnosing ME is that many doctors still fail to recognise it as a real illness. This is partly because there is no single diagnostic test and partly because of a lack of physical evidence that there is any underlying or organic abnormality. Despite this, some 150,000 people in Britain are thought to have ME, and the average doctor will have as many as 40 patients on his list suffering from it at any one time. Women seem to be more prone than men, although it affects all ages and social classes. One in six cases develop before the age of 18.

If you suspect you may be suffering from ME, you first need to find a doctor who believes in the existence of this condition and who will listen to your symptoms in order to put a clinical picture together.

Conventional Treatment

Unfortunately at the present time there is no cure and no absolute consensus by the medical profession on how the disorder should be best treated. The majority of sufferers should fully recover within 2–5 years, but the longer it seems to last the worse the outlook is. Once a diagnosis has been reached, support both psychologically and physically is as much as conventional medicine can offer. However, this is not so in the field of complementary medicine.

Nutritional Healing

Nutrition is often underestimated or neglected as a healing aid. ME calls for high-quality food, fresh and whole, unadulterated and organic if possible. The rules of the basic eating plan (p. 5) need only a little adjustment here. Have plenty of complex carbohydrates, whole grains, nuts, seeds and protein from soya, tofu and beans. Use plenty of onions, garlic and ginger in your cooking, making nutritious, easily digestible soups with fresh vegetables and a little fish, chicken or turkey. Try including some seaweed to add iodine to help your thyroid gland and some reishi mushrooms. If desired, you could add some fish, preferably salmon, herrings, sardines, tuna or mackerel. Fresh vegetables can be juiced and drunk whenever you wish, boosting your immune system, cleansing your system and giving you energy. Fresh juices are an instant source of nutrients, which can be easily digested. Try carrot, celery and beetroot together, or something more exotic like dandelion leaves, cucumber and spinach or cabbage. However, dilute it well since it's potent stuff and will detoxify your whole system. Drink it in small quantities throughout the day to boost your immune system.

Although you might feel that the caffeine in coffee helps lift your energy, it only makes things worse in the long run, so wean yourself off it and replace it with purified water and herbal teas or a little aloe vera juice. Try to have small frequent meals with a snack in between and try to choose something like oat cakes, rice cakes or cereal and fruit (particularly kiwis and other fruits high in Vitamin C) to maintain a good blood sugar level, rather than chocolate bars or biscuits which will lead to a slump in energy once the initial 'sugar high' has gone. Try keeping a food diary to see what suits you and helps you feel better and, equally important, what doesn't. Watch for food sensitivities and allergies and cut the offending substances from your regime for at least 3 months to see what happens.

Vitamins and Supplements

No doubt your GP will have checked all your systems thoroughly, although there's a lot of evidence that even the most modern techniques can sometimes miss an underactive thyroid. We usually suggest that patients take their temperature every morning before they get out of bed for at least 2 weeks. Often, despite normal thyroid function tests, there is a problem. If your core temperature is consistently around or below 36°C, then you may have an undiagnosed thyroid problem which will leave you tired much of the time and exhausted the rest! If so, try adding some kelp to your regime and you may even persuade your GP to give you a tiny dose of thyroid hormone on a clinical trial basis to see what happens. Sometimes people are completely turned around by this. Echinacea taken on an intermittent basis will help, especially if there is a viral basis for your problem. You need a multivitamin and multimineral daily of course, with very high doses of vitamin C – and we mean high. Some people find they can tolerate 5, 10 or even 20 g (yes, that's 20,000 mg) daily, but build up very slowly since you may find your digestion can't cope with this. Add also Vitamin E at the dose of 800–1200 iu per day, a strong Vitamin B complex tablet and not more than 50 mg of zinc picolinate which is the easiest form of zinc to absorb. Magnesium, CoEnzyme Q10 and the less readily available CoEnzyme 1, along with some ginseng and liquorice which is antiviral and supports adrenal function, complete your supplement regime. Watch your blood pressure if you take liquorice and limit it to 3 times a week.

Exercise and Lifestyle

We know you're feeling tired, but believe me, exercise will help even if you're feeling so weak that the only exercise you can take is passive exercise – that is, with someone else helping to move your body for you. Start with just some breathing exercises and some stretching (gently and only when your muscles are warm if you haven't exercised for a while). Don't go all out to do aerobics; you'll only end up feeling awful and convinced that this was a stupid idea and determined not to try it again. Put some music on at home and just let your body move to it, swaying gently. Try some Chi gong which is so gentle and yet so healing. Find a good yoga teacher and explain your problem. She will provide a regime that will help ease your body, mind and spirit, improve your mood, self-esteem and energy levels to say nothing of your immune function. Be aware of the toxins in your environment (see p. 7). We're not suggesting that you become a fanatic here, but just be aware of what might be draining your precious energy, and that includes toxic people! These are the ones who leave you feeling drained and exhausted even if you were feeling quite good when you met them. Are they really adding something positive to your life? If not, this might just be the time to offload them. There's little point in detoxifying your body to then allow yourself to be infected by others' gloom.

Take care of yourself, give yourself permission to rest when you need to but try to make it a rule to spend at least a little time outdoors each day. Agoraphobia is a problem you could do without, and becoming a recluse and relying on others to visit and fulfil your needs is an easy but dangerous route to follow. Lastly, try to avoid late nights and look at the suggestions about sleep (p. 468) to help you make the most of this healing process. If you need bed rest, then so be it. Some patients have been known to need artificial feeding although we hope that will never be the case for you. Divide your daily tasks into short episodes, resting between.

There are self-help groups both locally and nationally including Action for ME, the ME Association, and the Persistent Disease Research (see Useful Addresses).

Complementary Therapies

There are a host of complementary therapies that have good things to offer you. Trying them all simultaneously, apart from being expensive, is somewhat confusing. Look through the list and see what feels right for you to start with. Meditation is so good for everyone. It will destress you, make you feel more alive and refresh you while leaving you calm and serene. It's also something you can do at home without the need for a therapist once you've learned how. Relaxation therapy with some guided imagery will also soothe you. Massage, including shiatsu and aromatherapy, is wonderful and you might like to try an Ayurvedic massage which deeply relaxes, detoxifies and leaves you feeling initially like a wet noodle, the benefits becoming more obvious over the next few weeks. Try following it the next day with an ancient Ayurvedic remedy for fatigue. Blend some peeled almonds with hot milk and a pinch of ginger, cardamom and sugar, then drink it slowly with your hands wrapped around the cup. Especially good while wrapped in a blanket with your feet up! If you want to use aromatherapy oils at home try rosemary or basil (see caution on p. 48) to increase your energy, citrus oils such as orange to energise without over-stimulation, lemongrass to wake you up, and sandalwood to relieve tension, promote a sense of wellbeing and give you good restful sleep. Tea tree, peppermint and ylang-ylang are also good, but try to get an aromatherapist to mix a blend for you. Homeopathy has Anacardium for the four 'Fs' – brain fog, fatigue, forgetfulness and fixed ideas, Arsenicum and Kali phos for exhaustion, as well as Gelsemium and Lycopodium. A homeopath would probably give you a constitutional remedy, so go and see someone. You might be surprised at how much you'd benefit. As far as herbs go, astragalus and legustrum taken together can be very effective.

Acupuncture, autogenic training, naturopathy, biofeedback and clinical ecology can all be helpful. And last but not least, try some acupressure. The do-it-yourself version may convince you of its efficacy. When you're feeling exhausted, run your finger down your breastbone from the notch at the top of it just below your throat (the suprasternal notch). About 2 inches down, press firmly for about 15 seconds (it might feel a little tender but keep on pressing), then run your finger down another inch and repeat the process. Feel better? Don't forget psychotherapy and possibly the need for antidepressant medication. St John's Wort may help to elevate your mood.

Emotional and Spiritual Healing

Obviously if you're feeling exhausted and physically unwell, it's difficult to be bright and cheerful. But there's an old saying that pain is inevitable, but misery is optional. That's certainly so here. You are uncomfortable but your attitude can still be positive and upbeat or you can really make the most of your problem and become an unpopular burden to those around you. Positive thinking and a positive attitude will make you feel better and create a happier reality. Whatever might befall us, we can take control and improve it if we choose to do so. We are all familiar with stories of those who are handicapped or even dying who still enrich the lives of those around them, while there are others who never forgive life for having given them a cross to bear. Try having some healing and counselling to help you deal with the anger, resentment, disillusionment and disappointment you're feeling. Opening up your spiritual life may make all the difference to your being able to see your life as still rich with many gifts instead of feeling joyless. The more you shift your attitude, the more you'll shift your illness and let go of the despair, depression and helplessness that often accompany ME. However, if you have slipped into a deep depression, feel hopeless and despairing or that you'd rather be dead, then it's time to have a proper psychiatric assessment and possibly some conventional antidepressant medication.

Integrated Approach

1. Be properly diagnosed to make sure that there is no underlying illness that requires medical care.

2. Take adequate rest along with a good diet and supplementation.
3. Pace yourself, especially with exercise and other activities.
4. Have regular detoxification and rid your environment of toxins as much as possible and that includes toxic people.
5. Ensure that you have emotional and spiritual support.
6. Use complementary therapies as above.
7. Have counselling or psychotherapy.
8. Should you become hopeless, despairing or suicidal, have a full psychiatric assessment.
9. Don't forget support groups.

Memory Problems and Dementia

Memory problems may occur at any time of life and have a variety of underlying causes.

Ileni is 15. She has always been a bright girl and up until the last year she was in the top grade and had few problems with her studies. Lately, however, her grades have fallen and she finds herself unable to remember what should be easily within her grasp, bearing in mind her high IQ. Her teachers are concerned about the apparent decline in her performance. Questioning reveals that she has been desperately trying to lose weight and has been following a strict diet, skipping breakfast and eating very little at lunchtime. Her concentration is not very good and she feels less energetic in general. Ileni's memory problems are secondary to malnutrition.

Margaret, a marketing consultant, is 50 and menopausal and has recently been prescribed medication for her high blood pressure. She has always prided herself on her good memory and came to the surgery feeling anxious and worried about her embarrassment in meetings when she could not remember the facts of her presentation. She would sometimes stumble over simple words and be unable to follow her thread of thought in her usual articulate way. Margaret's memory disturbance is precipitated by menopause and her blood pressure medication.

Dementia on the other hand refers to an overall and progressive decline in mental ability and intellectual powers often accompanied by changes in personality and behaviour.

Harold, a retired accountant, has lived alone since the age of 68 when his beloved wife died of breast cancer. Although initially he was independent and capable, some 3 years later his daughter and son-in-law became increasingly concerned about his behaviour. His memory was appallingly unreliable, he was confused a lot of the time and on two occasions had to be escorted home by the police because he had apparently forgotten where he lived. The house was a tip, his appearance was dishevelled and slovenly and his personal hygiene dreadful. Harold has Alzheimer's disease.

Dementia has become a huge problem today, especially in modern developed countries like Britain, because as people are living longer, more and more are falling victim to this incapacitating illness. About 10 per cent of people aged over 65 and 20 per cent of those aged over 75 are touched to some extent by dementia.

Symptoms of Dementia

Loss of short-term memory is one of the earliest signs of dementia with inability to recall recent events, becoming lost in the neighbourhood or forgetting to turn off the oven or the gas fire. In severe cases even the names of the people closest to them may totally escape the sufferer.

Disorientation means often there is confusion about the time of day so sufferers sleep during the day and then wander about at night wondering why nobody else is around. They are bewildered by unfamiliar surroundings and may easily muddle up their medication.

Personality change is the symptom that close relatives often find the most distressing. Sufferers may lose all interest in their usual activities and pursuits, may withdraw socially and become moody, irritable, aggressive and ungrateful. The situation is sometimes compounded by a seeming preference to live in squalor and indulge in antisocial behaviour such as deliberate incontinence.

Loss of everyday practical skills such as cooking, shopping, dressing and washing.

Communication difficulties become apparent when conversation and conveying messages deteriorate as dementia sufferers struggle to find the words they are looking for or wander off the subject and fail to comprehend what is being said to them.

Causes

Contrary to popular belief a number of different conditions may lead to dementia but regrettably only a small minority are curable. The key lies in identifying which cases may successfully be treated and seeking such help quickly. Examples of treatable dementia include an underactive thyroid gland, the delayed effects of head injuries, Vitamin B_{12} deficiency, chronic alcoholism, the side effects of certain medications and depression.

Ralph, who lives in a back ward of the local psychiatric hospital, is 52 and was a heavy drinker for much of his life, beginning when he was only 13. Prior to his admission to hospital he was treated for some years for his alcohol addiction, although he was unable to heed the warnings about the progressive damage to his brain. For some years he had failing memory and now is unable to remember what he did only minutes earlier. He no longer recognises his family nor those who care for him, nor can he leave the hospital since he cannot remember directions and gets lost. He is quite happy in his way. Ralph has Korsakoff's disease, a specific type of dementia.

The commonest forms of dementia at the moment remain incurable. These are Alzheimer's disease, stroke or 'multi-infarct' dementia, and a rarer hereditary disease of the nervous system. Stroke dementia is due to gradual nerve cell damage caused by furring up of the blood vessels that supply the brain with oxygen.

Hannah has Alzheimer's disease. At 83 she lives alone following the death of her husband 7 years ago. She has good support from her 2 daughters and her son comes to visit her once a week. However, just lately they have noticed that she repeats herself a lot and seems absent-minded. Sometimes she forgets that they have even been to see her and from time to time makes phone calls to tell them some news that she has already told them about only days before. Nevertheless Hannah can recount stories from her childhood in great detail. She was seen at home by a geriatrician, after she was found by her son sitting outside in a thin dress despite the cold, having locked herself out.

Despite it being the commonest type of dementia and the disease at which the vast majority of research into dementia is directed, the causes of Alzheimer's disease remain unknown. What we do know, however, is that Alzheimer's disease is hardly ever inherited, so just because a parent may have suffered certainly does not mean that their offspring will as well.

Conventional Treatment

Those dementias which are due to identifiable causes are treated appropriately. With Alzheimer's disease conventional treatment is based on the symptoms. First of all the GP needs to look into the patient's medical history in detail and carry out a full examination. A visit to the sufferer's home is often useful to learn what is going on there and how the patient is coping from day to day. Investigations including blood tests, X-rays or scans may be called upon to reach a diagnosis of the exact type of dementia and then various specialists such as the psycho-geriatrician and neurologist will be involved. Alzheimer's disease is generally diagnosed after extensive tests have eliminated all other treatable possibilities and obviously this will take some time. Meanwhile the patient will need social and practical support in all sorts of ways to enable them to cope as efficiently as possible until an appropriate solution to their situation is found. Ultimately in severe and unmanageable cases permanent residential care may be required, but generally speaking, relatives, carers and the patients themselves prefer to remain within the community as long as they are realistically able to, with the help and support of all concerned. These support services include family, friends and neighbours, the GP and psychogeriatrician, district nurse, community psychiatric nurse, local day centre, respite care in hospital, church, Citizens' Advice Bureau, Alzheimer's Disease Society, Age Concern, Social Services and support for the carers themselves (see Useful Addresses).

Nutritional Healing

Brain function, like that of the rest of your body, relies upon a steady and constant supply of nutrients in order to perform well. Ileni's problems at school were a direct result of needing more brain fuel than she was taking while her body was trying to continue to grow. A better diet giving her all the nutrients she needed in a regular stream throughout the day soon solved the problem.

The basic nutritional recommendations given on p. 5 will generally keep you healthy, but as your brain ages, it becomes less efficient at utilising nutrients, mainly because of poorer, slower circulation. There are things you can do to help. First of all it would be better for you to have 6 mini meals spread out through the day rather than 3 major ones, thus ensuring a more steady supply of nutrients. A mineral assessment would be useful (there are dietitians and laboratories which would do this for you) and if necessary your levels can be topped up. In particular, you may need iron which is necessary for the production of haemoglobin and hence oxygenation of the brain as well as other tissues, boron which is essential for hand/eye coordination and memory, and zinc which is essential for learning and maintaining memory. Low iron not only results in anaemia, but can also affect attention span, concentration, and performance – part of Ileni's problem and also a factor for Margaret who had suffered very heavy periods in the pre-menopausal time. Meat, peas and beans, dried apricots and green leafy vegetables provide iron. Zinc is found in wheatgerm, yogurt, cooked peas and beans and dark green leafy vegetables. Choline, found in whole wheat bread, peanut butter, cauliflower, egg yolks and lettuce, will help your memory too. The B vitamins, found in milk, yogurt, wheatgerm, bananas and seafood as well as green peas, form part of the basic eating plan.

Animal fat tends to clog the cells and small vessels making for poor inter-neuronal communication and poor transport of oxygen across cell walls, so try to get what fat you do need from vegetable sources such as flax seed (linseed) oil or olive oil. Reducing your salt intake (watch out for the salt content of processed foods) and trans fatty acids found in margarine will also help. It has been said that saffron improves memory so using it in cooking or adding a little to some yogurt daily would be useful. Garlic improves learning ability and memory and is good for circulation. On the other hand, alcohol causes memory problems, the most classical and severe of which is Korsakoff's syndrome, from which Ralph suffers. Do be aware of food sensitivities which may contribute to your failing memory. In particular watch out for monosodium glutamate, often added to pre-prepared foods, and tyramine in cheese especially if it's matured. Adding nutmeg, bay leaf and black pepper to cooking may have a positive effect on memory.

If your elderly relatives are in residential care, do be sure to see that they are being properly fed, and top up their diet with some of the above to add essential nutrients.

Vitamins and Supplements

Even if you have a good diet, a daily supplement of B vitamins including folic acid (folate), Vitamin B_6 and B_{12} (probably much more commonly deficient than previously realised) will help preserve or improve your memory. Add Vitamins A, C and E to really improve thinking and memory, especially in the older age group. As we've said iron improves brain oxygenation and therefore cognition, so a lack of it can lead to poor attention span, poor memory, low energy levels and of course anaemia. Although up to 25 per cent of teenage girls like Ileni are iron deficient and many older women (and men) too, do have your GP check your iron level before embarking on an iron supplement except as part of a multimineral tablet. Free radicals cause damage to brain cells just as much if not more than to other tissues, since the brain has a high proportion of fatty acids which make it a good target. Antioxidants are therefore a must. Green tea and flax seed (linseed) oil are good, as are Vitamins C and E and carotenoids. Alpha lipoic acid is a rather special antioxidant which protects brain cell membranes from damage. Selenium, although present in your multimineral, can also be found in proprietary preparations combined with Vitamins A, C and E – ideal for the mid-life age group with memory disturbance.

Ginkgo biloba is the most exciting of the supplements for memory problems. It is a nootropic agent (that is, something that stimulates the intellect). However, it also improves blood circulation (some studies have linked it to an improved bloodflow of up to 70 per cent), increasing the availability of oxygen to the brain and other tissues including heart and legs, and it has beneficial effects much more widespread than on memory alone. It improves reaction time, recall, short-term memory and the ability to learn new information. It increases mental alertness and can have a marked effect not only on Alzheimer's disease, such as Hannah suffers, but on all of us. And as memory improves so does self-esteem, self-confidence and mood, with better social functioning and quicker response times. Some would say it would be useful to start to take it in young adulthood to prevent memory deterioration from starting in the first place! It may take 6–8 weeks or longer for the effects to show. A word of caution, however. Don't take gingko biloba along with blood-thinning medication as it may cause bleeding.

CoEnzyme Q10 is another powerful supplement which is useful here, protecting the mitochondria which are the powerhouses of your cells. Ginseng has also been said to help prevent memory loss and improve concentration. Choline is a Vitamin B-like compound that is a building block for acetylcholine, a chemical messenger (neurotransmitter) without which the brain can neither store nor retrieve information efficiently. Lecithin provides a rich source. Phosphatidyl serine (PS) is present in large quantities in brain cells, is essential to their health and is necessary for every phase of the memory process. It helps with judgement, memory and concentration. It may take 4 weeks before you notice much improvement but the benefits last up to 3 months after stopping supplementation.

The amino acids, precursors of neurotransmitters, are useful too, especially acetyl-l-carnitine which promotes repair of damaged DNA and delays the progression of Alzheimer's. However, amino acids should be taken with caution. Phenylalamine can cause insomnia and also brain damage in those with phenylketonuria, a congenital metabolic defect. L-cysteine shouldn't be taken by children or pregnant women. If you are going to take amino acids, start as early as possible, because older people may not show the same degree of improvement as those younger, and prevention is better than cure. DHEA (a hormone produced by the adrenal gland, the production of which reduces with age) is also found in some plants such as yam. It may help restore short-term memory and improves mental function in general. However pregnolone may well be the best of them all, although it is still undergoing tests. Tiny amounts boost memory and performance. Melatonin supplementation may also be useful since elderly people without Alzheimer's generally have twice as much melatonin in their brains than similar-aged Alzheimer's patients.

Gotu kola, used extensively in Ayurvedic medicine, has an overall rejuvenating action, although its effects are most marked on the nervous system where it helps memory, improves concentration and appears to improve intelligence. It is also said to aid longevity and boost the immune system. Beta carotene improves recall. There are also fairly recently developed so-called 'smart drugs' although these are not widely available in the UK. These include Depranil, Hydergine and Lucidryl. Lastly, if you want your brain to be working well, the filtration systems of the body which remove the toxic substances that may harm it need to be cleaned regularly and kept in good order. That means taking care of your liver and kidneys. See p. 7 for detoxification regimes.

Exercise and Lifestyle

If your memory isn't as good as it was, then try to adopt strategies that will help you, such as making lists and carrying them with you, or saying things aloud to yourself to make sure that you have actually registered the memory in the first place. Sometimes what seems like a memory problem is actually only poor concentration and a memory has not really been stored. For example, you're halfway down the road thinking about something else and wonder if you locked the door. You don't remember because you weren't concentrating on this mundane task at the time. If you were to actually say to yourself aloud, 'I've locked the door', you are more likely to remember that you have done so. Tony Buzan's wonderful little book *Use Your Head* suggests that you make name associations and think in pictures. For example, if I wanted to remember to buy 10 screws to put up a shelf, I could associate the 10 with hen since it rhymes, and visualise a hen wielding a screwdriver dodging under a shelf. If you don't take proper rest, your brain won't function as well as it might. Teenagers like Ileni often have this problem, but so do the older age group whose sleep is disturbed. Learning to power-nap in the day can have a marked effect on your alertness, concentration and memory (see Insomnia, p. 468). Reducing stress will also help improve short-term memory, concentration and attention span. Physical exercise as well as mental exercise (everything from reading to chatting with friends and doing the odd quiz) helps keep the mind alert and reduces stress. Mental stimulation is essential in older people, and attendance at day centres, drop-in clubs and visits from family and friends will keep brains working. Remember the old adage, use it or lose it. An accumulation of aluminium in the brain may be a cause of Alzheimer's, so remove all aluminium from environment, including canned drinks, some deodorants, cooking pots, baking powder and some table salt. Absorption of aluminium can be reduced by giving a magnesium supplement. Other toxins may cause some damage in all age groups. See p. 7 for a toxins checklist. Tobacco, alcohol and cannabis all have effects on memory, as do some blood pressure drugs, antihistamines, hormone preparations, and over the counter drugs such as cough suppressants, sleeping tablets and analgesics.

Complementary Therapies

Aromatherapy using geranium and rosemary together can be a powerful brain stimulant while the effect of the massage can be healing in itself, promoting relaxation and a feeling of wellbeing. Homeopathic remedies include Lycopodium which can be useful where the memory disturbance is accompanied by agitation and anxiety and Argentum nit which will help if memory is just generally weak. Atheus helps where poor concentration is the problem, whereas Barium carb will help those with problems of inattention and absent-mindedness. Your homeopath will prescribe for you.

Music has been found to have the ability of making contact with both autistic people and Alzheimer's patients, and it may help access memory which otherwise appears to be lost. Playing soft gentle or big band music while Alzheimer's patients are trying to learn tasks will sometimes help them both retain and recall their new skills. Ayurvedic medicine offers Ashwagandha, which is reported to promote relaxation mental function while acting as a rejuvenating agent.

Emotional and Spiritual Healing

It's a frightening situation to be aware that you can't remember as you used to do. Although often poor memory becomes a bit of a joke for those around you, it's certainly no laughing matter for the person who's suffering the problem. First of all, however, try to be gentle with yourself and ask others to be gentle with you also. Getting upset and angry with yourself, or having others be angry with you, are only likely to worsen the situation. The more you can focus and concentrate, the more likely you are to be able to lay down the memory trace in the first place and recall it later. Also be self-assertive enough not to let anyone hurry you so that you get flustered and can't think. Often you can aid your memory by adding some visualisation to your efforts. If you've forgotten where you've put something, for instance, apart from trying to retrace your steps, why not sit down for a few moments and imagine a clear screen, allowing whatever you've lost to start to appear on it. You may be surprised that you are suddenly aware of where the lost object is.

Touch, spiritual healing and gentle communication with the elderly can raise their self-esteem and self-confidence, making them more present and accessible on all levels, and thus increasing their ability to utilise their mental capacity. But please don't reserve this only for the elderly. The same can be said for children and anyone else. Gentleness and patience will often provide an atmosphere in which a great many more things are possible than would be otherwise.

Care for the carers

Adjusting to the fact that a member of the family is suffering from a serious and progressive form of dementia, like Alzheimer's, is never easy. The emotional impact can be immense and relatives need help with it. Anger, guilt, embarrassment and a sense of isolation are all regularly experienced. Sharing the burden with other family members and friends at this time is important, and a practical action plan, involving all professional avenues of support, is essential in facing the future.

Integrated approach

1. Proper assessment is needed which will often include a home visit.
2. Treat any underlying causes.
3. Ensure adequate nutrition and supplementation.
4. Beware of toxins in the environment such as tobacco smoke, aluminium, etc.
5. Use complementary therapies and healing.
6. Provide emotional and spiritual support for sufferers and carers.
7. Communicate in all ways possible – speech, touch, music.
8. If you're a carer, take time out when necessary to look after yourself.

Menopause

Cathy looked tired and said she felt exhausted. Over the last few months she has been sleeping poorly, often waking in the night with her nightie damp from sweat. She would often take a while to get back to sleep and felt that during the day she was never as alert as she used to be. Over the last couple of months she has also started to have embarrassing sweating during the day. She reported that the wave of heat would begin often around her head or neck and would then engulf all of her, resulting in her face being flushed and often with rivulets of sweat running down her neck. Even though the hot flushes would sometimes last only a minute or two, they would be severe enough to put her off her stride at work and render it impossible to continue to cook the dinner or be in a stuffy room. Lately she has started to avoid things she used to love such as going to the theatre or even doing the supermarket shopping, since she couldn't bear to be in a place where she would feel confined and unable to get out and get some fresh air. Cathy is suffering from the common symptoms of menopause.

Menopause occurs when the production of oestrogen from the ovaries slows down and then stops. In fact the strict medical definition describes the menopause as officially having occurred when a full year has elapsed without any menstrual periods having been experienced. It usually happens in the late forties or early fifties but it can occur much earlier, as young as 35 and up to the age of 60 in extreme cases. The change in oestrogen levels generally develops fairly slowly so that the effects of the menopause may be hardly noticed.

Isla is 52 and is enjoying her life. She is at the beginning of a new relationship, is feeling wonderfully happy, loves the freedom now that her family have become settled with their own partners. She hasn't had a period for 14 months, has had very few symptoms of menopause and came to the surgery to talk about whether or not she needs to worry about contraception.

However, for some women there can be dramatically unpleasant symptoms lasting from a few months in some cases to more than 10 years in others.

Symptoms

There are a large variety of both psychological and physical symptoms which cause many women to turn to their doctor for help. However, menopause is not a disease and therefore doesn't need a cure. But as the old term for menopause suggests, it is a time of major change that is best handled by understanding it well and by managing the changes in physiology which can otherwise be quite disconcerting.

The physical symptoms of the menopause include hot flushes, night sweats, heavy irregular periods, vaginal looseness, weight gain, backache, unwanted body hair and drier skin with coarse thin hair. Breasts tend to become smaller and less well supported. There may be an increase in the number of vaginal infections or dryness resulting in pain when making love, and gradual thinning of the bones leading to osteoporosis with the potential for fractures. In addition there may be psychological symptoms including insomnia, intense mood swings, depression, lack of concentration, short-term memory loss and irritability. Not everybody develops these symptoms, but many women have several of them to one degree or another, and some women have most of them to a severe degree.

Conventional Treatment

By and large, conventionally trained doctors regard the menopause and its treatment rather simplistically. Since falling oestrogen levels are the fundamental cause of the menopause, the simplest approach is to reverse the trend by replacing the oestrogen artificially by the use of HRT.

There is no doubt that HRT has revolutionised the treatment of the menopause and vastly improved the quality of many women's lives. However, inappropriate use of HRT in women who didn't really need it, partially explains the more recent development of the resistance to the use of HRT. This springs partly from the fact that women using HRT inappropriately suffered side effects and partly from a trend towards natural treatment at this stage in a woman's life.

When Dorothy came to the surgery she couldn't believe what was happening to her. She had only had one period in the last 5 months and she felt that she was going mad. She could not concentrate, she was irritable and moody and had totally lost any desire to make love with her husband. She ached all over, could not sleep at night and was plagued with hot flushes and night sweats. In fact Dorothy had many of the psychological and physical symptoms of the menopause, and when she had considered all the options, she elected to take hormone replacement therapy. She gained a little weight initially and felt a little nauseous for a week or so, but once an alternative preparation has substituted she was free of side effects and found a new lease of life.

Since every possible symptom listed above can be alleviated through HRT, doctors are understandably enthusiastic in prescribing it. After 40 years of use it has become widely regarded as safe, effective and possessing numerous short- and long-term advantages. It protects against osteoporosis (brittle bone disease) and heart disease for a start. In the long term this undoubtedly saves lives and dramatically reduces the number of fractures sustained by elderly women since the bones remain much denser and stronger. In the short term all of the commonest symptoms such as hot flushes and night sweats can be reversed almost overnight and the skin regains much of its former lustre, with toning up of muscles of the body into the bargain. Vaginal dryness improves, libido is restored and many of the psychological symptoms which can cause such distress, not only to the patient but to her family, revert to normal.

However, there may be disadvantages, common side effects

being nausea, irritability, weight gain, breast enlargement and abdominal cramps. Some women may not welcome a return to monthly periods although there are now continuous combined preparations which prevent this. Every women should understand the pros and cons, and make a decision with the help of her doctor based on the severity and duration of her symptoms and the likelihood that they will be improved by HRT.

IS HRT SAFE FOR YOU?

Some women should not take HRT. These include women with a history of breast cancer or cancer of the womb; women with certain types of liver or gall bladder disease, and those who have recently had a deep vein thrombosis. Women who suffer from migraine, diabetes, high blood pressure or epilepsy should take HRT with caution and under close supervision.

Different types of HRT range from skin patches, creams or tablets to implants which are inserted just under the skin. The type of preparation should be carefully selected to suit the individual. Every woman should be screened, both before starting HRT and regularly during such therapy. Her blood pressure and weight are measured, and the doctor may wish to carry out a general examination including a breast check to make sure all is well. Ideally regular mammograms, cervical smears and bone density measurements should be carried out, all of which can detect any abnormalities early, enabling effective treatment to be carried out. HRT is not comparable with the oral contraceptive pill in that the types of hormones and their strengths are different. And every woman should continue to use a form of contraception for at least one full year after her last menstrual period. Fertility is much reduced at this time, but there is nevertheless a theoretical chance that pregnancy could occur.

It is important to realise that only a minority of women require HRT and that those who regard it very favourably represent this group, all of whom have suffered so much before being started on the therapy. For many women with mild symptoms, no treatment whatsoever may be required. For those with mild to moderate symptoms, there are alternatives to HRT which should be considered.

Despite regular scare stories in the media, HRT can be regarded as very safe and well tolerated, provided it is individually tailored to your needs. It may take several months with 2 or 3 changes of preparation, but do persevere because most women with symptoms can be adequately accommodated. Sometimes your family doctor may refer you to a special menopause clinic so that someone who has more experience in prescribing HRT can help you achieve the best result.

Contrary to popular belief, HRT does not significantly raise the risk of breast cancer when taken for 5–10 years although when used for more than 10 years, there may be a slightly increased risk. However, this is less than the risk associated with not having breastfed a baby in the past or from having a significant family history of breast cancer (that is, two first-degree relative – mother, sister, aunt or grandmother – of any age or one first-degree relative who had breast cancer before the age of 45). Clearly those women with a family history of breast cancer would be well advised to avoid any further increase in risk by avoiding HRT. Women who might consider using HRT should also know that by taking it they would be protected against endometrial and ovarian cancer to a greater extent than if they did not take it.

Beth finished her periods at the age of 48 and initially felt a little tired and lethargic. She seemed to have lost much of the tone in the muscles of her body. Her breasts sagged and she did not sleep so well. She was, however, keen to avoid HRT so she contacted the Women's Nutritional Advisory Service and arranged for some aromatherapy and acupuncture. She increased the amount of exercise she took, and bought a variety of herbal and other health supplements to improve her wellbeing. Beth sailed through her menopause thereafter, and the only form of HRT she took was in the form of vaginal cream which helped some dryness and irritation she had experienced after love-making.

Nutritional Healing

It has long been observed that Japanese women experience fewer hot flushes and less breast cancer and osteoporosis than other women around the world, apparently due to the high proportion of soya in their diet. Indeed a study in *Obstetrics and Gynaecology* reported that women taking 60 g of soya protein daily for 12 weeks suffered 15 per cent fewer hot flushes than control groups. Oats, nuts (especially cashews and almonds), alfalfa sprouts and apples all have phyto-oestrogens in smaller amounts and can help hot flushes. Oats, brown rice and some other grains contain gamma oryzonol (ferulic acid) which has also been found to be very effective for hot flushes. The recommendations on p. 5 will give you a well-balanced diet. However, increasing your fibre intake even more will not only help constipation but can often ease irritability. Sunflower seeds, walnuts and hazelnuts are good added to salads, while cabbage, asparagus and broccoli can be taken either cooked or raw. Have cereal at some time of the day. Muesli or porridge made with oats can be very comforting. If you find dairy produce difficult to tolerate, remember that goat's or sheep's milk, yogurt and cheese contain a lot of calcium but rarely trigger the kind of sensitivities caused by cow's milk. Sprinkle sesame seeds on salads or cereal for another good source of calcium, essential to help prevent osteoporosis (see p. 399). Cut down on canned drinks and avoid caffeine as much as possible, taking herb teas instead. If you must have coffee or ordinary tea, have it only in the morning. Chinese green tea makes a good substitute and can be found flavoured with orange (our favourite) and other delights. Most importantly, drink plenty of water and reduce your alcohol intake to no more than one unit of alcohol daily. Eating small frequent meals will leave you feeling light and more energetic. Be aware that hot, spicy food may trigger hot flushes. Pumpkin, sesame seeds and safflower oil will give you your omega-6 fatty acids while fish will provide you with the necessary omega-3 fatty acids, all of which are good for preventing ageing and vaginal dryness. Salmon (and sunlight) will give you your Vitamin D. Have plenty of fruit. Citrus fruits, strawberries and kiwis will not only give you Vitamin C, but citrus fruits also contain hisperidin, a flavinoid which is effective in controlling hot flushes. If you're not eating enough fruit, make sure you have a supplement. We believe that we can rarely have too much Vitamin C and always take a supplement anyway.

Vitamins and Supplements

This is a time of rapid physiological (and psychological) change, so even though you're not ill, you need to take extra care of yourself. A daily multivitamin and multimineral will give you your basic requirements as long as you're also eating a healthy diet. A strong Vitamin B complex tablet daily will give you the full range of B vitamins including folic acid (folate). Vitamin E prevents vaginal thinning and drying and also keeps your skin soft and smooth. The *Journal of Clinical Oncology* (1998; 16: 495–500), in a study that loked at reducing menopausal symptoms in women who couldn't take HRT because of previous breast cancer, reported that Vitamin E reduces hot flushes. Flax seed (linseed) oil contains both omega-3 and omega-6 fatty acids and is also a good source of phyto-oestrogens. Oil of evening primrose gives you gamma linoleic acid (GLA). A calcium supplement is a good idea – look for carbonate or citrate for easy absorption. Calcium and magnesium are often found together nowadays and are usually formulated in exactly the right proportions. Boron is a mineral that we often neglect. Check that there's some in your multimineral. Wild yam cream can take care of night sweats, irritability, anxiety and bloating associated with menopause while DHEA from yams has had quite amazing press as a supplement which invigorates and helps one feel young. Aloe vera juice taken last thing at night can cool you and prevent night sweats and hot flushes while cleansing your whole system. Black cohosh (cimicifuga) is the supplement that many women swear by because of its capacity to decrease hot flushes and prevent vaginal dryness. It may, however, slow your heart rate a bit and cause mild nausea or vomiting. If so, stop taking it. If you want to try it, do so for 6 months, then stop for a month and resume. If forgetfulness is your problem, then gingko biloba is your supplement. Liquorice will help your hot flushes but don't take it if you have high blood pressure. Carrying some Bach Rescue Remedy in your handbag is sensible and try some Bach walnut essence if you tend to be emotionally unstable.

Exercise and Lifestyle

It's important for life to be as normal as possible, although there are measures you can take to make yourself more comfortable. Choose natural fibres for clothes and have extra garments you can add or take off as necessary. When exercising, synthetic fibres which carry moisture away from your skin are preferable. Carrying a fan in your handbag may be seen by some as laughable, but is very useful. Sex can become painful if you're dry and get sore, so buy a lubricant and use it.

Julia had always enjoyed a happy relationship with her husband which included a good sexual life. She said that her libido had gone down a little since she had become menopausal, but that that wasn't the main problem. She now found that sex was not only uncomfortable but downright painful, and that often she was sore for a good while afterwards. She was now avoiding sex which was causing sadness for her and some irritability in her husband. Julia didn't want to lose that physical intimacy which had been so important to both of them, but had heard from her friends that they had also lost enjoyment in sex around menopause. She was eager to find out if there was something seriously wrong and what she could do to reinstate the intimacy.

Myths about women not enjoying sex around menopause are generally unfounded. The advice to Isla about contraception was that having been free of periods for over a year, she should be fine. Exercise is a must, but start gently if you haven't been used to much activity. Although weight-bearing exercise such as walking or dancing gives you the best protection from osteoporosis (see p. 399), find something you enjoy, whether it be swimming or riding your bicycle, and make it part of your routine. Why not make 'the change of life' exactly that? You can make new choices, change your outlook and dedicate your life to being healthy and having fun!

Complementary Therapies

There are several herbs that you might find useful, among them black cohosh, which we've already discussed. Red clover contains phyto-oestrogens, and chaste berry (agnus castus) reduces mood swings, hot flushes and dryness but may take 1 or 2 months to start to work. It also helps keep progesterone levels steady. Herbs which contain significant amounts of phyto-oestrogens and progesterone include wild yam, don quai, alfalfa and blessed thistle. Skullcap, motherwort, valerian root, ginseng and passion flower are all useful, although a herbalist would prescribe the best herbs for you depending upon your symptom profile. Homeopathy has several effective remedies. If you have flooding with dark clots, China would be appropriate. Secale and Phosphorus could help with heavy bleeding without clotting. Phosphorus can also help if you have memory difficulties and feel frightened about what's happening to you. Try Sabina if you're irritable and Sepia if you have an itchy, dry vagina. If you get even more upset when someone tries to console you and into the bargain you have a sore dry vagina, then Natrum mur is for you. But as always, have a proper assessment to get the best results. Don't forget aromatherapy. Clary sage or basil can help your hot flushes and other symptoms (put a drop on your handkerchief or carry some in your handbag) and treat yourself to a massage where your therapist may choose either one, fennel, peppermint or a combination. Acupuncture, acupressure and reflexology are also worth a try.

Emotional and Spiritual Healing

Menopause used to be regarded as an unwelcome event to be feared – the end of one's reproductive life and the beginning of the descent into grey-haired old age. Now there is a growing movement to encourage us to view the menopause as one of life's natural passages to the next calmer stage, where the burden of childbearing and rearing has ended and women can concentrate on their own lives. Such positive outlook undoubtedly has a major bearing on how you may adapt through your menopause and how you tolerate any symptoms you may have. It's sad that menopause has had such bad press and that we're often bombarded with horror stories about it. Bearing in mind that we create our own reality, the more we expect bad things, the more likely they are to happen. However, a positive attitude such as that of Isla can make all the difference to whether or not you view this as an amazing time, freeing you from many of the ties of the past and moving you into a time of growth. Certainly there is room for grief for some women, especially if for one reason or another they have not borne children and now their biological clock has struck its final hour, or if menopause occurs ahead of time due to surgical intervention. Whatever feelings you have about it are valid and you have a right to experience them. However, when you've done so perhaps you could start to take the focus off the fact that childbearing is over and see the joys that now lie ahead. This is the time when many women become aware of or intensify their intuition and spirituality. For many, it is the first time that they have been free to follow their own desires regarding education, career and hobbies. This entry into senior womanhood can bring with it a new wisdom and comfort. Women will discover the wonderful feeling of being no longer fettered by many of the social and cultural expectations that they live with and of becoming elder stateswomen with the courage to speak their truth.

On a physiological level, once our hormones settle down we have higher levels of testosterone than we had before. This stimulates the emotional and spiritual development of the more masculine side of us, the inner male, which gives us courage, allows us to feel more independent, self-assertive, powerful and where appropriate, fierce. What an amazing time, full of zest, positivity and growth with opportunities for change on all fronts – career, hobbies, and sometimes partners. If you need support, find a women's group or have some counselling. Don't forget that some cultures see older women as sages holding the wisdom of the tribe. Hold your head up high as you become one of these.

Integrated approach

1. Remember that menopause is not an illness.
2. See it as an exciting time of your life leading to more freedom and growth.
3. Talk with your doctor about the pros and cons of HRT so that you can make an informed choice.
4. Remember to use contraception until at least 1 year after your final period.
5. Eat well, being sure to include soya and other foods containing phyto-oestrogens. Add supplements when necessary.
6. Keep active to prevent heart disease and osteoporosis.
7. Use complementary therapies where appropriate.

Menstrual Problems

Margaret, 49, was at her wit's end with heavy irregular periods which left her feeling exhausted. She lost a lot of blood with clots, and her periods always started at unpredictable and inconvenient times. She was found to have a very enlarged uterus because of fibroids and when hormonal treatment failed to reduce her blood loss, she was offered a hysterectomy. She welcomed the operation after adequate counselling and within 6 weeks she was a different woman, full of life, vibrant and energetic once more.

Menstrual difficulties are experienced by most women at some stage in their lives. They may be abnormally painful, heavy, absent or irregular, and are often a source of great worry and inconvenience. There may also be psychological problems related to periods, including premenstrual syndrome (PMS). Some women are reluctant to seek help either because there is embarrassment involved in seeing a male doctor or simply because of the tremendous variation of blood loss at period times between different women, making it difficult for example for women to know what constitutes a heavy period when they have no benchmark. Broadly speaking, a light period involves the loss of about 2 teaspoons of blood, whereas a heavy period may involve the loss of half a teacupful. Conventional doctors tend to regard heavy periods of blood loss as being over 80 ml, but this means little if anything to most women, and not all the loss will be made up of blood. It is useful to look at the different problems in turn.

Painful Periods

The pain experienced during a period is usually described as a dull ache in the lower abdomen of a cramping or dragging nature. The ache can radiate through to the lower back and even spread into the top and front of the thighs; in severe cases there may be fainting or sickness as well. The pain tends to begin a day or so before the period is due. There are two main types of painful periods, primary dysmenorrhoea, which tends to start at a young age when periods first start, and secondary dysmenorrhoea, which tends to occur as a result of some underlying abnormality in the reproductive organs. The first type tends to occur in the first 3 years after periods start, and generally eases off, disappearing by the time the woman reaches her thirties. Generally speaking having a baby cures the problem but this is not universally the case. Women who develop painful periods later in life in their twenties and thirties may have underlying problems such as fibroids, pelvic infection or endometriosis.

Lee has complained about backache during the latter half of her periods for several years and has seen her doctor on several occasions. She usually comes away with the impression that she is complaining about nothing and should just put up with what is a normal part of being a woman. Having talked to some of her friends, however, she asked for a second opinion and has now seen a gynaecologist who did a laparoscopy in which she inserted a tiny camera through a small incision in Lee's navel to inspect the organs of her pelvis. What she found were small patches of cells from the lining of the uterus which had become embedded in her pelvis and which react in the same way each month as her uterus. It is these patches of endometriosis that cause her dragging pain and leave her feeling so ill before her periods. Lee has endometriosis.

In both types of painful periods, there seems to be a sensitivity to prostaglandin, a hormone-like chemical secreted by the lining of the womb, which results in very powerful muscular contractions and pain. Medical treatment involves prostaglandin inhibitor preparations such as ibuprofen or mefenamic acid although sometimes a synthetic progesterone may be used, particularly in the 10 days before a period is due, to change the hormone balance and prevent prostaglandin release. Another alternative solution is to prescribe the oral contraceptive pill which at the same time as preventing an unwanted pregnancy regulates the sex hormones in such way as to significantly reduce period pain.

Heavy Periods

Different women lose different quantities of blood during their periods, and what some would define as a heavy period may be light for others. Broadly speaking a woman comes to seek help from her doctor when the heaviness of her periods becomes an inconvenience in her life or when the amount she is losing suddenly increases drastically. The conventional approach to treatment lies in identifying the cause, which can be anything from fibroids, pelvic infection, endometriosis or endometrial infection to an underactive thyroid, a blood clotting disorder or polyps, which are fragile benign fleshy growths in the lining of the uterus or womb that can easily bleed. Other causes of heavy bleeding include the presence of an intrauterine contraceptive device, a coil, or an injectable form of contraceptive known as Depo-Provera which is given at 3-monthly intervals. An overall health check would include an internal examination and a cervical smear. One solution if appropriate would be the prescription of the oral contraceptive pill to regulate hormone levels. Mefenamic acid (Ponstan) can reduce bleeding in up to 50 per cent of women. Failing that, hormonal treatment such as danazol can be effective although side effects of unwanted hair and weight gain can occur. If there is a blood clotting problem, drugs such as Epsikapron can be useful, and if there is iron deficiency as a result of heavy blood loss, iron with Vitamin C can help. Some women, who have completed their family and who are plagued by the weariness and exhaustion induced by heavy irregular periods, welcome the suggestion of a hysterectomy as this can effectively alleviate all their worries. However, you may not wish to undergo such a drastic procedure, in which case you could consider a transcervical resection of the endometrium (TCRE). This operation, similar to a D&C, involves the permanent removal of part of the lining of the womb, which cuts down the bleeding and the pain and allows only minor blood loss at period time. Have your thyroid checked since there's an association between heavy periods and low thyroid function.

Absent Periods

Known as amenorrhoea, absent periods can be present right from the beginning of a girl's reproductive age (primary amenorrhoea) or can occur secondary to some underlying disorder. Primary amenorrhoea may be familial, in that a girl's mother may have started periods late or always had very light periods, or it may be that a girl is under a critical weight which inhibits the hormonal control of normal periods. At weights below about 48 kg, the hypothalamus gland situated at the base of the brain is unable to kick-start the ovaries into action and periods cannot occur. Once weight is gained, however, periods can be triggered if necessary with the drug Clomid (clomiphene). In women who once had normal regular periods but then cease to have them, it is imperative to exclude the possibility of pregnancy which is the commonest cause of periods that suddenly stop. An alternative cause might be significant weight loss, which is seen in professional dancers and athletes, for example, but also in women with anorexia nervosa.

Jenny, 25, was a dancer/choreographer who was obsessive about her weight and kept herself extremely slim. She was in an ongoing relationship and took the oral contraceptive pill. Bizarrely, although she experienced regular periods for the previous 10 years, they suddenly stopped. A pregnancy test on two occasions was negative, but she worried about her future fertility, and consulted a doctor. In fact her diminutive weight of 49 kg, along with the contraceptive pill, was preventing her ovulating and resulted in absent periods. When considering the options for treatment, she decided to continue with her current lifestyle without having periods as she was not prepared to sacrifice anything for her career at that time.

Women who have experienced emotional shock or constant stress may also find that their periods cease temporarily. Taking the oral contraceptive pill can significantly reduce the amount of blood loss or even stop it altogether, and women who are anaemic or have an underactive thyroid or large fibroids can also suffer from secondary amenorrhoea. The conventional approach to treatment here is to identify any underlying cause and treat it appropriately. Remember that you remain fertile and should continue to take precautions against pregnancy.

Sal, 38, had had difficulties with her periods since her late teens. Never having had any children, a personal decision because of her career in an international bank, she had finds that both the pain and the emotional turmoil before her periods have become steadily worse. During the last few day before her period is due she feels as though she is going crazy, with sudden changes of mood, tearfulness, irritability and fatigue. Sometimes she feels so angry that she is scared of becoming violent. Her physical symptoms include backache, cramps and bloating. Water retention results in the swelling of her fingers, ankles and breasts. Her bleeding has also become heavier over the last few years. Now one of her colleagues has made a complaint about her rude and irritable behaviour which he feels is no longer tolerable.

This is a classical picture of premenstrual syndrome, although it is by no means only the province of the childless. It can become so pronounced that there is little of the month that is pleasant, since the woman and her family are usually just recovering from the effects of one period when the next one is upon them. The conventional approach includes treatment with serotonin boosting antidepressants (such as Prozac) which seem to be fairly effective in some patients, since these women have a deficiency in their brains of the neurotransmitter, serotonin, in the premenstrual phase. However, there is a considerable amount of help that the complementary field can offer, which we shall look at later.

Where to Find Professional Help

Perhaps the first port of call would normally be the family doctor, but there may be reasons why you might prefer an alternative source of help. For example, you may wish to see a woman doctor, or even the practice nurse might prove helpful. There are often well-woman clinics within GP practices or run by the Family Planning Association. A referral to a specialist gynaecology clinic may be in order and organisations such as the Women's Health Concern are also a good source of advice (see Useful Addresses).

But let's look now at what you can do to help yourself.

Nutritional Healing

The basic diet (see p. 5) will help give you the nutrients you need for self-healing. However, there are some important additions here. Organic food is best, if expensive. Wash everything carefully to remove pesticides and other toxins. And filter your water. You need to keep your blood sugar levels steady by eating a complex carbohydrate snack every 3 hours or so through the day and keep a snack by your bed to eat if you wake at night. Celery and fennel made into juices will help with fluid retention. Try to reduce dairy products, animal fats, salt, caffeine, alcohol and refined sugars in your diet to a minimum and if possible get rid of them altogether, but take your time. You may need to cut down your caffeine slowly to prevent a withdrawal problem. Increase your intake of whole grains and vegetables. Although you should reduce dairy produce, warm milk contains tryptophan, a natural sedative with mild antidepressant action, which can be comforting before bedtime and will help you sleep. Tryptophan is also found naturally in turkey so you could choose this if you eat meat. If you're overweight, losing a little would be helpful, since oestrogens are stored in fat and they exacerbate the problem. Watch for oestrogens also in food and in your environment – we're bombarded by them in water, plastic containers and bags, etc. (see p. 7). If heavy periods are your problem, much of the above still applies to you. However, you may need to have your iron checked, and you should add to your diet dark green leafy vegetables such as spinach as well as an iron supplement.

And period pains? Add plenty of greens, grains and vegetables. Soya products will also help. Green tea will not only soothe but will give you lots of antioxidants, while aloe vera juice will ease the pain when a small, diluted amount is sipped over a period of an hour or so.

Vitamins and Supplements

Don't forget to take plenty of Vitamins C and E with a good multimineral and multivitamin daily. Chlorophyll as a supplement or as a natural algae product can help with heavy periods, and shepherd's purse made into a tea is beneficial.

If you have premenstrual syndrome the B vitamins, especially B_6, are a must, and taken properly with oil of evening primrose they can have a dramatic effect, even though this may take 3 or more cycles to reach its maximum benefit. We usually recommend that oil of evening primrose is taken as follows:

TAKING OIL OF EVENING PRIMROSE

Count the first day of your period as Day 1. Mark Day 14 in your diary and take 1000 mg oil of evening primrose and 50 mg Vitamin B_6 each morning from Day 14, up to and including Day 1 of your next period, then stop. Start again on Day 14 of the next cycle. If you have a particularly bad day, sit down with a warm drink such as nettle tea, have another 3000 mg oil of evening primrose as a single dose and rest for half an hour, by which time you should feel much better.

Natural progesterone will help and can be obtained as a cream or supplement to be taken internally, whereas synthetic progesterone can have so many side effects that it can make matters worse. Vitamins C, D and E are essential, as is selenium. Magnesium levels are often low (alcohol and caffeine precipitate a loss of magnesium) and an antioxidant supplement will help.

Exercise and Lifestyle

Most women with PMS feel alone and helpless and think that no one really understands the problem. Usually they know that they're behaving irrationally and yet are unable to do anything about it. It will help if you understand that if your breasts and fingers are swelling, then your brain is also probably squashing your mood centres and producing your volatility. Learn some relaxation and meditation techniques and do some gentle exercise. This will help with fluid retention and other irritating problems such as constipation. Reduce stress as much as possible (see p. 48) and leave stressful jobs and social commitments until times in the month when you're feeling more like doing them. Most women with PMS find that there's some point in the month when they have a flood of energy and a bit of a high. This is the time to get those jobs done, but don't overdo it! If low mood is your problem, make use of as much natural light as you can by exercising outdoors, and if necessary invest in a SAD lamp (see p. 204) since full-spectrum light will help regulate your moods and reduce stress. Try to structure your days, get a good night's sleep and try an Epsom salt bath before bedtime to truly relax you.

Complementary Therapies

Herbs can be very useful and there are a lot to choose from. For water retention, you could try alfalfa, nettle, uva ursi or dandelion tea. For cramps, try cramp bark, black cohosh, squaw vine or passionflower. Black cohosh is also useful for normalising your periods, as are nettle, motherwort and rosemary. Nettle restores iron lost in menstruation and has lots of trace minerals such as calcium, iron, magnesium, potassium and silicon as well as Vitamins A and C. Don quai is useful for all menstrual problems.

Geranium oil is perhaps the classic aromatherapy oil to use and it will help alleviate irritability, relieve mood swings and settle your nervous energy. It also induces mental harmony and brings calm while refreshing body and spirit. Feverfew may help with menstrual cramps, as will aloe vera gel taken with a pinch of black pepper.

If you'd like to try homeopathy, Lycopodium may help if there's bloating and bowel disturbance and if you're irritable and tetchy; try Colocynth for pain, and Natrum mur is indicated if you're depressed and weepy with headaches and salt cravings. Mag phos, Belladonna, Lachesis and Pulsatilla also have their place, but do get a homeopathic opinion. Bach Flower Remedies or Australian Bush Essences can give gentle but effective relief. Try pomegranate.

Get your partner to gently rub your lower back and massage your abdomen using lavender oil diluted with almond or castor oil. Castor oil itself applied as an abdominal pack can work wonders. Soak a soft cloth in castor oil and place it over your tummy and then add a hot pad – either a hot water bottle or a heating pad. Or place a plastic cover on the bed and lie tummy-down on the oil pad which will allow some pressure too. Sometimes some gentle pressure to your lower abdomen will help. You can stimulate the acupressure points in your groin by lying on your tummy with your hand curled into a fist and placed under the crease between your thigh and your lower abdomen. Reflexology can help with menstrual problems, as can acupuncture, yoga and meditation.

For period pains (dysmenorrhoea), the herbs that are particularly effective include gardenia and corn silk, the latter being helpful if there's associated bloating. Homeopathic remedies include Colocynth, Mag Phos and Pulsatilla. Aromatherapy oils you might like to try include clary sage, marjoram and lavender. As always make sure you get enough exercise (outdoors whenever possible) and enough rest. Yoga will help heal mind, body and spirit.

Emotional and Spiritual Healing

Often by the time a woman goes to her GP for help, the whole family is dreading period time as they lurch from month to month with little respite between. Sometimes women have learned from their female relatives that nothing can be done or they have no wish to be patronised and have all their problems attributed to their periods. However it will help alleviate the problem immediately, if you start to talk openly about your difficulties, so that your partner and family can understand why there are times when you are simply not able to function as well as you might. Good communication between you and your doctor and between you and your partner and family will relieve the feeling of isolation, while the good news is that family members are usually so eager for the situation to get better that they're supportive of your efforts. Try to explain everything to them and ask for their help. It's amazing how co-operative others can be if you give them a chance. If you need to lie down for half an hour with a cup of warm milk or herb tea, they'll get used to that and prefer it to having you haring around the house screaming at them. Most of all, however, communicate with yourself, listen to your body and be gentle with yourself. Feeling guilty and hating yourself for your behaviour will only make things worse. But of course the onus is on you to do all you can to help yourself and to refrain from manipulating situations for your own benefit by blaming your periods for behaviour that has nothing to do with them. Sometimes menstrual problems can be so severe that the concern about the next time prevents you from enjoying the good times in between. Try to stay in the present and exact every bit of enjoyment you can from every day. On bad days if you need to withdraw and rest, then tell those close to you what's happening and accept what help's available. Take the time you need to minimise your difficulty. Some cognitive therapy may help you to become more positive in your thinking and attitude as you overcome the feelings of helplessness and dependency which often dog those with menstrual problems. Realising your own power as a woman will often make otherwise draining physical problems bearable. As you'll see from p. 540, menstrual problems are the province of the sacral chakra and doing some work here will often alleviate them. Have a look at the exercises and meditations that are appropriate for this chakra and try them. You will need to do them over a period of time and if you should unearth something painful that happened around the ages of 5 to 8, find yourself a good therapist to work with. If you're ambivalent about something, try to sort it out and resolve it. You may be surprised at the difference that releasing tension will make in what you may have seen as a purely physical problem. Learn some self-healing and do this regularly, while also having some spiritual healing.

INTEGRATED APPROACH

1. Talk to your GP and have appropriate investigations.
2. Orthodox medication includes prostglandin inhibitors such as ibuprofen and mefenamic acid.
3. Adopt a low fat, high-carbohydrate, high-fibre diet with lots of green vegetables, eaten in small regular meals.
4. Take Vitamin C and E supplements along with a daily multivitamin and multimineral.
5. Herbs, homeopathy, aromatherapy and reflexology are beneficial.
6. Open up good communication between yourself and those around you to help them understand the situation.
7. Psychotherapy or cognitive behaviour therapy can help you become more positive.
8. Have some healing and in particular look at sacral chakra issues and your empowerment as a woman.

Multiple Sclerosis

Multiple sclerosis is the most common disabling neurological condition affecting young adults and there are some 85,000 sufferers in the UK alone. This represents 1 in 700 people. Fifty new patients are diagnosed each week, translating to 2500 every year, a very significant number when you consider that this is a progressive, cruel and unpredictable disease. The average onset is between the ages of 20 and 40, affecting people in the prime of their life when responsibilities to their families and jobs are greatest. There are 2 men to every 3 women affected, and although it is not hereditary, there does seem to be a familial susceptibility, perhaps because a sufferer's genetic make-up makes them more sensitive to some environmental factor which triggers MS itself.

The Cause

The underlying cause of MS remains unknown, but at a microscopic level it is possible to see the resultant scarring and degeneration in the myelin sheaths that cover and protect nerve fibres. Without healthy myelin, these fibres cannot function properly, transmitting electrical impulses along the nerve. The damage to the myelin sheath is patchy, scattered throughout the body, affecting several nerves at any one time. The resultant symptoms are responsible for the name multiple sclerosis. The cause remains unidentified but of the various theories, a slowly progressive virus infection or a deficiency in the immune system remain favourites. Many scientists believe that MS is an autoimmune disorder whereby for some unknown reason the sufferer's own antibodies target and destroy their own myelin. The body may have been exposed to some micro-organism with characteristics similar to that of myelin which causes the antibodies that are produced in response to that micro-organism to inadvertently damage the myelin. There may well be a genetic predisposition to such an autoimmune disorder, and this would explain the familial susceptibility.

Several viruses have been isolated from patients with MS. These include: rabies, herpes simplex, scrapie, parainfluenza, measles, subacute myelo-opticoneuropathy virus and coronavirus. All MS patients have high levels of antibodies to the measles vaccine in their blood and cerebrospinal fluid.

Symptoms

Because damage to the myelin sheath is patchy, symptoms can be very varied and widespread. In fact no two people will have identical symptoms, and initially the symptoms can be reminiscent of many other nervous disorders, as MS mimics other diseases. It has been referred to as the great mimic.

Diana noticed one day that when she walked, her right toe kept scraping along the pavement and she had actually worn a small hole in her shoe as a result. It seemed such a minor thing that she was shocked at the thoroughness of the medical examination she received from her family doctor. The doctor in fact diagnosed the condition foot drop, where the muscles pulling the front of the foot up while walking had stopped functioning properly. When she asked why she was being referred to a neurologist for such a simple symptom, the doctor replied that in the absence of any other logical explanation, he wanted to have multiple sclerosis ruled out as this was a not uncommon presenting symptom of the disorder.

Dysfunction of different components of the nervous system causes disorders of sensation, of coordination, of movement, of vision and even of involuntary functions such as bladder and bowel. Patients may complain of numbness, pins and needles, tingling and weakness with heaviness of the limbs, double vision, slurred speech, fatigue and facial pain, difficulty in walking, dizziness and loss of balance. In more advanced cases, muscle spasms and spasticity, frequent urinary and respiratory infections, constipation, skin sores, and mood swings ranging from wild euphoria to deep depression can occur. Symptoms may arise fairly suddenly for no apparent reason or can come on gradually following some injury, infection or general stress.

There are a number of different patterns of symptomatology in MS, and each of the different patterns carries a different outlook. In one pattern, the person has a sudden onset of symptoms followed by a complete and permanent recovery, never experiencing another episode. These are the luckiest ones. In another group, the initial symptoms resolve almost completely, but leave a 10 per cent neurological deficit overall. The person then carries on living a normal life until a second bout which again results in a flare-up in the symptoms with a small permanent loss of function thereafter. This pattern then continues with relapses and remissions throughout life. In a third group of sufferers, the initial onset of the symptoms is steadily progressive, with gradual and uninterrupted loss of function over the course of time. In another group, the onset of symptoms is rapidly progressive and the results devastating, but the number of patients in this category remains very small. The vast majority of sufferers of MS develop a manageable disability that can be treated, although about 20 per cent eventually become severely disabled.

Diagnosis

The diagnosis of MS is difficult on two counts. First the diagnosis is often made on clinical grounds, and only when every other possibility has been excluded. It is very difficult in the early stages to distinguish tingling or a visual problem from part of some other disorder, and it may only be when other symptoms develop in distant parts of the body that the clinical picture of MS emerges. Second the question arises of when to tell the patient that the doctor suspects MS. Unnecessary worry can be damaging to the patient and yet to withhold information from a patient who desperately seeks answers to their problems may appear equally insensitive and arrogant. Such was the dilemma for the doctors in Peter's case.

Peter aged 23 woke up one morning unable to see properly. Part of the right-hand side of his vision appeared to have been lost and he also experienced some tenderness and pain when moving the eyes or touching them. Having always been a fit sportsman, he went to see his doctor somewhat concerned. The doctor used a special viewing instrument called an ophthalmoscope to look at the back of his eyes and saw some inflammation of the head of the optic nerve. He prescribed some steroids and referred Peter to a neurologist. The neurologist could not tell what the problem was, and Peter remained puzzled even after seeing him on three occasions. In fact both doctor and neurologist were suspicious that he had developed MS, but were reluctant to give him this diagnosis until they had definitive proof.

In fact so great is this clinical dilemma in the treatment of patients with MS that it has prompted the MS Society, along with the National Hospital for Neurology, to publish their own standards of care which set out guidelines and advice on how to counsel and approach patients suspected of having MS (see Useful Addresses). The diagnosis can be achieved eventually by a combination of the clinical picture, lumbar puncture and through visual evoked responses (that is, an investigation involving tracing electrical activity within the brain in response to visual stimulation). CT and MRI scans can also show evidence of patchy loss of myelin throughout the nervous system.

Conventional Treatment

Regrettably at the current time conventional medicine has no cure for MS, although many of the symptoms can be treated in one form or another. Medications can modify many problems such as constipation, depression, muscle spasms and infections. Pain can be alleviated with analgesics, and coordination and movement disorders can be helped with physiotherapy and the provision of various aids. Indeed physiotherapy, occupational therapy and general nursing care are vital in keeping MS sufferers as healthy as possible. The use of steroids and Vitamin B_{12} injections has long been advocated to reduce the severity and duration of relapses, and this treatment continues in most centres.

Conventional medicine has been using interferon beta with reductions in symptoms of about 30 per cent. In some studies using natural interferon alpha which is available in some places as a supplement, up to an 80 per cent improvement has been reported and sustained by the majority of participants for 2 years or more.

However, a great deal of work goes on in the complementary medical field to find a solution to MS while the search for a cure for MS continues unabated. The MS Society is currently spending £60 million on 60 different research projects.

Nutritional Healing – The Remarkable Effect of Diet

Dietary measures can be extremely important in limiting the disease and reducing the incapacity it causes. For over 40 years there has been compelling evidence from around the world on the effect of diet on MS. Norwegian studies have shown that those who live inland and eat more animal products including dairy produce have a higher incidence of MS than those who live in coastal areas and eat more fish. Japanese studies have shown that the higher the levels of saturated fatty acids in the diet, the higher the rate of MS, whereas a diet high in seafood and soya results in a lower incidence. Another study showed that those who stuck to a diet high in natural polyunsaturates and low in saturated fats had minimal disability for 30 years or more, whereas those who discontinued the diet developed symptoms again. Changing your diet is not going to bring overnight results, however. You need to look at this as a long-term healing project that can eventually result in some repair of the nerves which have been damaged by your illness. It can also reduce the stickiness of your platelets, lower the autoimmune response and normalise the essential fatty acids in your tissues, blood and cerebrospinal fluid, leading to a general reduction in the frequency and severity of attacks. So, the rules are: avoid solid fats, red meat, dairy produce and eggs. Beware the high fat (and salt) content of some ready-prepared foods. The usual cautions apply to alcohol, refined sugars and salt. Chocolate, shellfish, yeast and food additives are best avoided too including monosodium glutamate. Instead try to take plenty of seeds, grains and nuts, fruit (especially pineapple) and salad. Try oat or rice cakes as snacks and have soya products, fish and organic poultry to top up your protein if necessary. Add plenty of garlic to your cooking or take a supplement.

Vitamins and Supplements

Physicians practising an integrated approach to MS may require investigations – such as a sweat mineral test to detect possible heavy metal toxicity, a test for antioxidant capacity, and an adrenal stress index to see how well the adrenals are working, as well as the more common urinalysis, glucose tolerance test, full blood count and biochemistry – in order to prescribe a complete regime. Flax seed (linseed) oil will help in rebuilding your myelin sheath and is better than evening primrose, safflower or sunflower oil. Linoleic acid reduces both the frequency and severity of attacks. You'll need extra Vitamin E because you're having more fatty acids in your diet and selenium would be good to add too. In Japan they use huge quantities of Vitamin B_{12} since levels are almost invariably low in those with MS. You may be able to take up to 60 mg daily with no ill effects. Most Vitamin B_{12} on the market is cyanocobalamine. However, look for methylcobalamine which is more active and more easily absorbed. Pancreatic enzymes are also usually low, so add to them with supplements of papain, bromelain (you'll be getting some of this in fresh pineapple) and pancreatic extracts which will help malabsorption and which may help reduce the levels of the products of autoimmune reactions (immune complexes) in your blood. Gingko biloba will improve your circulation and the B vitamins and some CoEnzyme Q10 will help your energy. Colamine phosphate (Calcium AEP) is registered as a treatment for MS in Germany.

Exercise and Lifestyle

Whether you have a mild case of the illness or are more seriously affected by it, you need to learn to pace yourself, avoid getting overtired, and generally be kind to yourself. Try to be aware of what's good for you and what isn't and choose your activities wisely. You don't have to apologise for yourself or your illness, but letting others be aware of what the problem is and what you don't feel comfortable doing will lead you to be much less stressed in the end. Although of course it's important to do what you can, do accept offers of help with shopping, housework, etc. and save your energy to do the things that you really enjoy. Talk to your dentist about the possible removal of amalgam fillings since there have been reports of an association between these and MS. Avoid hot baths and saunas.

Complementary Therapies

Many of the complementary therapies such as relaxation, hypnosis and guided imagery will make you feel better, raise your spirits and your self-esteem. Breathing exercises at the beginning and end of every therapy session will oxygenate your tissues and carry healing to every part of you. Have a word with a good aromatherapist and get her to mix a blend of calming oils such as lavender, sandalwood and ylang-ylang. Homeopathy can also help. Yoga will keep you supple and flexible while strengthening your muscles and improving your posture. Tell your teacher about your illness so that she can set up the best programme for you. There are some encouraging studies on the use of magnetic products to help heal damaged nerve and muscle tissue (see p. 23). Some people selling magnetic products will lend you items such as a magnetic mattress for a trial period to see if it helps before you make an investment. Colonic therapists may suggest oil instillation into your bowel followed by chamomile enemas.

Emotional and Spiritual Healing

The families and carers of people with MS can obtain a great deal of help from the MS Society, and there are of course a number of healthcare professionals who can advise, counsel, prevent and treat many of the symptoms and complications of this disabling and unpredictable disorder.

Feelings of anger, despair and grief often accompany the diagnosis of this illness. Added to that is the loss of self-esteem, the isolation and the loneliness that some people with

MS suffer. It doesn't have to be like that! You need to get in gear emotionally and spiritually to deal with it, since being in what we call 'alarm mode' all the time isn't good for you. Adopting a more laid-back attitude and accepting the illness will lead you to more peace. Psychotherapy or counselling will help both you and your partner to live with the illness and stop fighting against it. It will also allow both of you to voice your disappointment about the things you feel you've lost because of it. Use these sessions to communicate fully about how you feel. As always, healing is an active process in which you need to take part. Have Reiki sessions (see p. 25) or spiritual healing and learn self-healing techniques also. There are some who claim that if we had only worked harder, done better things, had better karma, we would not suffer as we do. There may be some truth in that, but there's also the fact that we came here with certain tasks to complete, and for whatever reason, MS is part of that for you. Wherever we are in our life right now is where we're supposed to be, but that doesn't mean we have to stay there. So with a good grace try to learn whatever lesson you're meant to and take care of yourself.

INTEGRATED APPROACH

1. See your GP if you have any of the symptoms mentioned above but be patient about the length of time it may take to make a diagnosis.
2. Changes in your diet can have a profound effect over time.
3. Ask for nursing care, physiotherapy and occupational therapy where appropriate.
4. Steroids and Vitamin B_{12} as prescribed and other vitamins and supplements can be very helpful.
5. Develop a positive attitude and reduce stress as much as you can.
6. Pace yourself and avoid overtiredness while living as normal a life as possible and taking gentle but regular exercise.

7. Relaxation, aromatherapy, and a variety of other therapies will help.
8. Counselling or psychotherapy for you and your closest relatives will help you voice your feelings and come to terms with negative emotions you may feel.
9. Try spiritual healing, Reike sessions and self-healing techniques.

Osteoporosis

Catherine tripped over her back door mat while picking up her morning paper, and although she rolled to the floor rather than fell, she still ended up with a fractured hip. X-rays in hospital revealed a very brittle skeleton with much loss of density, especially in the spine, the long bones of the limbs and the ribs. She took several months to recover from her surgery and despite medication, suffered a further fracture of her wrist a few months later. Catherine has osteoporosis.

Osteoporosis is a condition where bone becomes porous and brittle, and susceptible to fracture. Often there are no symptoms even though the process may have been progressing slowly for years. Fractures, spinal curvature, back pain or lessening of height may be the first signs. Post-menopausal Caucasian and Asian women have the greatest risk of developing osteoporosis due to the changes in hormonal balance which occur at menopause. Hormone replacement therapy (HRT) may correct the balance and prevent further bone loss, though for some, HRT may cause unpleasant side effects as well as increasing the risk of uterine and breast cancer. Inadequate intake or absorption of calcium, especially in childhood can also predispose to the development of osteoporosis.

The risk is increased if you

* have a relative who had osteoporosis
* smoke
* are thin
* drink alcohol excessively
* have low calcium intake
* don't exercise regularly
* are a childless woman
* have had a hysterectomy

Some medication, such as steroids, the anticoagulant heparin and some anticonvulsants (drugs for epilepsy), can accelerate bone loss. Men can also have osteoporosis. Particularly susceptible are those who take corticosteroids for asthma or other conditions.

Diagnosis and Treatment

The best way to find out whether you are suffering from osteoporosis is to have a special DEXA scan which measures the total amount of calcium in your skeleton, especially in your hips and spine. Unfortunately these are not available to everyone on the NHS and tend to be reserved for those at extra risk. Ordinary X-rays are easier to obtain but less certain.

In addition to HRT, the conventional treatment for osteoporosis includes etidronate, calcitonin and other therapies which are all available to slow or reverse bone thinning. Surgical treatment for fractures or pain are on hand if necessary. Osteoporosis is very much a silent epidemic as far as many women are concerned as the condition begins to develop at about the age of 35 and gradually progresses thereafter until the menopause when rapid acceleration of bone thinning occurs over the next 10 years. The National Osteoporosis Society offers information, practical advice and prevention guidance for all potential sufferers, and is an active and enthusiastic organisation which is well worth joining (see useful Addresses).

Nutritional Healing

It is essential to have a calcium-rich diet throughout life, but especially in childhood, during pregnancy and when breastfeeding. The body loses four times its normal calcium loss during lactation. If you are in a high risk group, ensure that you take plenty of foods containing calcium (see p. 544). Also be aware that high-fibre diets tend to bind calcium and prevent its absorption, increasing your calcium requirement. Cutting down on dairy produce reduces the usual intake which must be replaced by other calcium-rich foods such as sesame seeds, broccoli, spinach, almonds and figs. Cola drinks contain phosphoric acid which draws calcium out of your bones and can cause an osteoporotic picture, so it would be as well to refrain from these. Brussels sprouts and scallions contain vitamin K which has an action vital in the maintenance of bone density, so add these to your diet regularly.

Vitamins and Supplements

Choose a supplement which is easily absorbed, such as calcium citrate which doesn't require stomach acid to break it down and can therefore be taken at any time of the day. Calcium in this form also doesn't become bound to fibre and get lost. Calcium carbonate is less well absorbed. All women should take a magnesium supplement which helps calcium absorption and cell repair, and maintains energy production. But it can also help reverse osteoporosis, help protect heart muscle, relieve migraine, backache, constipation and depression. Taken at night it will help you sleep. It can also have the beneficial effect of lowering high blood pressure and easing premenstrual syndrome. It is best taken in citrate form, and a good way is to take a tablet combining magnesium and calcium (ideally the magnesium should be 50 per cent of the level of the calcium). Vitamin D builds and strengthens bones and teeth and aids the absorption of calcium. In addition to spending at least a little time in sunlight to synthesise your own vitamin D, taking a supplement is a good idea. Boron slows down the loss of both calcium and magnesium from bone and can significantly raise oestrogen levels; it can therefore be useful taken during menopause and also in the premenstrual phase at the dose of 2 mgm daily.

Lifestyle and Exercise

Sedentary occupations tend to worsen osteoporosis and it is essential to have exercise, especially weight-bearing exercise such as walking or dancing. Stress can worsen the condition, so see the chapter on stress (p. 481) and ensure that you take time to relax regularly. Since smoking and alcohol consumption make it worse, do try to stop these and talk to your doctor about any drugs you may be taking which may interfere with calcium absorption.

Complementary Therapies

Acupuncture, naturopathy, osteopathy and Traditional Chinese Medicine have all been found useful in the treatment of osteoporosis. There are also several herbs which are beneficial. Rose hips are filled with vitamins and minerals and are good for bone building and overall health. Herb teas made from alfalfa, dandelion, horsetail, lemon grass, nettle, oat straw and red clover are helpful either singly or in combination. Shatavari (asparagus root) helps oestrogen production and incidentally also helps lactation. It is also good for healing gastritis and ulcers. Vidarikanda promotes progesterone formation and helps prevent osteoporosis while also easing symptoms of PMS and menopause. Shiatsu and yoga can be helpful in both promoting relaxation and also giving gentle stretching of the muscles at the points where they insert into your bones.

Emotional and Spiritual Healing

Osteoporosis can be such a destructive condition that there are often associated emotional symptoms such as depression and anxiety, fuelled by the concern about what is happening to our bones and whether or not we shall fall and sustain fractures. Like any other illness, however, it is important to keep positive and to do all that we can to take care of our bodies and heal them as much as possible. Do have some spiritual healing or Reiki which can help promote calm as well as allowing the body to heal itself. If necessary, avail yourself of some counselling or psychotherapy.

Integrated approach

1. Prevent osteoporosis by eating a high calcium diet and by taking plenty of regular weight-bearing exercise from your teenage years onwards.
2. Consider supplements after the age of 35, especially if you are in a high-risk group.
3. Avoid smoking and drinking.
4. Ask your doctor about HRT if you are menopausal.

5. Concentrate on nutritional therapy if HRT is not for you.
6. Have a bone density scan if you are in a high-risk group and consider taking etidronate, calcitonin or other medications to maintain bone density if the results warrant it.

Pregnancy

For many women pregnancy is a wonderfully happy time during which they have never felt better in their lives. Others have a few predictable discomforts, and others can be incapacitated by one thing after another for the entire 9 months. No two women are alike nor are any two pregnancies. Most problems arise from the huge change in the levels of sex hormones in the body, namely oestrogen and progesterone, which trigger the production of up to double the usual amount of blood and fluid, which adds to the increasing weight of the growing baby and the enlarging size of the uterus. Many symptoms require no intervention whatsoever, but when they become severe, it is not helpful to be told that they are normal and will disappear, and that nothing can be done until the pregnancy is over. In fact there are a number of treatments, both preventative and active, that you may wish to try.

Preconceptual Care

This is designed to ensure that you are in peak physical health before you embark upon your pregnancy. Good advice about a healthy diet, about stopping smoking, about taking regular aerobic type exercise and keeping alcohol intake to within moderate limits are all important, as is avoidance of certain micro-organisms which potentially might affect not only your health but that of your planned baby. Bugs such as those responsible for listerosis and toxoplasmosis may be avoided by wearing gloves when emptying cat litter trays and washing hands after handling pets, and by keeping soft cheese, pâté and undercooked eggs off the menu. It is important to make sure that you are immune to rubella via a blood test, and taking folic acid (folate) in a minimum dose of 400 mcg per day has been shown to significantly reduce the possibility of spina bifida in the baby, once conceived. Because it is critical that the baby has sufficient folic acid in the first few days after conception, the folic acid must be taken from the moment you first try to conceive.

Antenatal Checks

Antenatal care is designed to make sure that any serious problems are detected at an early stage of pregnancy so that your health and that of the baby can be protected. Generally speaking you will be encouraged to visit the clinic to see the midwife or doctor at least once a month until you are 28 weeks' pregnant, when the visits increase to fortnightly, becoming weekly from week 36. At your regular antenatal visits your urine will be checked to see if any protein is present, indicating the start of high blood pressure and a disease called pre-eclampsia, and also to look for sugar in the urine which could indicate the presence of diabetes. Your weight is monitored because excessive weight gain can produce problems, and the size of the womb is measured to ensure adequate fetal growth. Blood tests are carried out to exclude anaemia and to test for any germs and abnormal antibodies. Many symptoms arising during pregnancy may require medical help, so do discuss with your doctor anything that concerns you. In particular diabetes, pre-eclampsia, heavy bleeding and severe abdominal pain require urgent medical care since these complications could affect the safety of both you and your baby.

Symptoms

Despite the number of symptoms listed below, however, pregnancy is not an illness, and many women feel particularly healthy and happy at this time. The following symptoms when severe can be treated in the following ways.

ANAEMIA

Anaemia can creep up unexpectedly, especially if you are not getting all the nutrients you need from your diet, or have excessive blood loss (see p. 145). The capacity of your blood to carry oxygen is decreased and a number of other symptoms occur.

Tracy, a vegetarian, was delighted to be pregnant for the first time, but within a few weeks she felt breathless, had palpitations and couldn't sleep at night. Her midwife noticed that she looked pale and when her blood results came back after her first antenatal appointment at 3 months, she was shown to be iron-deficient and anaemic. She was treated with a diet rich in iron and was also prescribed some iron and Vitamin C tablets. Within 2 weeks she began to feel better and her next blood tests confirmed that the problem had been corrected.

Backache

Not only does your posture change as the baby grows towards the end of pregnancy, but the ligaments in the spine become more flexible, allowing the bones in the back and pelvis to slip out of alignment more easily, which leads to backache. It is advisable to avoid gaining too much weight, to keep your back as straight as possible, to wear sensible footwear such as flat or low-heeled shoes and to sleep on a firm mattress. Swimming is an excellent exercise to help prevent backache, and care should of course be taken with any lifting or bending. Having a small cushion in the small of your back is helpful and in severe cases, some gentle manipulation by a chiropractor, physiotherapist or osteopath is useful.

Vaginal bleeding

Any significant blood loss during pregnancy could possibly indicate either a miscarriage or a cervical erosion. A cervical erosion occurs as a result of raised oestrogen levels and merely means that the neck of the womb has become softer and more likely to leak a little blood. A threatened miscarriage can first show itself through vaginal bleeding, and if there is any form of abdominal pain whatsoever, an urgent examination is required. Often the bleeding settles down and the pregnancy continues normally, but where the bleeding continues and examination confirms that the neck of the womb is opening, a miscarriage may become inevitable, resulting in the loss of the baby. Consequently any bleeding should be reported to the doctor urgently. Recurrent mid-term miscarriages may be prevented by the insertion of a special circular stitch called a Shirodkar suture which prevents premature opening of the neck of the womb.

BLEEDING GUMS

Just as bleeding can occur from the neck of the womb as it becomes softer, softer gums can bleed more easily, especially when there is gingivitis (gum disease resulting from plaque). Having regular dental check-ups is important and they are free during pregnancy. Using a soft toothbrush and flossing regularly is advisable.

CONSTIPATION

This is common especially towards the end of pregnancy, so eating plenty of dietary fibre in the form of fruit and raw vegetables, adding bran to bran-rich cereals and relying on wholemeal bread and pasta can help, providing that plenty of extra water is drunk to lubricate the passage of this fibre through the intestine.

CRAMPS

These are common during pregnancy, particularly in the calves, thighs and feet. Poor circulation is partly to blame, but calcium deficiency can be partly responsible too. Massaging the affected area and taking plenty of calcium in the diet will help.

CRAVINGS

The taste for bizarre food and drink during pregnancy is due to changing hormone levels. However, eating what you fancy may be just what you need even though some of the combinations you choose at this time may be rather strange. Try to eat little and often and have plenty of complex carbohydrates such as pasta, fresh fruit and bread which avoid rapid swings in blood sugar levels. In this way cravings can be kept to a minimum.

FAINTING

Because blood vessels relax under the influence of female sex hormones, blood can pool in the skin and legs, resulting in temporary drops in blood pressure which cause a feeling of faintness. This is best avoided by not standing for long periods, not wearing tight clothes or underwear, not lying flat on your back but on your side, and by putting your head between your knees when you feel faint.

FALLEN ARCHES

The arches under the soles of the feet can fall a bit as ligaments become laxer. It can be prevented by wearing arch supports and keeping your weight gain to within recommended limits.

FLUID RETENTION

The hormonal changes of pregnancy lead to the build-up of fluid, causing puffiness in the feet and ankles (oedema) and some bloating. Very salty foods should be avoided, as should long periods of standing. Sometimes elasticated support stockings can be helpful.

FREQUENT URINATION

This is caused partly by pressure on the bladder from the growing baby and can get worse towards the end of the pregnancy.

Elisabeth was expecting her baby in 3 weeks' time, but was plagued with the need to pass urine several times during the night. Sometimes she leaked a little urine when laughing or coughing. She also complained of an ache in her lower back. Her doctor, aware that there is a tendency for infection to ascend from below leading to cystitis, sent off a urine sample for laboratory testing. This revealed a heavy growth of E-coli bacteria and required treatment with antibiotics. Within a few days the frequency of urination settled very markedly, the backache disappeared and the stress incontinence cleared up completely, despite the fact that a very large baby was still pressing on the bladder. She was advised to keep to a minimum caffeine-containing drinks such as coffee and tea, as these are diuretics.

HAIR AND SKIN

Skin can become greasy and hair rather oily due to the extra hormones being produced, but all you need to do during the pregnancy is to have a more regular cleansing and toning routine and to shampoo more frequently. The situation is reversed immediately after childbirth.

HEARTBURN

Heartburn and indigestion are caused by acid coming back up the gullet from the stomach. Eating little and often, avoiding fatty foods and taking antacid tablets or liquids will help. Raising the head of the bed slightly will also discourage acid reflux.

HIGH BLOOD PRESSURE

The blood pressure should be monitored regularly during antenatal care by your doctor or midwife, and if it is found to be too high, especially if it is associated with protein in the urine and oedema, it must be urgently treated to prevent pre-eclampsia (see p. 412). High blood pressure on its own does not cause symptoms and is therefore a silent problem.

INSOMNIA

Many women find that they are not able to sleep well during the last 3 months of pregnancy because they are uncomfortable. The growing baby is more active and there may be an increasing desire to pass urine as the baby's head presses on the bladder. A hot milky drink at night, some relaxation exercises with calming music and wearing light cotton clothes in bed to avoid overheating will help. Sleeping pills should not be taken as all drugs should be avoided during pregnancy if possible.

ITCHING

Itching skin merely requires the application of some calamine lotion or the addition of half a cup of bicarbonate of soda to your bathwater. Oat-based emollient soaps such as Aveeno will help.

Morning sickness

This is something of a misnomer since the sickness of pregnancy can occur at any time of the day or night. It is due to increased levels of oestrogen and progesterone. Medication should be avoided wherever possible. Sweetened drinks and natural ginger are helpful in small quantities. Eat several small meals daily, avoiding rich and spicy foods. Taking ginger either in food or as a tea will help. Try having papaya mid-morning as it has the capacity to settle queasy tummies. And while out and about carry a lemon with you and sniff it if you feel nauseous. Be sure to drink plenty of water and keep well hydrated.

Nasal congestion

Nasal congestion with a stuffy blocked-up nose is another symptom caused by high hormone levels. The inhalation of steam with or without eucalyptus oil and the short-term use of nasal decongestants can help, although once again the symptoms will disappear as soon as the baby is delivered.

Piles

The blood vessels responsible for piles relax and dilate under the influence of progesterone, and the situation can be made worse by constipation (see p. 407). Eating plenty of fibre, avoiding hot baths and putting ice packs on the affected area or using creams or suppositories from the chemist will help. In severe cases, antihaemorrhoid suppositories are available on prescription, and these work better than creams as they can act on the dilated veins within the rectum rather than just on the skin outside. Cypress oil in your bath will help, but it should only be used after 5 months of pregnancy.

Rashes

The skin is more sensitive during pregnancy and allergic or fungal rashes are common. If skin folds are kept clean and dry, fungal infection such as thrush may be avoided, but if it happens, antifungal and anti-inflammatory creams can ease the symptoms.

SKIN-COLOUR CHANGES

In response to the changing hormone levels you may develop areas of pigmentation particularly around the nipples and in a straight line below the navel. Sometime a classical facial distribution of pigment known as chloasma develops. The pigmentation tends to fade after the baby is born but using a sunblock and keeping out of strong sunlight will help keep pigmentation to a minimum.

STRETCH MARKS

Stretch marks occur when the elastic tissue beneath the skin becomes irreversibly stretched. Keeping your weight down during pregnancy can help. Mandarin and lavender oils together in a carrier oil (3 drops of each to a 100 ml bottle of almond oil or similar) are good to prevent stretch marks and should be applied to breasts or abdomen from early on in the pregnancy even before stretch marks could start to appear. Wheatgerm oil and Vitamin E oil can be applied similarly.

THRUSH

Up to a third of women develop vaginal thrush during pregnancy, partly due to the increased sugar content of the cells of the vagina. There are many preparations available, perhaps the most convenient being a fungicidal pessary such as Canestan which can relieve symptoms with just one dose.

TIREDNESS

It is natural to feel tired especially in the early and late stages of pregnancy, so rest as much as possible and delegate as much as possible to your partner or relatives.

VARICOSE VEINS

These occur because there is an increased amount of fluid circulating in the body and the muscular walls of the blood vessels relax, allowing them to dilate and distend. Sadly the blood vessels may never return to their pre-pregnant state. Firm support stockings can help, as can putting up your feet during the day even if only for a few minutes. Avoiding standing for long periods is preventative and regular swimming will help. Also do ankle exercises, making circles with your foot by flexing your ankle, and remember not to sit with your legs crossed. You could make up a massage oil with 3 drops of cypress oil (only after 5 months of pregnancy) and 3 drops of lemon oil in 100 ml carrier oil and massage it gently into your legs as a preventative measure.

Nutritional Healing

Now let's have a look at your nutrition. Obviously you're going to choose a healthy diet (see p. 5) rich in fibre and it's best to avoid raw fish or meat products such as sushi, smoked salmon, Parma ham, proscuitto, etc. Take lots of green leafy vegetables, broccoli, cauliflower and cabbage (all contain Vitamin B_6 and Vitamin K) and plenty of fruit and vegetable juices. Try cucumber, fennel and celery juices well diluted and with a little lemon and honey if you prefer. Dairy produce, broccoli or sesame seeds will give you calcium which is essential not only for your bones but also for those of your baby. Also low levels of calcium have been associated with the development of pre-eclamptic toxaemia (PET).

Vitamins and Supplements

A calcium supplement would be useful along with Vitamin C and other antioxidants which may help prevent PET. Obviously you'll be taking folic acid (folate), and Vitamin B_6 will help with nausea and vomiting if taken at the dose of 25 mg 2 or 3 times a day, although check with your doctor first and don't take for more than a few weeks.

Exercise and Lifestyle

As we said before, pregnancy isn't an illness and adhering as much as possible to your daily routine may be seen as a good thing. However, it's also a time which is very short and you can't put off until later all the wonderful things that you can do now. So how about changing your lifestyle a bit. You aren't an invalid, but how about taking time out to sit and ponder and be with your baby even before it's born. Bonding begins right now so talk, sing or play music to your baby and enjoy this precious time. And do remember that your blood supply is the same as your baby's. If you're dashing around in alarm mode, your baby is having the same anxious time – and he or she doesn't have a choice as you do. Also get plenty of exercise, outdoors as much as possible, with good breathing exercises at the beginning and end to really oxygenate your (and your baby's) blood. If you're at the nausea stage, avoid strong smells! Beware toxoplasmosis . . . Let your partner take out the cat litter.

Complementary Therapies

Be careful about do-it-yourself complementary medicine during pregnancy, especially if you tend to see such therapies as simply feel-good factors and may not therefore respect their potency. There are several oils which you should avoid (see below) although aromatherapy given by a well-qualified professional can still be wonderful. It would be wise to avoid saunas and steam baths and to take care when using flower remedies without professional advice, except Rescue Remedy for emergencies and walnut for emotional harmony. Red raspberry leaf tea is a good for pregnant women, and chamomile will be calming especially at night or in the afternoons when you put your feet up (you *will* be resting in the afternoons, won't you?) Homeopathic remedies could help with every one of the discomforts you may experience. See a professional.

WARNING

The following aromatherapy oils should be avoided during pregnancy:

- Basil
- Calamus
- Cedarwood
- Clary sage
- Hyssop
- Jasmine
- Juniper

Marjoram
Mugwort
Myrrh
Pennyroyal
Rosemary
Sage
Thyme
Wintergreen

Spiritual and Emotional Aspects

It would be ideal if all prospective parents could spend some time sorting out their own personal issues and those within the relationship into which the baby is about to be born, as well as dealing with issues of their own birth and childhood. Avoid listening to the many myths that surround pregnancy and childbirth and if you are worried by any you have heard check out the reality with a professional. If you have suffered sexual abuse and feel like a powerless, helpless victim, try to sort out some of those feelings so that you can feel gently in control and able to work alongside the health professionals to deliver your baby happily and safely. Unplanned and unwanted pregnancies undoubtedly lead to the most problems, physically, emotionally and spiritually. And yet many pregnancies that began that way can have the most wonderful outcomes, provided the issues are addressed while there is time. Women who were born prematurely are more likely to have premature babies, but counselling during the pregnancy may help prepare you for the eventuality and help you deal with it.

The bonding process with your baby begins long before the birth. In fact the practice of scanning and giving the parents a photograph of the baby in the womb, of being able to know the sex if you wish and to start choosing names, all add to the deep attachment. Hopefully it also makes women aware of the great responsibility of carrying a child and the fact that this little being is totally dependent upon you for its welfare. Everything that happens to you will be happening to your baby also. Its blood supply is the same as yours, therefore if you want to be gentle with your baby you have to be gentle with yourself. Toxic substances as in smoking will affect your baby too. Time taken to talk to the baby in your womb, singing to it, playing music, and just being still and reflecting upon the wonder of it all, will be richly rewarded by a deepening bond, usually a more pleasant delivery and easier parenting of a more placid child. Don't forget to include your partner in this wonderful experience. The sooner he can bond the more mutually supportive the two of you can be when the child is born.

This is a miraculous time and if you allow yourself to relax and tune in to your body (and your baby), you will find that even if this is your first baby, you have a wisdom that is ancient and you will know how you want to deliver the child, what you need, who you want to be there, etc. If you're socially isolated and have neither a partner nor family close by, then do ask a friend or even someone from a local church or similar to be with you as your birthing partner. Should you develop PET or the delivery has to be rushed for some other reason, having someone with you who loves you and understands you is a great help. Try to keep focused on the fact that there are greater forces at work here and that the timing of the birth will be exactly as it should be, and the birth itself will be exactly as it is meant to be. You and your baby have made an ancient and spiritual pact to be at this place and time together, and all will work out just as it is meant to.

This can be one of the most empowering times of your life when you naturally, as women have always done, go through the process of labour to bring your child into the world. It is not meant to be a time of controlled sterility but of natural spiritual beauty when out of pain and sweat you produce the greatest work of your life. Although pain control during labour is available and you may choose to have whatever you wish, you may like to look at natural childbirth, seeing the whole process from conception to birth not as a crisis but as a gift that no one can take away from you. Should there be complications, then trust the team working with you to do their very best for you and your baby, try to keep calm and talk to your baby as you have always done. Women are transformed by pregnancy and giving birth. Enjoy.

Integrated approach

1. Care needs to begin as soon as you start to think of getting pregnant.
2. Always have regular antenatal care and ask as many questions as you wish.
3. Report all symptoms to your doctor. Some of them may only require reassurance. Others may herald the onset of some condition requiring urgent medical care.
4. Remember that many of the discomforts of pregnancy will reverse as soon as the baby is born.
5. Take adequate rest and remember that your baby has the same blood supply as you and doesn't have any choice over what you subject it to.
6. Remain active within reason and check the safety of sports with your doctor.
7. Take time to bond with your baby and involve your partner as much as possible.
8. Prepare psychologically and emotionally as well as physically for delivery and have someone you love and trust to be your birth partner.
9. Complementary therapy and healing can help both you and your baby but heed the warning about what NOT to use.

Prostate Problems

The prostate gland is a mystery to many men and most of them are entirely unaware of their prostate until something begins to go wrong with it. In fact the prostate gland is a chestnut-shaped organ located at the base of the bladder surrounding the urethra, the tube which drains urine from the bladder down the penis to the outside. Its function is to produce secretions that form part of the semen in which sperm swim. The gland enlarges at puberty under the influence of male sex hormones (androgens) and reaches its maximum size at the age of about 20, by which time it weighs about 20 grams. After the age of 50 it enlarges very slowly.

The major disorders include prostatitis, benign enlargement of the prostate (BPH) and prostatic cancer.

Prostatitis

This inflammation generally occurs in men between the ages of 30 and 50.

Len is 48 and as an accountant spends much of his day sitting at his desk. He admitted on routine questioning that he drinks rather too much alcohol in the evenings and compensates the next day by drinking lots of coffee to help keep himself alert. Living alone, he tends to cook fast food or have takeaways and has little fresh fruit or vegetables in his diet. The only exercise he takes is to look after his garden where he has been using some quite toxic pesticides. He has had recurrent urinary tract infections over the last couple of years and now has pain in his left loin area. He said that he has some discomfort in passing urine which is cloudy with occasionally some blood. Len has prostatitis with a complicating urinary tract infection that is now affecting his left kidney.

The infection usually finds its way to the gland through infection in the urethra and this may be sexually transmitted.

However, that is not always the case, and the presence of a urinary catheter can predispose to prostatitis. Symptoms include pain when passing urine and a more frequent desire to do so (frequency). Discomfort around the rectum and scrotum, blood in the urine and discharge from the urethra may or may not be present.

Critical Tests

A sample of urine is examined and any discharge from the urethra can be swabbed and cultured in the laboratory to identify any organisms. The doctor can also examine the prostate gland with a gloved finger in which case it may feel tender, 'boggy' and enlarged.

Conventional Treatment

Treatment consists of antibiotic drugs, the selection depending on the micro-organisms responsible, which may need to be taken for a prolonged period in order to completely eradicate the infection.

Benign Prostatic Hypertrophy (BPH)

This term refers to the non-malignant physiological enlargement of the prostate gland which occurs in all men over the age of 50. One in three men over this age will develop symptoms which are medically referred to as 'prostatism' and which are indistinguishable from many of the symptoms of prostatic cancer.

Harry is 60. He complained that over the last year or so he has had some difficulty with his waterworks. The first thing he noticed was that he wanted to pass urine more often than usual, but that when he got to the toilet, he often had to wait a while and strain a bit before the urine would start to flow. Lately the stream of urine stopped and started and even though he desperately wanted to go, there was little force and he felt that he never really managed to finish. He has no pain, but in the last day or two he started to have a burning sensation while passing urine. It was this that prompted him to go to the surgery. Harry has benign prostatic hypertrophy (BPH).

Men like Harry with an enlarged prostate complain that they need to go often (known as frequency) and that they need to go urgently (known as urgency). Frustratingly, however, they find it difficult to start (known as hesitancy), the flow is weak and dribbling, and it continues even after they have attempted to stop. They have to get up at night to empty their bladders, and they may be prone to regular bladder infections or even incontinence. Occasionally the outflow from the bladder becomes completely obstructed by an enlarging prostate, and acute abdominal pain and a swollen bladder may occur. This constitutes an acute medical emergency, and some patients require the passage into the bladder of a fine, flexible tube called a catheter, in order to bypass the obstruction. All these symptoms arise because enlargement of the gland compresses the urethra at the base of the bladder and prevents the proper outflow of urine.

Critical Tests

A rectal examination by the doctor using a gloved finger will confirm that the prostate is enlarged. A urine sample can reveal if any urinary infection is present, and a blood test can measure kidney function which can be detrimentally affected if chronic outflow problems have led to back-pressure to the kidneys, jeopardising excretion. At the same time the blood sample may be analysed for an enzyme known as prostate specific antigen (PSA), which helps to distinguish between benign prostatic hypertrophy and prostate cancer (see p. 421). Urinary flow tests can measure the strength of the urinary stream, and give extra information about the degree of any obstruction. Finally, ultrasound scanning using a probe placed within the rectum can help to identify any suspicious areas within the prostate gland which, together with the digital rectal examination (DRE) and the PSA test, can help confirm that the enlargement of the gland is benign.

Conventional Treatment

SELF-HELP

Good advice to men with BPH would be to look carefully at their nutrition and follow the recommendations given later in the chapter. A policy of watchful waiting is sometimes employed by doctors. This merely means that a doctor re-examines his or her patient from time to time to assess whether the symptoms are getting worse or not. Sometimes the condition remains static. It may help to avoid drinking copious quantities of fluid at any one time or having drinks before bed. Adjustments to the lifestyle and taking any supplements (see below) are helpful.

DRUG THERAPY

When symptoms are only mild or moderate, medication can be used. There are two main types known as alpha blockers and 5-alpha reductase inhibitors, both of which are capable of delaying the progression of symptoms so that surgery can be postponed or even avoided. The alpha blockers relax the muscle in the prostate and relieve the pressure on the urethra as a result. They cannot prevent enlargement of the prostate, but they do relieve the symptoms. If no benefit is derived within a month, it is unlikely to follow thereafter. There are of course side effects occasionally which you should ask your doctor about. The 5-alpha reductase inhibitors stop the production of a hormone known as dihydrotestosterone which is believed to be the main hormone responsible for prostate enlargement. These drugs may slow the enlargement of the gland and in some cases may even shrink it. Improvement of symptoms occurs in more than 50 per cent of cases, but again there may be side effects including reduced libido and impotence. One drug, finasteride, has the potential to cause damage to unborn babies, so men taking it should wear a sheath during intercourse.

SURGERY

Surgery to remove the prostate (prostatectomy) is still generally regarded by most doctors as the best way of relieving symptoms. There are many different types of surgery, but the gold star treatment is generally regarded as being a TURP (trans-urethral resection of the prostate). This is carried out under a light general anaesthetic, and it takes about an hour to perform. Urinary flow rate is much better following the operation, but it may take several weeks before frequency subsides. Up to 80 per cent of men having a TURP are satisfied with the outcome, but all patients should be fully aware of the possible complications of such surgery, which may include bleeding after the procedure, sub-fertility, possible erection difficulties and a small risk of incontinence. One of the most common side effects is retrograde ejaculation where semen flows back into the bladder instead of being ejaculated through the penis at sexual climax. The sensation is similar to a normal climax, but no semen emerges from the penile tip. There are alternatives to this commonly performed operation, including an open prostatectomy which is done through an abdominal incision rather than through the penile urethra, but this is usually reserved for very large prostate glands. Other treatments are also possible, using metal coils or stents to hold the urethra open or to burn, laser or microwave away parts of the large gland, but these are operations you need to discuss with your specialist urologist. The information is complex and confusing, and a sympathetic and well-informed GP is ideally placed to advise you as to which treatment is best in your own individual case.

PROSTATE CANCER

Believe it or not, cancer of the prostate is the second most dangerous cancer in men. It accounts for some 9500 deaths every year in the UK. Nobody knows what the underlying cause is, although there is a growing feeling that a Western diet, too rich in saturated fat and too low in vegetables, could be responsible. There is a familial tendency to develop it, the risk being greater if an affected relative was young, and if more than one close relative in the family was affected. A gene has been identified which predisposes to a greater risk of cancer of the prostate. One unsubstantiated myth is that having a vasectomy increases the likelihood of developing cancer of the prostate. There is little evidence that this is true. The symptoms of prostate cancer are almost impossible to distinguish from those of benign enlargement of the gland, and like BPH they become increasingly common with the patient's advancing age. It is known that over 70 per cent of men in their eighties will have small areas of prostate cancer, yet only a few of them will ever develop problems.

Alex, aged 74, has been complaining for some time of difficulties with urination. He cannot get through the night without having to go to the toilet 3 or 4 times and yet on each occasion he can pass very little urine. He has no pain, but occasionally a dragging ache in his lower abdomen and lower back. On rectal examination his prostate was found to be hard. He tested positive for the prostate specific antigen (PSA, a protein found specifically in those with prostate cancer) and a biopsy confirmed that Alex has prostate cancer.

Of course prostate cancer can coexist along with benign enlargement and it is no surprise therefore that many men undergoing the TURP operation for BPH are informed afterwards that cancer was detected in their prostate.

To have the PSA test or not?

Whether or not to introduce national prostate screening is a controversial issue. The PSA test is useful, but as well as worrying some men unnecessarily when their slow-growing cancer would cause them no harm if left alone, the test also may prove falsely positive in men who never had cancer in the first place. A new form of the PSA test which measures free PSA, unattached to protein in the blood, appears to be more sensitive and will undoubtedly be more widely adopted in the future. In the meantime, the screening debate will continue. Your GP and specialist urologist will be your best advisers as to whether you have a PSA test done, along with the other two important parameters of prostate health, namely the digital rectal examination and the rectal ultrasound test. If you are to have the PSA blood test it should always be conducted prior to a rectal examination as the latter can falsely elevate the PSA level in the blood as a result of manual pressure on the gland.

Critical Tests

Rectal examination, the PSA test and a rectal ultrasound test, together with the tests described in the section on BPH, are the important tests in this disorder. X-rays may be taken to see if any spread of cancer has occurred in the bones. Occasionally an isotope bone scan is conducted as these are even more sensitive than X-rays. MRI or CT scans can provide greater detail about the prostate with images from many different angles and will show the presence of small cancers.

Conventional Treatment

Treatment will vary depending on many factors including your general health, your age and the type, size and spread of any cancer. The tests described above are important in helping the physician and urologist come to an appropriate conclusion about the best form of treatment for you. There will always be alternatives to the treatment recommended and particularly with the treatment of prostate cancer it is sometimes helpful to have a second opinion so that a decision can be made more easily. It is essential that the consequences of treatment are discussed with the patient because some of them can be fairly unpleasant. These include occasional urinary incontinence and impotence as well as infertility. These problems are unpredictable and vary in degree, but it is important that all patients are prepared in case they occur. The pros and cons of any kind of treatment must always be weighed up, and there are many men who have refused treatment and have lived long and fruitful lives, eventually succumbing to some unrelated health problem.

In older men whose cancer is confined to their prostate, a decision may be made to merely carry out regular examinations and checks on PSA levels, as this type of cancer is unlikely to cause problems for at least 5 years. Lifestyle and dietary changes during this time would be advisable. Radiotherapy is also commonly used for localised cancers. This treatment kills off cancer cells but as a side effect can also destroy some of the normal cells with the consequence that diarrhoea, discomfort in the rectum and bleeding may occur. Pain when passing urine and frequency are also reported alongside impotence and incontinence. Furthermore, radiotherapy cannot guarantee that the disease will not recur although it is thought that up to 60 per cent of men survive up to 15 years after treatment.

A radical prostatectomy is an operation that removes the whole of the prostate gland and offers the best likelihood of a cure, provided of course that the cancer is completely restricted to the prostate gland itself. The success rate is similar to that of radiotherapy in the same circumstances. Again the risk of impotence and incontinence must be borne in mind. It is probably best used in younger men with aggressive tumours that have not spread beyond the prostate and in whom there is a long life expectancy. For the older man its benefits probably do not outweigh its side effects.

Hormone treatments are particularly important when cancer has spread beyond the prostate because the cancer cells are dependent largely on the male sex hormone, testosterone, to keep them growing. If testosterone levels can be reduced, then the growth of the tumour can decelerate or it may even shrink. Such treatment involves injecting under the skin a hormone that prevents testosterone being released in the body, and tablets that block the action of testosterone on the cancer cells. A combination of the two types of medical treatment is often referred to as total androgen blockade. Sometimes this kind of hormonal treatment is used together with radiation or surgery and again there may be inconvenient side effects such as impotence and hot flushes, similar to the kind women experience during menopause. When prostate cancer has already spread to other organs in the body including the bones, hormonal treatments and radiotherapy are usually prescribed together.

THE PATIENT AS AN INDIVIDUAL

Prostate problems in men are notoriously difficult to sort out. Because of this, it is essential that a good relationship is established between the patient and the doctor, and that the patient has every opportunity to discuss the options and the current situation. A second or even third opinion can be helpful in reaching a decision. There is a reluctance among many men to talk about health issues below the waist, and attitudes have got to change before this situation improves. Men must develop the habit of talking about their sexual health among their peers just as women do, and doctors must make advice in this department much more accessible. It is important to remember that men can feel just as threatened about the effects on their sexuality of treatment for prostate disorders as are women when faced with hard decisions about treatment for breast disorders.

Nutritional Healing

Len's diet couldn't have been much more unhealthy. Eating too much fat, drinking too much caffeine and taking too much alcohol all predispose to prostate problems. The basic dietary recommendations on p. 5 would be good for him to adopt, but there are some extras that would be useful. Tomatoes are a great standby for all men and should be eaten in some form every day, whether raw or as a pasta sauce, for example. Tomatoes contain lycopene, the most powerful of the carotenoid antioxidants which help to prevent prostate cancer, while also protecting the immune system and helping its fight against infections. Other carotenoids, the phytochemicals which can cut the risk of cancer, are found in carrots, sweet potatoes, yams, pumpkins and leafy green vegetables. Raw nuts and seeds help add fibre and also act as detoxifying agents for pesticides and other noxious substances that have been found to be implicated in the development of prostate cancer. Be very careful about washing fruit and vegetables to remove any pesticides, and where possible, buy (or grow your own!) organic food. Pumpkin seeds or sunflower seeds should be added to salads or cereal since they can help reduce not only the size of the prostate but the amount of urine that otherwise gets left in the bladder to form a perfect medium for infections. Pumpkin seeds also tone the muscles of the bladder wall and relieve congestion and inflammation. A handful of dandelion leaves or parsley added to a salad will not only provide a lovely flavour but act as a natural diuretic. Asparagus, full of minerals, is also a natural diuretic. Cranberries are natural antiseptics for the urinary tract (see the section on UTIs, p. 514). Garlic appears to slow down the growth of cancer cells in the prostate. It's a good move to get your cholesterol down, since according to some studies, the products of cholesterol breakdown have been found to accumulate in the cells of the prostate, may be carcinogenic and can cause swelling. Soya milk or protein has a protective effect on the prostate, reducing the risk of cancer.

Vitamins and Supplements

Zinc is rarely found in our diet in sufficient quantities for our needs as we get older. It's worth having your zinc level checked (see Screening, p. 11) since not only does zinc help with wound healing, but it has a specific action on the prostate. Oil of evening primrose, sunflower seeds or borage oil may also help to reduce swelling and make passing urine easier, while Cernilton, an extract from flower pollen, has been found to reduce the size of the prostate and decrease residual urine.

Exercise and Lifestyle

If you are in a job that involves a lot of sitting, stand up, stretch and have a little walk if only around your office at least every hour or so. Getting good exercise, preferably outdoors, is as essential to prostatic health as it is to the health and wellbeing of the rest of your body. Hydrotherapy, which involves alternating hot and cold bathing of the area, is useful for both prostatitis and BPH. Ideally sit in a hot bath for a couple of minutes, having close by a receptacle large enough to sit in, filled with cold water. Alternate between them every 2 minutes or so for about 15 minutes in all. This helps to improve circulation and the tone of the pelvic muscles. Prostate cancer in later life has been linked to the human papilloma virus and therefore safe sex is important, with the use of condoms throughout adult life, as is the careful choice of sexual partners. Your GP will advise you about check-ups and screening, but if you're over 50 you would be wise to have an annual test for the prostate specific antigen (PSA), a useful predictor of prostate cancer, and a routine rectal examination. If you're of African descent, then you'd be wise to ask your doctor to start these screens earlier than 50. The PSA blood test can give false positives in about 60 per cent of cases. You can reduce these odds by refraining from intercourse for 48 hours before the test. Also, you should stop smoking. Not only is it adding noxious substances to your system and having adverse effects on your heart and lungs but it is bad for your prostate. It really is time to give up if you haven't done so already.

Complementary Therapies

Herbs that are effective include saw palmetto which has long been used in the treatment of problems associated with the urinary tract. In many men, its effect on the prostate can be marked after a month or so of use. It can relieve the constriction of the ureter and make passing urine easier, also reducing inflammation. Pygeum can reduce the feeling of urgency, decrease the need to pass small quantities of urine frequently and is also anti-inflammatory. An extract from the root of stinging nettles can help urinary flow and reduce the amount of urine that gets left behind in the bladder (residual urine) as well as reduce frequency. Other herbs your herbalist may prescribe include diuretics such as couchgrass, hydrangea and buchu, and antiseptics such as uva ursi. Homeopathic remedies having an effect upon the prostate include Conium, indicated where there is night-time frequency, worse after alcohol; Iodum, when the prostate is hard and possibly cancerous (make sure you see your GP and have a full investigation); Sabal, where there is stinging or burning as urine is passed. Barium carb and Calc carb may also be effective, but always see a good practitioner who will prescribe for you on the basis of the whole picture and not only isolated symptoms. Acupuncture may help if you feel particularly distressed. Stay calm and count your breathing if you become panic-stricken about not being able to pass urine. This helps by relaxing the tissues. As with all illnesses, you can help yourself with creative visualisation, a relaxing process whereby you use the power of your mind to envision your cells becoming healthy, a reduction in swelling and your tissues having a good blood supply, bringing essential nutrients into the area.

Emotional and Spiritual Healing

Any illness that suddenly makes us aware of the inevitability of old age can have a marked effect upon our self-confidence and self-esteem. Where this may involve sexual performance, especially in men, the perceived insult to the psyche can be considerable. As with all illness or change in our physical state, it's important not to neglect the emotional and spiritual effects. Try to talk about your problem to your partner if you have one or to a trusted friend, or join a support group where you can also obtain practical advice and alleviate some of your fears should surgery be necessary. Prostate problems are a first (root) chakra issue, and doing some work to clear and heal this area will help (see p. 539). Have some healing with a healer who can talk through issues with you, especially the events of very early childhood (birth to 5 years old) which is the time when this chakra would be developing.

INTEGRATED APPROACH

1. Develop a good relationship with your doctor that will allow you to talk openly and honestly about your prostate and whatever worries you.
2. Make changes to your diet and lifestyle even before you could develop problems.
3. Take supplements as above to protect the health of your prostate.

4. Look into the complementary therapies available. These may form a good alternative if you and your doctor decide upon a conservative watchful waiting strategy.
5. If you plump for surgery, make sure you are aware of the potential post-operative problems that might occur.
6. Practise safe sex throughout your life to protect against infection. No matter how old you are, it is never too late to start to protect yourself.

Schizophrenia

To most people, schizophrenia has come to mean a split personality, a sort of Jekyll and Hyde character who sometimes behaves quite normally and at other times is evil or mad. Unfortunately this is not just a simplification but a misinterpretation of a term which literally means 'split mind'. Schizophrenia is not a single entity but a collection of illnesses which have some aspects in common, mainly the loss of touch with reality. People with schizophrenia may exhibit a spectrum of symptoms which are beyond those normally experienced by the rest of the population. This feature distinguishes the psychotic illnesses, to which the schizophrenias belong, from the neurotic illnesses where the symptoms may appear bizarre but are in fact only exaggerations of feelings we all experience from time to time. As you will see, the people we shall mention, Rhoda, Sam, Sally and Mable, all present in slightly different ways, but all are experiencing things which the rest of us generally do not. Sally's case is slightly different, however, and will be discussed later. Some 1 per cent of the population is affected by schizophrenia and this seems to be fairly constant among different populations around the world. Men and women are affected equally. The age of onset varies with the type of schizophrenia, some young people in their late teens and early twenties being affected, and others not until comparatively old age.

Sam is 19, was a high achiever at school and was expected to do very well at university. He was always a bit of a loner, spending more time studying than being with friends. He had difficulties living in a hall with lots of other young people where he found it hard to make friends. In the second term he left abruptly, appearing very depressed and being unwilling to discuss with anyone his reasons for dropping out. He took to staying in his bedroom and eating. His sleep was erratic while his level of self-care deteriorated to the point that sometimes he would refuse to wash or bathe for days. He appeared less articulate and sometimes seemed unable to think clearly. Sometimes he would stop in the middle of a sentence, appear to be listening to something and would then smile, laugh or appear angry. Sam has hebephrenic schizophrenia.

Rhoda, however, is 46 and works as a librarian. She is well respected in her job and copes with it very well. She has never married and lives with her ageing mother. About 4 years ago she started to complain that her neighbours were threatening her life and that of her mother. She had some treatment as an in-patient for a few weeks and has stayed on medication. She still believes that she was under threat but that her neighbours have now stopped their campaign of terror against her. Rhoda has paranoid schizophrenia.

Sally's situation is different. At 28, she works in a bookshop and is popular with her colleagues for her quiet gentle ways. Over the last year or so she has lost a considerable amount of time at work because she has been having frightening experiences and thinks she's going mad. She has always been a religious young woman with a deep sense of something spiritual and has been studying philosophies and religious beliefs from around the world. She feels from time to time that she can hear strange noises, sometimes voices, talking to her. Sometimes she has a strong sense that she receives messages from another planet and feels very confused about what is happening to her. This has led her to become more isolated because she doesn't want to tell anyone about what's happening in case she is mad.

Although Sally needs proper professional assessment and may be developing schizophrenia, it's more likely that she is having a spiritual awakening which she doesn't understand and for which she is unprepared.

And then there's Mable who is 82 and has lived alone since her husband died. She is deaf and really needs some extra help, either to continue to live at home or to move into accommodation where she can have more support. Over the last few months she has become increasingly angry and now sometimes refuses to let her daughter into her house. She complains that people are talking about her and harassing her with loud music. Sometimes she has been heard shouting from her doorway for people to get away from her house and leave her alone. Mable has paraphrenic schizophrenia.

In acute schizophrenia, such as Sam is experiencing, there are hallucinations where the person has a physiological response but without an actual stimulus. Sam hears voices talking outside his head when actually there is no one there. Delusions are common to all the schizophrenias. Rhoda's belief that there is a plot against her is a delusion, and although it's a false belief, no amount of reasoning will be able to shake her conviction that it is true. Often the sufferer will be preoccupied with voices, frightened by their delusions and feel that they are being controlled by external forces such as laser beams or gods which control their actions and make them do things. In chronic schizophrenia, there are problems with social interaction as the person becomes more and more withdrawn, with little motivation and drive, speaking little, neglecting themselves and often being quite depressed. Although sometimes there seems to be the impression that those suffering from schizophrenia are violent, this is rarely the case. Occasionally, however, people do respond to the voices by being frightened or angry, or on occasion by doing what the voices tell them to do, which may be of a violent nature.

Sometimes diagnosis can be difficult and may take a while to evolve.

Drug-induced psychosis

Psychotic states similar to schizophrenia in their symptomatology and presentation can be induced by the use of cannabis, ecstasy, amphetamines, magic mushrooms, LSD and some other illicit or recreational drugs. If such a state has occurred, then repeated use of the substance at any time is likely to precipitate a further psychotic episode.

Causes

Schizophrenia is multifactorial in origin. Scientific evidence from family, twin and adoption studies shows that a vulnerability to develop schizophrenia is probably inherited. Environmental issues then compound the problem and precipitate the final development of the illness. Trigger factors include family dynamics, excessive expression of emotion, stressful life events, birth trauma and infection. Changes in the levels of chemicals in the brain known as neurotransmitters (e.g. dopamine) play a part.

Conventional Treatment

The treatment of schizophrenia relies on physical, psychological and social methods. Since one of the characteristics of schizophrenia is that insight is lost, often the person suffering the illness doesn't ask for help and is brought to the doctor's surgery by a relative or friend. Most people will need medication during the acute phase and will then be maintained on this for a considerable time to prevent relapse. These drugs are useful to reduce hallucinations and delusions. A wide variety of such medication is available and should be tailored to the patient's needs, taking into account side effects and personal preference. Some are quite sedative and useful when someone is agitated, and others help to lift the more negative symptoms of withdrawal. Sadly many people with schizophrenia refuse to take their medication and relapse fairly regularly. Sometimes the doctor or psychiatrist will suggest a depot medication, perhaps every 2 or 3 weeks, where the drug is given by injection deep into the muscle and gradually released into the bloodstream, maintaining a level of the drug sufficient to keep the patient well. Unfortunately most of the medication for schizophrenia has side effects and often therefore another drug such as procyclidine or benzatropine will need to be given simultaneously to offset these unwanted symptoms.

Very occasionally the psychiatrist may also suggest electroconvulsive therapy (ECT) where there is coexistent excitement or depression. Supportive psychotherapy helps the person to deal with their confusion, depression and fear. Social management involves environmental stimulation which needs to be carefully controlled in the acute phases. Occupational therapy and attendance at day centres and halfway houses – or Care in the Community as it is now called – can be planned. Attendance is encouraged while stress is kept to a minimum. Work with families is also an essential part of the management since they are often under considerable stress and need to try to understand what is going on.

Community care

The decision to close large mental hospitals was partly due to the desire to prevent the institutionalisation of chronically ill people. The intention was to provide high-quality, community-based residential and recreational centres for them which were thought to provide better, more personal care than the old lock-up institutions. It is still unclear how successful this approach is, however. Education of the general population about this dreadfully debilitating illness is necessary if vulnerable individuals, already handicapped by their illness, are not to remain isolated, become vagrants or end up in prison. Adequate finance and resources and better communication between health professionals are essential. The future outlook depends upon the continued development of the social aspects of treatment and the provision of enough rehabilitation units, both in hospitals and in the community, while the search for new and better drugs continues, the aim being to provide safe medication free from debilitating side effects.

Nutritional Healing, Vitamins and Supplements

Sadly people with mental illness tend not to take proper care of themselves and so those who are in positions to care for them should try to ensure that they have a proper diet. It is worth looking at the possibility of food allergies and environmental toxins which may be playing havoc with the delicate balance of the mind. However, the main thrust must be to get them to eat well, drink plenty of water and have as many nutrients as possible. When in the florid state (actively psychotic) it may be impossible for them to eat well so vitamins and supplements play a very important role here. Of course it may also be difficult, because of their paranoia or other strange beliefs, to get the person with mental illness to take these either. Between attacks, however, everything must be done to encourage proper nutrition. Please see p. 4 for the basics.

Exercise and Lifestyle

Encouraging the person who suffers from schizophrenia to live what the rest of us may see as a normal life is often difficult and sometimes impossible, since they feel controlled by other forces which tell them to behave differently. Sadly some social decline and isolation from the rest of the world is often unavoidable. However, the newer medications address this aspect of the illness and make it easier for patients and their families to return to normal. Too much expressed emotion will only push the person away and therefore to be angry, tearful or anxious about the situation is counter-productive. Better to encourage where you can and accept it when your intervention falls on stony ground. Often when a routine is established, however, it will be rigidly adhered to, so obviously the more healthy components it can have the better. Sometimes having a dog will encourage the person to take walks, but it may be too much to expect that someone having difficulty with taking care of themselves can adequately take care of a pet, so you may find yourself having to do some of the work. Attendance at a day-care centre will often make a great deal of difference as a routine is established, professional carers are on hand, meals can be supervised if necessary and there is the opportunity for as much socialisation as the person can manage. Don't forget that one of the essentials of living with someone with a chronic illness is that the carers need to take care of themselves, so in the midst of all this, don't neglect yourself.

Complementary Therapies

Homeopathy is perhaps the complementary therapy with most to offer in this illness. There are a number of remedies that may have quite a marked beneficial effect. Where there is agitation, swinging moods, alternating withdrawal and hyperactivity, Tarantula hisp may help. Thuja occidentalis is more appropriate where there is depression and irritability with the complaint that some external force controls the person and makes them do things. Anacardium orientale can sometimes help where there are hallucinations, inappropriate moods, obsessional features and a feeling of outer controlling forces. Lachesis is indicated where paranoia is a prominent symptom and where things seem to be considerably worse in the mornings. Your homeopath may well begin treatment with a constitutional remedy. Other remedies that may be helpful include Belladonna, Stramonium and hyoscyamus. Schizophrenia is not an illness that lends itself well to do-it-yourself treatments and we would strongly advise that you see a homeopath who is versed in treating mental illness. Aromatherapy oils such as lavender and clary sage will help with relaxation, and lemongrass burned in the home in the mornings either as incense or oil may help where there is lack of motivation and drive. Sadly depression and the desire to die are not uncommon in young people with schizophrenia so using the complementary therapies discussed in the section on depression could be useful. Music and movement as well as art therapy may help the person unlock some of their inner pain. The art of those with schizophrenia has been written about over many years and can often be a diagnostic tool in itself. It can also predict the onset of an attack as well as herald the end of one as the images return to normal. Looking at the art of someone in the depths of a psychotic illness can often give us a glimpse of their suffering and hopefully increase our compassion in dealing with this illness.

Emotional and Spiritual Healing

Schizophrenia does exist. However, there is a theory which is that of spiritual emergence and emergency where sudden spiritual changes including the unexpected raising of the kundalini can thrust the person into a state which appears foreign and frightening, during which what they report and experience is hardly distinguishable from schizophrenia. What is of great concern in such cases is that if the state is wrongly diagnosed and the patient is put on medication that is inappropriate, it is difficult to the reach the person to help them return to a more normal state. If you, either as a sufferer or carer of someone diagnosed with schizophrenia, have any doubt about the diagnosis and feel that there may be a spiritual explanation for the mental state, then do ask for a second opinion from a spiritual psychiatrist. The International Association for Spiritual Psychiatry could help you find someone in your area, and the Royal College of Psychiatrists is being encouraged to set up a special section for psychiatrists who specialise in spiritual states. The Scientific and Medical Network has several members who are psychiatrists who may also help you to contact someone to give you another opinion. Do try to do this through the proper channels, however, observing medical etiquette by going to your GP and asking for a referral or by asking your consultant psychiatrist to refer you. In the meantime, having some healing, especially working on the root chakra and grounding exercises, will help. If you're a relative, then do take care of yourself too. Try some healing for yourself that will help you to relax and accept things as they are. Your anxiety, anger, disappointment and resentment about the situation can do no good and may well be harmful. It's natural, of course, to feel all of those things, especially if you're a parent. Sam's mum and dad were devastated by his illness and the loss of their expectations about their son. However, these emotions needed to be dealt with separately and privately, not expressed to Sam for whom it would only make things worse.

INTEGRATED APPROACH

1. Make sure that an accurate diagnosis is made and if necessary ask for a second opinion.
2. Medication may be essential, not only in the acute phase but longer term to prevent relapse.
3. Rule out possibilities such as food allergies, drug abuse, etc. and correct where necessary.
4. Nutrition is often neglected so try to ensure that it is optimum by a good diet and supplementing where necessary.
5. Try to ensure adequate communication between professionals on the health-care team who may be spread between hospital, community, Social Services, GP's surgery and home. If you are a carer, ask for an interview when you need one so that you can get the information you need to help you in your role.
6. Complementary medicine has a considerable amount to offer and healing can help.
7. Expressed emotion, both positive and negative, may be too much for the person to take and may precipitate further illness, so try to keep it to a minimum to prevent relapses.
8. If you are a carer, take time out to look after yourself.

Sexual Problems

Sexual problems can arise for a number of reasons but most of them relate either to a problem of sexual performance or sexual behaviour. These difficulties can affect either or both partners in the relationship. Sometimes the underlying cause is psychological but there may be an organic physical disorder or hormone imbalance, or the situation may be due to the side effects of certain medicines or pollutants in the environment.

COMMON PSYCHOSEXUAL PROBLEMS

These include:

* Performance anxiety, where one partner feels that he or she cannot match the expectations of the other.
* Failure to achieve orgasm, as a result of fear, inhibition or guilt, and lack of sex drive due to problems within the relationship such as mistrust and stress.
* Generalised stress, which can have a major effect on sexual desire and performance.
* Vaginismus, which is the involuntary contraction of the vaginal muscles. This may have a physical cause such as thrush, endometriosis, salpingitis (inflammation of the fallopian tubes) or pelvic inflammation, but the cause may be deeply psychological, causing entry to be blocked and making penetration difficult if not impossible.

Peyronies disease, where the penis becomes angulated on erection, balanitis (inflammation of the foreskin) and hardening of the arteries all produce their own problems. People disabled by spinal cord injuries, or diabetes, or who have had prostate surgery, also have their own special problems. Examples of medications causing sexual difficulties are found on p. 446.

For sexually transmitted diseases, see p. 447.

Conventional Treatment

Whatever the sexual problem, your family doctor is probably the best person to approach first. A full history of the problem will be taken, followed by a physical examination. If the problem is physiological, rather than psychological or performance-related, further tests may be required.

Sex therapy can help both partners learn specific techniques such as sensate focusing, designed to decrease anxiety about performance and increase awareness about each other's needs by focusing on sensual rather than sexual sensations for much longer periods before actual love-making is attempted. Premature ejaculation, one of the commonest sexual problems in men, responds to a different technique.

Patty and Harris came to the surgery for some marital therapy. Patty complained that she was unhappy and irritable and was having thoughts about leaving the marriage after 10 years. Initially there appeared to be little reason for this, but then she angrily accused Harris of knowing the reason why and not doing anything about it. He eventually disclosed that he had a problem in that he would ejaculate almost as soon as he became sexually aroused and that this had been a source of pain between them for a number of years. During this time she had tried to persuade him to get help and he had refused, thinking that nothing could be done and also feeling embarrassed to talk about the problem with anyone. Both were greatly relieved to learn that there is a fairly simple technique that could cure this as long as both of them were willing to come to psychosexual counselling together. Patty was taught the squeeze technique and this, along with some counselling for them both, resolved the problem.

Other forms of sex therapy can help women with vaginismus who find reaching orgasm very difficult or whose sex drive is low, whether or not this is a recent phenomenon. Psychotherapy, either on an individual basis, in couples or in a group setting, can be extremely beneficial for women and men who have suffered any form of sexual abuse in the past or who, for whatever reason, have never been able to enjoy a full sexual relationship as a result of the emotional scarring they have suffered. Your family doctor can refer you for this form of therapy which can be helpful for both you and your loving partner. Knowing that you are not alone with your problem can be very comforting.

VIAGRA

This much-publicised treatment needs to be approached with care. Do have some counselling before you think of using it since your expectations may be unreasonable. It does not increase desire, nor enhance performance where there is already normal function. But it can help even where there has been poor functioning for many years due to diabetes, prostate operations, and other conditions. There are, however, side effects which include flushing, stomach upset and mild headache. Talk to your doctor about the dangers of using it while taking other medication, especially glyceryl trinitrate or other heart nitrate preparations.

Nutritional Healing

Food and water free of contamination with pesticides and other toxins help all of your systems to be healthy, including your sexual function. Foods such as soya, brown rice, chicken, dairy produce and nuts will help to enhance arousal in women. Brightly coloured fruit and vegetables will give you Vitamin A which will help your vitality, while foods rich in Vitamin B_2 (in oatmeal, peanuts, pork, liver, kidney, milk, yeast and cheese) have a beneficial effect on the whole reproductive system. Vitamin E (in green leafy vegetables, wheatgerm, whole grains, avocados and eggs) has long been associated with sexual function and improves your stamina. The diet for heart disease (see p. 295) is ideal for impotence since it keeps the blood vessels in good repair and therefore improves the ability to get and sustain an erection. Garlic is a great aphrodisiac but needs to be taken in large quantities over a period of time. Oysters have traditionally been known as an aphrodisiac and this may have some validity since they are a good source of zinc, essential for male fertility and for a proper level of testosterone.

Vitamins and Supplements

Arginine may be taken as a supplement, 2–5 mg in the evening or an hour before attempting intercourse. All of the vitamins mentioned above may be taken as supplements although as always it's better to obtain them from natural sources as much as possible. Kava may help to lower your anxiety about your performance.

Complementary Therapies

There are a host of complementary therapies which can help your sexual function including acupressure, aromatherapy, massage, meditation, psychotherapy, relaxation, Traditional Chinese Medicine and yoga. Stress management also plays a part (see p. 481). For men various herbs can help sexual function. Yohimbe, gingko biloba and ginseng can all assist blood flow and may therefore may help your erection. Yohimbe can have a positive effect in about a quarter of men who try it but beware of using too much since it can cause prolonged painful erections as well as nausea, vomiting, dizziness and anxiety. It's best to start with a small amount to test the effect and never take more than 40 mg. Usually about 60 mg of gingko biloba taken daily over several months will have the effect of restoring potency in about 50 per cent of men. Ginseng needs to be taken on an intermittent basis at the dose of 100–200 mg daily for about 6 weeks, then 1 or 2 weeks off to give the best results. Muira puama taken as a tincture will strengthen erections in 50 per cent of men after only 2 weeks of taking it daily. Testosterone injections can sometimes be prescribed. DHEA, a hormone produced by the adrenal gland and a precursor to testosterone, is useful in those who have had their level checked and found to be low.

For women one of the best aphrodisiacs is a lovely clean body, with music coming in a close second. Men complaining about their partner's frigidity would do well to check their own hygiene first. Taking care of bad breath etc. may go far to sorting out what is not really a sexual issue but one about their not being nice to be close to. However, don quai is an all-round sexual tonic (but must not be used during pregnancy). Damiana tea from Mexico has had a debatable press. The chaste berry (agnus castus) can balance hormones but again this must not be used during pregnancy or if you're trying to become pregnant. Men may like to carry in their trouser pocket a piece of black obsidian, a crystal which has been said to have effects on male potency.

Exercise and Lifestyle

Exercise can tone up your sexual function as well as everything else. Often when our bodies feel good, are toned and honed, buffed and bronzed, we feel sensual and sexual and many of our inhibitions about sex disappear. However, often it isn't as easy as this, and it is important that we can appreciate ourselves as sexual beings even if we are overweight and not in the shape or condition we would prefer. Try to make time for a special routine incorporating toning and stretching, nevertheless, since the very act of doing this will make you feel better.

Stress is a depressant of sexual function and needs to be dealt with. There is little point in trying to deal with issues of a sensitive nature if you are tired and stressed – or feel pressed for time and that there are a host of other things you need to be doing. Is it possible for you to set aside a particular time to be with your partner without the children running around and when you can relax? So often, not having sex becomes a habit because there never seems to be a good time. Often couples hardly seem to have the time to sit and talk to each other, and even less to make love.

Sometimes there is an underlying incompatability about the sexual preferences of the other partner, or indeed questions about the rightness of the relationship or even whether you would prefer a partner of a different gender. If any of these issues trouble you then do try to talk about them, though you may find it easier in the first place to talk through your feelings with a professional before confronting the issue with your partner. If in truth you know that you require a total change in your lifestyle and in particular that you are not being true to your natural sexual orientation, do get some help with this since the sexual problems you suffer may disappear when you have done so.

Having said that, most relationships go through periods where sex is not as good as it could be, and these are times that need to be gently worked on by both partners with patience, gentleness and compassion for the other's needs.

Emotional and Spiritual Healing

For many sexual problems, sex therapy and psychotherapy can be extremely helpful. Pyscho-sexual dysfunction is experienced by about 50 per cent of the population at some time in their lives, and sex therapy is intended to help people alter their attitudes, to help couples understand each other and their needs, and to teach specific techniques to overcome particular problems. Often both partners in a relationship suffer the consequences of any problem and therefore it is often helpful for the therapist or doctor to see you together. The emotions surrounding sex are perhaps the most complicated of any of our functions as human beings. Our experiences in the years from birth until the age of about 8 can affect us in this area for all of our lives, moulding our sexuality and our ability to enjoy sex and good relationships. Any form of abuse, loss, abandonment, etc. may leave us with unhealthy views on sexuality, and we may find ourselves being promiscuous, using sex as a tool to control others, feeling that sex is dirty, seeing others or ourselves as sex objects or associating pain, shame, masochistic or sadistic feelings with what can be the most wonderful crowning of the love of two human beings. If you're already having sexual problems, or if you're aware of childhood problems, then psychotherapy could help you (and your partner) to heal those areas. If you could have such therapy with someone who also has a healing background and can do some work with your first and second chakras, that would be ideal.

Peter has been married for 17 years, and during that time he and his wife have had a happy and healthy sex life. At 52, he reported feeling depressed, since over the last few months he had had difficulty in getting an erection. Sometimes he managed, but could not sustain it to penetration. Although his wife was very patient and eager to allay his anxieties, Peter is now so anxious about whether or not he can make love that he tends to withdraw from her. Peter's impotence needs to be investigated, but meanwhile his wife's gentle encouragement, her continued statements of love for him and her willingness to find other ways to please them both do a lot for his confidence.

For men who have lost their sexual potency, whether temporarily or a permanently, there are issues about your ego that need to be addressed since so much more of your self-esteem is wrapped up with your sexual performance than it is for of women. Hopefully your partner will treat you with compassion and understanding, as Peter's wife did, as the more you can relieve your anxiety about the situation, the greater the possibility of recovery. However, you may be being prompted to look at other aspects of yourself which are perhaps more important but which you have valued less. Although there may be physical reasons for the problem, do have some healing. You may be pleasantly surprised with the result.

MEDICATION WHICH MAY CAUSE IMPOTENCE OR OTHER SEXUAL DYSFUNCTION

Drug	Effect
Some antidepressants	Impotence or delayed ejaculation
Fluoxetine (Prozac)	Loss of libido in both sexes, difficulty in reaching orgasm particularly in women
High blood pressure medication	Impotence
Some appetite suppressants	Impotence
Some anti-psychotics (e.g. thioridazine)	Urine retention, difficulty in ejaculating
Alcohol	Impotence
Heroin, cocaine, amphetamines	Loss of libido or increased sexual drive
Oral contraceptives	May reduce libido
HRT	May reduce libido

(Most of these effects are transient and disappear when medication is stopped. If you have to continue on your medication, ask your doctor about 'drug holidays' where you may not take medication at the weekends for instance. Please take proper advice on this.)

INTEGRATED APPROACH

1. Don't neglect the problem – find someone you can trust to be honest with and have the necessary investigations and treatment.
2. Let go of guilt, shame, etc. as quickly as possible and if necessary get some therapy or counselling to help you.
3. Have proper nutrition, exercise, etc. to look after the rest of your body.
4. There are several complementary therapies that can help but don't try them all at once – take your time.
5. Value the whole of yourself and not just your sexual prowess. Love, companionship, trust and humour may well be more important in the long run.
6. Have some healing for your whole self and relax.

Sexually Transmitted Disease (STDs)

While most sexually transmitted diseases are short-lived as well as socially and physically inconvenient, a few untreated varieties can become major problems, causing sterility, damage to unborn children and even death. The commonest STDs these days are chlamydial infections, responsible for urethritis (inflammation of the tube leading from the bladder) and fallopian tube inflammation, and which account for 25 per cent of all cases of STDs in genito-urinary clinics, and is a major cause of both male and female infertility. Chlamydia is caused by a parasite which lives in the human cells and may do so for long periods seemingly without causing any problems. However eventually there may be vaginitis and pelvic inflammation in women and painful inflammation of the urethra and prostate and low sperm count in men. Other infections include trichomonas infection, genital herpes, genital warts, gonorrhoea, syphilis and of course HIV and AIDS. Hepatitis B and candida infections may also be transmitted through sexual contact but this is not invariably so since the former can be passed on through blood-to-blood contact, for example by sharing dirty intravenous needles. Since herpes infections can be recurrent (see below) and since both hepatitis B and AIDS can prove fatal, it is clear that promiscuous sexual behaviour is a high-risk activity.

Sally is 33 and has been in a new relationship for about 6 months. She came to the surgery complaining of feeling generally ill, having swollen tender lumps in her groin and a fever. She has severe pain around her vulva and inside her vagina and can hardly bear to pass urine because of the burning sensation. Sally has a primary infection of genital herpes.

Rachel on the other hand had primary herpes about 6 years ago. She has been celibate for about 3 years since leaving her last partner. Lately she has been under a lot of stress at work, has just moved into a new flat and has recently had a major row with her best friend with whom she still remains very angry. She recognises the early symptoms of a flare-up of her herpes with tingling around her labia and pain down the inside of her thighs.

Sally and Rachel have a lifetime infection with the Type II herpes simplex virus which may lie dormant for years and then reoccur at times of stress (see Eileen's story on p. 453).

Symptoms

Early symptoms of STDs are generally noticeable in men, although women may have no symptoms at all, their first clue being that their partner is diagnosed. The more you change partners (or your partner has sex with others) the more at risk you are, so don't neglect regular check-ups and learn as much as you can about STDs, especially about the early symptoms your partner might have since they can be very different from your own.

Conventional Treatment

Your family doctor is probably the best person to approach first. However, some people who have an STD may prefer instead to attend a genito-urinary clinic or STD clinic where they can be treated anonymously. You don't even need an appointment and the service is free. You'll be treated with respect, courtesy and utmost confidentiality even if you're very young, and your parents don't have to be told. Assessment of symptoms includes taking a full sexual history and having a full physical examination, if necessary with smears, swabs and samples for laboratory investigation. Sometimes a blood test will be required also. Once any infecting organism has been identified, appropriate treatment often with antibiotics will be prescribed and you will then be followed up to see that the problem has completely cleared. If necessary, contact tracing, where recent sexual partners are confidentially approached, is conducted to ensure that they too are adequately treated and do not become asymptomatic carriers who are able to pass on the disease to anyone else. This is clearly in their own best interests and that of the community as a whole. Where there is possible contact with the human immunodeficiency virus (HIV), full counselling prior to blood testing should take place so that the implications of the test results can be fully understood (see the section on AIDS, p. 63).

Most STDs can have a good outcome, so get help as soon as you can. It's important that your partner is treated as well, or else you can continue to reinfect each other for a long time. It's better to see a doctor than to treat STDs yourself in case you miss something more serious. For instance if you have repeated thrush infections, you need checking for diabetes. If your symptoms disappear without treatment, this doesn't necessarily mean that the illness is cured. The symptoms may come and go but without treatment the illness often gets worse, as was the case for Diana (see p. 453).

For herpes sufferers, the more you know about your infection, the better-equipped you will be to deal with it. The virus may remain dormant sometimes for years before erupting at times of increased stress such as illness or bereavement. Allergies may precipitate an attack, as may drugs that affect your immune system such as antibiotics, steroids and antidepressants. Anything that will reduce your stress levels (see p. 481) will help reduce both the frequency and severity of attacks. When you have an attack, try to rest and take it easy. Although genital herpes doesn't necessarily cause problems in pregnancy, if it is active at the time of delivery, most obstetricians would probably opt for a Caesarean section since should the baby become infected, the infection can be very severe. However, try not to worry about it since this will only stress you and increase the risk. Why not talk things over with your doctor well ahead of time.

Obviously safe sex is a must both to protect you and to be responsible towards your partner and it would be unwise to have oral sex, whether you have Type I or Type II, if you're at the tingling stage. It would be wise to have no sex at all if your herpes is active, that is, while you have a sore.

Loose-fitting cotton underwear will be most comfortable and will allow the area to breathe. Try to avoid contact with the sore. It's highly contagious, so it's wise to boil or destroy towels after use or better still dry the area with a hairdryer and use either cotton buds or swabs to apply any medication. To avoid contamination, change your toothbrush regularly, dry it between use and don't share. Soak it in some antiseptic or bicarbonate of soda now and then, especially after you've used it if you have a sore.

Often people feel very angry with and blame their current partner, but the actual infection may have originally occurred years ago. However, as with all sexually transmitted diseases, both partners usually need to be seen, so try to involve your partner if you have a flare-up.

Prevention

Condoms can block everything except the human papilloma virus (HPV). Diaphragms and caps are not so effective. Insist that your male partner wears a condom unless you're monogamous, have been together for a long time and know that you're healthy. Spermicides are effective against chlamydia and gonorrhoea but don't rely on them for complete protection, use a condom or cap too. Have regular pelvic exams, pap smears and screening for chlamydia, gonorrhoea, etc. Your GP can do this, or if you prefer to see a stranger, go to your local STD clinic. A vaccine is available for Hepatitis B. Douching will only increase your risk of spreading the infection into your pelvis, and in any case, washing with soap and water is sufficient to get rid of anything which hasn't infected you yet. Urinating after sex will help wash away germs which might otherwise enter the urinary tract.

Emotional and Spiritual Healing

If you have been diagnosed with an STD, you may be experiencing a whole host of feelings, including anger with your sexual partner, anger with yourself, resentment, guilt and shame. Although these are common and understandable to some extent, it would be worth remembering that you have an illness, not a stigma, and that you have simply been unlucky, if perhaps a little careless. Should this have happened within the context of a committed relationship, then there may be fences to be mended or perhaps a decision to be made about whether or not you wish to stay in the relationship. Whatever, do take time and counsel to help you assess the situation in the cold light of day and get the help you need for your own health and wellbeing.

Nutritional Healing

Food and water free of contamination with pesticides and other toxins help all of your systems to be healthy, so they have a role in STDs.

Herpes

Herpes is one of those illnesses where diet and supplementation can make a real difference. There are three main principles:

1. Increase your intake of garlic which is perhaps the most effective natural remedy (see Vitamins and Supplements), by adding more to your cooking or eating it raw if you don't mind being antisocial (chewing some raw parsley after it will help).
2. Increase your intake of lysine-rich foods such as potatoes, brewer's yeast (but not if you also get thrush), fish, beans and eggs. Ask your GP to check your cholesterol level since eating more of these may make it go up.
3. Keep the arginine–lysine balance in your diet right, so restrict your intake of arginine-rich foods such as cereal, chicken, chocolate, dairy produce, meat, nuts (especially peanuts) and seeds.

Adding cayenne pepper to your cooking, or taking it as a supplement, will also help, as will a more alkaline diet, so try to eat more fruit (except oranges), more vegetables, seaweed, kelp, millet and other seeds, while reducing meat, fish, eggs, dairy produce, bread, nuts, tomatoes and alcohol. Eat small light meals regularly and cut down on caffeine and sugar. Drink lots of water and herb teas – sage, rosemary, red clover and chapparel are helpful. You might also like to add live yogurt which contains acidophilus, a natural antibiotic.

Vitamins and Supplements

Dr Christianne Northrup in *Women's Bodies, Women's Wisdom*, recommends that herpes sufferers take 12 capsules of deodorised garlic at the first signs of an attack, followed by 3 capsules every 4 hours during the day for the next 3 days. L-lysine, an amino acid which inhibits the virus, can be taken as a supplement, as an addition to increasing your intake of lysine from the natural sources listed above. Vitamins B_6 and C are helpful and liquorice root may also inhibit the virus. Vitamin E can be taken orally or applied as a cream. Zinc, which aids healing, is useful taken as a supplement at night or applied to the lesions as a cream. Capsaicin in cayenne reduces the pain of post-herpetic neuralgia when taken orally or applied as a cream. Bee pollen (as long as you're not allergic to bee stings) and propolis have been found to be fairly effective. Supporting and improving your immune system (see p. 535) will help reduce the frequency of attacks.

Complementary Therapies

Tea tree oil, diluted with a little almond oil and applied directly to a herpes sore on a cotton tip or a swab, will act as a natural antiseptic. Try melissa (lemon balm), either in the form of oil or cream, or make a strong lemon balm tea and bathe the area with it 3 times a day. Myrrh oil can be applied directly onto cold sores, and bergamot, geranium and rose oils are also helpful. Calendula cream is soothing and ice held directly on the sore will often reduce the pain. Reflexology can help especially with post-herpetic pain. Homeopathy has several offerings including Natrum mur, Phosphorus, Apis and Petroleum for either Type I or Type II; Dulcamara for Type II. Herb teas have already been mentioned and aloe vera, either as juice or applied topically, is worth a try.

Diana is a fit young woman with a fairly active sex life and no health problems that she is aware of. At 34 and now settled with her partner, she started to have pain during intercourse and some abdominal pain. Occasionally she had a mild, odourless discharge and some burning, Since they wanted to start a family, they had not been using contraception for about a year, but Diana hadn't conceived. She wondered if the failure to conceive might be associated with the rest of her symptoms. On being tested, Diana was found to have chlamydia which she may have had for several years.

Exercise and Lifestyle

Education must be the mainstay of promoting sexual health. Information about the physical risks from promiscuity or dangerous sexual activity needs to be made widely available to all those who are sexually active or have the potential to become so. Emotional and spiritual guidance can help people to form loving, enduring relationships which enrich self-esteem and form a basis for ongoing rewarding sexual health. Many complementary therapies, especially of the ancient Chinese variety, pay much more attention to this as part of the holistic management of the whole person.

To get into a relationship that offers you partnership, love, respect and monogamy, in which you can both grow, will probably allow for the best possible love-making. However, although that may be the ideal for some, it just hasn't happened yet for many people. In the meantime, STDs are a fact of life for those who are sexually active whatever their age, race, occupation or sexual preference. Nevertheless, two thirds of cases of STDs occur in those under the age of 25, half of all women having contracted one before menopause.

Eileen, a widow of 53 who had had no sexual contact since her husband died 5 years ago, came to the surgery complaining of genital soreness and pain on passing urine. She had never had a vaginal infection of any kind to her knowledge. Recently she had been distressed by another family bereavement. Examination revealed 2 small discrete ulcers which were finally diagnosed as herpes. It appeared that Eileen has had asymptomatic herpes for some years.

Integrated approach

1. Don't neglect the problem – go to your GP or local STD clinic and have the necessary investigations and treatment.
2. Get enough information to protect yourself if you're sexually active. STDs can happen to anyone.
3. Let go of guilt, shame, etc. as quickly as possible and if necessary get some counselling to help you.
4. Have proper nutrition and follow good hygiene rules.
5. There are several complementary therapies which can help herpes.
6. Have some healing for your whole self and relax.

Shock

Shock can mean many different things in a medical setting. At one extreme it can refer to clinical shock, a potentially life-threatening emergency which occurs when there is a drastic reduction in blood flow through the tissues of the body leading to collapse, coma and ultimately death unless properly treated. At the other extreme, it can be an emotional response to any kind of bad news, whether a bereavement, the loss of a job, financial security, a relationship or even some real or imagined threat to one's health. Shock may be triggered by physical or emotional trauma, or may be the result of injury or illness and is often made worse in the presence of severe pain or anxiety.

Serious organic disorders leading to clinical shock would include septicaemia resulting from the powerful micro-organisms responsible for meningitis, poisoning, spinal injury, peritonitis, clots within deep veins of the body, heart attack and severe bleeding.

Severe allergies, leading to swelling of the lips, tongue and respiratory passages and the leakage of fluid from the circulation into the body's tissues, may be responsible for a different kind of shock known as anaphylaxis.

Post-traumatic stress disorder is another form of shock which arises in those who have been involved in or were witness to severely stressful situations such as war, natural disasters, violence, rape, physical assault and torture. It was formerly known as shell-shock when it was first recognised in military personnel in the field of battle. It is also suffered by those who have lived through traumatic times such as adult children of alcoholic families and those who have suffered incest and sexual abuse.

Symptoms and Signs

Emotional shock

This interferes drastically with normal mental function. After an initial period of numbness and denial that the trauma has actually taken place, there often follows a period of anger and resentment or even guilt that it has. The sufferer then becomes preoccupied with the event to the point that they are unable to function in their usual manner. The subsequent period of adjustment may last anything from hours to several weeks or even years in extreme cases.

Clinical shock

Frank was involved in a serious road traffic accident during which the steering column of his car fractured his breastbone and several of his ribs. In sustaining this injury, he suffered a small tear to one of the main arteries in his chest which slowly pumped out oxygenated blood, compressing his heart and lungs. His blood pressure fell alarmingly and he was transferred unconscious by the ambulance crew to the nearest trauma unit. He was treated for clinical shock in intensive care and eventually made a satisfactory recovery.

The symptoms and signs that Frank exhibited – rapid and shallow breathing, rapid and weak pulse, cold and clammy skin – are classical in clinical shock. The victim also feels dizzy, weak and faint and eventually when the blood pressure falls even further, the patient may collapse and lapse into coma.

Post-traumatic stress disorder (PTSD)

Sufferers of post-traumatic stress disorder complain of recurring nightmares and experience a growing sense of personal isolation with interrupted sleep patterns and poor powers of concentration. Often they report an emotional numbness or general irritability and sometimes there are feelings of guilt which may or may not be associated with a deepening depression. Some sufferers experience these symptoms acutely immediately after the traumatic event, whereas others may be seemingly normal to begin with, only developing the symptoms several weeks, months or even years later. Often those close to them will report a personality change which began after the event.

Tony returned from the Falklands conflict a very different man to the one his wife had waved farewell to at Southampton

Docks. Once outgoing and cheerful in disposition, he returned moody, pessimistic and full of gloom. He tossed and turned in bed at night, often shouting out in his sleep and sitting up startled in a pool of sweat. He had witnessed several of his friends being killed in action and felt particularly guilty that he had survived when they had not.

Vera's situation was different, although she also suffered from post-traumatic stress disorder. She is 42 and has had a very unhappy life. She was abused as a child both sexually and physically and she has never had a satisfactory relationship. She drank heavily, had few friends, lived alone and was sometimes promiscuous for favours such as cigarettes or beer. She had made several attempts to end her life, but had usually been too drunk to carry out her plans. Her sleep was harassed by nightmares and flashbacks of her childhood experiences. She hated herself and the world and was filled with fury and resentment about what had happened to her. She required a lot of therapy to help her gain some normal balance in her life and help her stop abusing herself.

Conventional Treatment

Adequate support from partners, relatives or friends will help most people come to terms with bad news. For those who have nobody on hand to listen and advise, or where what help there might be is not skilled enough or deep and persistent enough to resolve all the issues, professional counselling may be required. Talk to your family doctor who may refer you to a counsellor, a psychiatrist, a Macmillan Nurse (in the field of cancer bereavement, for example) or a group such as CRUSE.

FIRST-AID FOR CLINICAL SHOCK

First-aid measures must be instituted immediately to avoid a life-threatening emergency. The most important issues are:

* Summon professional medical help at once.

* Do not give anything to eat or drink until help arrives; anaesthesia may be required and food or drink make the risk of vomiting more likely.
* Stop any bleeding.
* Keep the respiratory airway open.
* Keep the patient lying flat.
* Reduce undue heat loss by keeping the patient warm.
* Reassure the patient to prevent panic or excessive anxiety.
* Reduce pain.

Expert medical treatment will include the transfusion of intravenous fluids and/or blood, oxygen therapy, and pain and anxiety relief in the form of morphine.

People suffering from post-traumatic stress disorder require time, emotional support and long-term counselling or psychotherapy. The outlook is better for those whose trauma was short-lived. Where there has been ongoing physical deprivation, torture or abuse, such as in prison camps, or childhood sexual or physical abuse, there may be deep-seated psychological scarring which can take many years to heal. Without proper help it is unlikely that it will ever heal at all.

Nutritional Healing, Vitamins and Supplements

In the past we physicians have not been very good at helping our patients in the aftermath of trauma, to replenish their stores and to help them have the optimum nutritional state to repair wounds both physical and mental. Yet it is at this time that good nutrition is of paramount importance and the guidelines in the section on surgery apply (see p. 29). The B vitamins, Vitamin C and beta carotene are absolutely essential, as are zinc, potassium, magnesium and chromium. A balanced diet will help, although initially only fluids may be acceptable. If so, soups, juices and puréed fruit would be fine. Try to include ginger, garlic, canteloupe melons, red peppers and strawberries for Vitamin C; ginger, parsley and carrots for zinc; highly coloured fruits and vegetables for carotenoids, and bananas and spinach for potassium.

Exercise and Lifestyle

The sooner a 'normal' life can be resumed after a state of shock, whether physical or emotional, the better. Returning to a point where days can be structured and there are regular hours in terms of mealtimes, exercise, sleeping and rising will help. Exercise should be gradual and gentle; follow the guidelines on p. 7. There should be no hurry to rush ahead; instead take things easy and rest as much as possible. The accent should be on taking care of yourself or allowing someone else to take care of you for a while.

Complementary Therapies

Rescue Remedy will often help deal with shock until some help is at hand. Arnica is the classical homeopathic remedy and will be useful whatever the cause, even after the initial shock has subsided. Ignatia will be indicated where shock is due to loss – for example, when someone has died. For emotional shock, music therapy, yoga, biofeedback and psychotherapy are useful to help open communication and soothe.

Emotional and Spiritual Healing

Both Vera and Tony need some help to change their lifestyle and begin to live a more normal life. However, it may take a long time and a lot of tiny steps before they or anyone else can appreciate that progress has been made. Sadly, if trauma continues for a long time, as was the case for Vera, the drama, pain and chaos eventually become the norm, along with the feeling that the person will always be a victim at the hands of some aggressor or another and that they are helpless to change the situation. Certainly, changing in Vera's case will need a lot of help and a lot of effort on her part. It will also require a long time working with someone who can be compassionate enough to hold her through the pain as she tries to make sense of all that has happened and come to a point of some resolution of her anger and fear. It would be good but perhaps unrealistic to expect her to get to the point of forgiveness. She needs a loving, patient and compassionate therapist who nevertheless can set good boundaries and put responsibility but not blame totally in her hands. This is the only way in which she will ever be able to feel a sense of control and power and also that her actions have consequences that she then has to live with. Traumatic incident reduction work will be a major part of her treatment to enable her to uncover the feelings of past events and deal with them until they lose their sting. The sooner this can happen after a single traumatic event, for example witnessing a tragic car accident, the quicker and more complete the resolution can be.

For all these people with their quite different presentations, healing can help. There have been cases documented where healers have stemmed bleeding, mended fractures and alleviated shock when on the scene before other help arrived. Similarly the person with PTSD will benefit from healing even though the process may still be a long one. Sometimes the outcome is that the person who has been struggling for a lifetime with horrendous life events can come to a point that they can accept that the people who hurt them did so because of the difficulties they themselves were suffering. Then sometimes we can move a step further and see that if our souls needed to learn a particular lesson, then someone had to come into our life to teach us. At this point there can be complete forgiveness and resolution of the emotional and spiritual pain. Work on both the heart and base chakras is essential, although usually all the chakras need work.

Integrated approach

1. Shock can be a medical emergency requiring urgent orthodox medical care.
2. Emotional shock needs time, patience and skilled handling.
3. Although helpful non-professionals are well meaning, you may find that you really need professional help.
4. Complementary therapies and healing can be very beneficial.
5. The earlier the treatment after the event, the more complete will be the recovery from it.
6. Try to see things from a spiritual perspective.

Skin Disorders

Few people regard the skin as an organ of the body, but in fact it is the largest and the most exposed. Disorders of the skin are rarely life-threatening, but many are cosmetically dramatic and some may be severely debilitating. Psychological difficulties commonly arise from skin conditions and even acne, common as it is in adolescents in their formative years, can often cause such severe depression that suicide may result.

A vast number of different conditions can afflict the skin:

* Birthmarks, which breech babies are born with.
* Leg ulcers, mainly in the elderly.
* Infections, such as measles, chickenpox, cold sores and shingles.
* Fungal infections.
* Inflammations, such as contact dermatitis and eczema.
* Psoriasis, a common and persistent dry flaking condition of the skin affecting up to 1 per cent of the population at some stage in their lives.
* Prickly heat, experienced by many when the sweat glands become blocked in very warm weather.
* Hormone disorders, which can lead to acne when the sebaceous glands produce excess oil under the influence of androgen.
* Allergies, which can arise due to a vast number of environmental factors.
* Injury, as a result of trauma, insect bites or burns.
* Autoimmune disorders, whereby antibodies are produced which damage the skin; including vitiligo, which produces white patches and destruction of the skin's pigment cells;

pemphigoid, which leads to large blisters, and lupus erythematosis, which produces a characteristic red rash.

* Tumours, benign (including moles and seborrhoeic warts or age spots) or malignant (see the section on skin cancer, p. 173).

The last condition to mention is herpes, a painful condition which led Geoff to come to the surgery (see also p. 447, Sexually Transmitted Diseases).

Geoff has been under a lot of stress. He was made redundant at work and is in financial difficulties. He has felt run down and now complained of severe burning pain down the right side of his chest and around his waist. He'd had an itchy rash for a few days which he tried to ignore and claims that the pain is much worse now that the rash has cleared up. Geoff has shingles (herpes zoster or Type II infection) with post-herpetic neuralgia. This is not a sexually transmitted disease.

Liz has a different kind of herpes infection. She had been working outside in very cold weather and developed a painful cold sore on her lip. She has had these before, sometimes when she'd had a cold or when she hadn't protected her lips in the sun. She knows that they are highly contagious and regrets having ignored the tell-tale tingling that she knows heralds the painful blister. Liz has herpes simplex (or Type I infection).

For both of them this is a lifetime infection with the herpes virus. Occasionally, however, Type I can infect the genital area and Type II (genital herpes) can infect the mouth or nasal area. For all sufferers, the infection may have lain dormant for many years. This is not necessarily a sexually transmitted disease.

Conventional Treatment

Because the skin is so accessible and easily visible, much skin diagnosis can be reached purely by observation by a GP or specialist. The character of the rash or marking, its distribution and its associated symptoms are often sufficient to determine the problem. Where the symptoms are non-specific and the signs vague, doctors will often prescribe anti-inflammatory preparations such as hydrocortisone or stronger steroids to suppress the inflammation and ease symptoms. Where infection appears to be present, antifungal, antiviral or antibacterial agents are used, either in cream, tablet or injectable form. Where a skin disorder suggests malignant change, a biopsy may be taken whereby a sample of the tissue is removed for microscopic analysis so that a definitive diagnosis can be made. Even birthmarks these days can be cosmetically removed with the use of special laser equipment and this may be done at an early age before the child becomes psychologically aware of their disfigurement, so that emotional consequences may never arise. As a rule of thumb, keep moist skin dry and dry skin moist.

Self-Care

If you want your skin to glow with health, then you need to start from the inside – that is, with good nutrition and detoxification to rid this largest of all organs of the toxins it carries, exposed as it is to atmospheric pollution from the outside and from all manner of things from within.

Nutritional Healing

Vitamin A is the vitamin of the skin and of all the surfaces of the body, even the inner ones. Your diet therefore needs to have plenty of it. The carotenoids are also important as well as Vitamin B_6, C, E and folic acid (folate). Zinc is necessary for healing, as is magnesium and potassium. So check for the natural sources of these on p. 545. Acne may respond well to changes in your diet, so cut out animal fats, shellfish, eggs, wheatgerm, iodised salt (all of which contain iodine which may exacerbate the problem), ice cream, cream, cheese, chocolate, wine, tea, sweets, processed foods, biscuits, cake and sweet drinks. Increase your fibre and use olive oil for cooking, adding some flax seed (linseed) oil daily to give you essential fatty acids. Cucumber cleanses the skin from the inside by acting as a detoxification agent for the liver. It is also healing if applied topically in lotions or even raw. Radishes may prevent skin eruptions, herpes, acne and boils. The same suggestions apply with regard to organic food and pure water. If you can't buy organic make sure that everything is washed well or peeled. For psoriasis, eliminate alcohol, caffeine and refined sugars from your diet while reducing meat and dairy products as they contain substances such as arachidonic acid which may be inflammatory. Herb teas will help cleanse your system while green tea, full of antioxidants, will help the health of your skin. Try juicing some carrots and beetroot which will cleanse your liver and make it more efficient as a filter of toxins. Celery, parsley, lettuce, lemons and limes are good for psoriasis so add plenty to your diet. Turkey is also said to be healing for psoriasis so eat it a couple of times a week. Aloe vera juice taken internally is as important as applying the fresh gel to skin lesions. If you have shingles, take extra garlic raw or in cooking, or as deodorised tablets. This will not only help reduce the length and severity of the illness, but also the neuralgia associated with it.

Vitamins and Supplements

Vitamins A, B_6, C, E, the carotenoids and other antioxidants are worth taking as supplements if you have a problem skin. However, don't take Vitamin A in large doses if you're pregnant. Try selenium and zinc, especially if your skin problem is associated with premenstrual syndrome (PMS) or menstruation itself. For acne, try taking brewer's yeast in the dose suggested on the container. Blackcurrant seed oil will give you essential fatty acids and you may prefer it to flax seed (linseed) oil. For psoriasis, try taking a probiotic supplement.

Exercise and Lifestyle

Although it's important for you to get as much exercise outdoors as possible, don't forget to adequately protect your skin with moisturisers and sunscreen. Daily sea salt baths are particularly good for psoriasis, after which you can treat your skin with one of the oils mentioned below. Your skin is the largest organ you have and part of its function is to rid your body of toxins, so if you ensure that there is adequate cleansing inside and out (see p. 7 on detoxification), your acne has a good chance of clearing. Poor liver function is a factor in the development of psoriasis, so dandelion and milk thistle will help. However, all skin disorders, especially acne, may indicate that there is an internal imbalance linked to stress, diet, heredity and hormones. Try keeping a diary and note when your skin problem flares up. Are there any substances in your environment that may be irritating or to which you've become sensitive? Detergents, perfumes, hairspray, deodorants, shampoos, plants, household cleansers and insect sprays, etc. may all have an effect on a delicate skin. Try to use the simplest and purest of products for your skin, such as rose water or witch hazel to cleanse and tone, and perhaps soap made of olive oil or beeswax. In general be gentle rather than aggressive with your skin. Natural products, such as papaya or apricots mashed and spread on your skin as a mask while you sit down and rest with a cup of herb tea, will do more to ease the problem than hours in front of the mirror picking and scrubbing. Although you may think that wearing your hair forward to hide troubled areas is better cosmetically, if you have acne it is better to keep your hair back as much as possible. Also make sure that you keep brushes clean and that you boil facecloths to ensure that they don't carry infection.

Complementary Therapies

Do try homeopathy since it can have amazing results unequalled by orthodox medicine. For psoriasis, Berberis, Graphites, Arsenicum, Petroleum, Sulphur or Lycopodium may help. For acne, Kali brom, Sulphur and Antimonium tart are worth trying. If you have shingles, try Arsenicum, Ranunculus or hypericum. Calendula, taken internally as a tincture or applied as a cream, can cool and heal. Neem, a herb from an evergreen in India, is traditionally used for eczema, psoriasis, rashes and other skin conditions. Milk thistle and red clover are good for acne and a tea made from cumin, fennel and coriander together can cleanse and detoxify. Try making tea from chamomile and letting it cool before using it as a lotion. Aromatherapy oils can be wonderful: tea tree oil is a natural antiseptic good for small wounds, cold sores, bites and stings. It has an antibacterial and antiviral action. It was because of the accidental discovery of the amazing effect that lavender oil can have on the healing of burns that the art of aromatherapy was reborn earlier this century, but lavender is also healing for dry sensitive skin, as is rose oil. Sandalwood and lavender oils can go a long way to healing acne. For more mature dry skin try jasmine, melissa (lemon balm) and patchouli preparations. Ylang-ylang will help oily skin and jojoba and rosemary can be useful for both skin and hair. Chamomile oil, which is antifungal and antibacterial, can soothe inflamed and sensitive skin, acne and psoriasis. Try it in your bath or diluted for external application. Cedar or juniper oil in the bath will help psoriasis. Organic honey is healing to small cuts and wounds and using products containing honey may also help. There are also lots of natural creams available using a variety of products such as kaolin and oatmeal, camphor, peppermint, arnica, sulphur, sage and zinc. Have a browse around your local natural remedy shop. And of course as a standby, Rescue Cream may work wonders. Reducing stress and anxiety will have a direct effect upon your skin (see p. 481). Acupressure, acupuncture and reflexology can also help.

Emotional and Spiritual Healing

Although your emotions and your skin may seem unrelated, emotional issues may affect your skin, trigger an outbreak or make it more severe. Stress has a marked effect upon every organ of our body and the skin is no exception. The depression and low self-esteem caused by chronic skin problems such as acne and psoriasis can't be overestimated. Often people avoid relationships that may eventually include intimate contact because of their embarrassment about their skin. Sufferers from psoriasis, for instance, can lead lonely and isolated lives, and young people suffering from acne can have their lives ravaged by social phobias. Sadly many of these are chronic conditions, so don't expect instant miracles. However, we have seen psoriasis remit very quickly with healing, although it will often recur unless other more long-term treatments are also used. Spiritual healing, Reiki or therapeutic touch can help, and do think about having some psychotherapy. The power of a good support group is borne out by the results of a study which showed that people with malignant melanoma who joined a 6-week support group lived years longer than those who didn't. It's important to see yourself as a whole human being and to see your beauty as coming from the inside as well as the outside. A beautiful quote from Antoine de Saint-Exupéry's wonderful book *The Little Prince* comes to mind: 'What is really important is invisible to the eye.'

INTEGRATED APPROACH

1. Remember that your skin is the largest and most exposed organ you have and therefore if it gets sick it can have a major impact on your life.
2. Although your skin is on the outside, healing often needs to start from within with good nutrition.
3. Cleansing should be thorough but that doesn't have to be harsh or aggressive.
4. Keep dry skin moist, moist skin dry, and if there's inflammation, treat it.
5. Symptomatic treatments of orthodox medicine may work quickly and yet still be surpassed by some complementary techniques such as homeopathy and aromatherapy.
6. Remember that beauty is not only skin deep, it comes from within.
7. Healing can sometimes have rapid results but you still need to look after the basics.

Sleep Disturbances

Sleep disorders are experienced by at least 1 in 3 people at some stage in their lives and account for many thousands of appointments with the doctor every year. Insomnia, which simply means having trouble sleeping, is by far the commonest complaint although it may mean different things to different people. Many people complain that they do not get enough sleep, but our individual requirements for sleep vary considerably. Some people are happy with 4 hours' sleep a night, famous examples being Margaret Thatcher and Albert Einstein, whereas others are not at all happy unless they have a routine 8 hours' sleep every night, without which they feel irritable and jaded all day long. People with insomnia may have difficulty falling asleep (initial insomnia) or may get off to sleep fairly quickly but then wake up frequently during the night, much to their annoyance. But there are a number of more specific sleep disturbances which require special consideration and these include sleep apnoea, jet lag, night terrors in children, sleepwalking and narcolepsy. Each requires different assessment and treatment and we shall look at all of these in turn.

Insomnia

Difficulty falling asleep or frequent interruption of sleep may be due to a number of things. Often anxiety and stress is the reason. Sometimes environmental factors such as too much noise or bright natural daylight may be responsible. This is especially true of shift workers who need to try to sleep during the day. Too little exercise, too much coffee or alcohol and irregular hours are often the culprits with drugs or medication adding to the list. Withdrawal from sleeping pills or antidepressants or even from illicit drugs can certainly cause insomnia. There are also a number of psychiatric conditions such as depression and mania which can lead to difficulties.

Rosalynn dreads going to bed and delays the event for as long as possible. She knows that despite every effort to go to sleep she will probably still be lying awake, tossing and turning until about 2 a.m., worrying about the fact that she will be so tired the next day. She feels resentful that her husband falls asleep so easily and that their considerable financial worries and her concern about the fact that their teenage son may be using drugs doesn't upset him. She cries more these days and eats compulsively, often having chocolate in bed while watching TV before trying to settle down to go to sleep. Rosalynn has initial insomnia as a symptom of depression.

In depression, patients often suffer from initial insomnia or early morning waking, in which they awake in the early hours of the morning feeling despondent and sometimes suicidal. In mania, the person is extremely stimulated and frenetic with a very active mind and excessive physical energy, and is unable to sleep. People suffering from dementia and schizophrenia may have an altered body time-clock so that they sleep during the day and wake during the night. There are also a number of physical conditions that can interrupt sleep, such as pain from some cause, and restless leg syndrome, which affects some 15 per cent of the population and leads to jumpy, twitchy limbs. The only answer for this is to get up out of bed and pace around the room to exercise the muscles.

As we get older our need for sleep often wanes. Such was the case for Eleanor.

Eleanor is 82 and sleeps very little these days. She goes to bed very early because she has little else to do and finds that by about midnight she's wide awake. She doesn't mind being awake, but her son and daughter-in-law with whom she lives get very upset about her wandering about in the night. Eleanor simply has less need for sleep at her age.

In chronic sleep disorders, investigations may be conducted in a sleep laboratory, which involve an electroencephalogram (EEG) to monitor brainwave patterns and tests to monitor breathing rates, muscle activity and other bodily functions. Many people with severe insomnia are shown to have more sleep than they believe they get but the sleep is frequently interrupted. For most people, in fact, it is the quality of sleep rather than the quantity that is important. Sometimes chronic sleep disorders are secondary to some other problem.

Angie had a cocaine problem for about 3 years but even 2 years after she shed the habit, she still cannot sleep well. She hates the night time and is awake wanting to eat every couple of hours. She then finds it difficult to get up in the mornings and has had difficulty holding a job down because of this. Angie has a chronic sleep problem precipitated by her drug abuse.

SELF-HELP FOR INSOMNIA

The initial treatment of insomnia involves simple self-help measures:

* Take plenty of regular physical exercise, allowing the body to secrete hormones such as the growth hormone which may have a profound effect on the quality of sleep.
* Try not to eat too late in the evening and avoid large meals late at night or your digestion will be stimulated, leading to heat production and heartburn.
* Avoid smoking and alcoholic drinks in the evening as these stimulate the brain and keep it active at a time when it should really be slowing down.
* Avoid stimulants such as coffee and other caffeine-containing drinks and foods (e.g. chocolate) in the evening.
* Some drugs may also stimulate mental activity or the heart rate, such as ventolin.
* Have a hot milky drink last thing – it contains tryptophan which will help you sleep.
* Make sure the bedroom is warm and quiet, but well ventilated, and that the bed is comfortable and supportive. Try to ensure that your mind is free of worry and stress – it helps to write down any concerns to externalise them before you settle down to sleep.

* Try playing some relaxing music or reading a soothing book.
* Have a regular routine for sleep rather than continually upsetting your body-clock by changing your bedtime.

Sleep Apnoea

This is a potentially serious sleep disorder where on a regular basis breathing may stop during sleep for periods of 10 to 30 seconds. Often sufferers are themselves unaware of the problem at night but they may be extremely tired during the day, with poor concentration and poor memory, and they may find that their occupation and social life suffer as a result. This condition is known to be associated with high blood pressure and heart failure and it has even been linked to heart attacks and strokes in some people. The condition seems to be more common in middle-aged men, especially in those who snore heavily and are overweight. The cause of the condition is usually floppiness of the muscles of the soft palate at the back of the roof of the mouth, which relaxes during sleep and allows the muscle to sag back against the airway walls. Snoring reaches a crescendo as obstruction of the airway becomes greater and greater and when complete obstruction occurs breathing stops. Eventually the brain gets the message that oxygen supply has been seriously reduced and an emergency arousal reflex operates which restarts breathing but wakes the person briefly in the process.

Treatment of Sleep Apnoea

Simple measures involve losing weight, cutting out smoking, avoiding alcohol, especially at night, and sleeping on one's side. It is also important to avoid large meals at night and any form of sedative medication. In severe cases, tests to monitor breathing during the night can be conducted and if the condition is confirmed, continuous positive airway pressure (CPAP) can be supplied to deliver air from a compressor via a special mask worn over the nose. There are now two very helpful surgical operations undertaken by ear, nose and throat specialists which can cure snoring. One is called a uvulo-palato-pharyngoplasty (UPPP) which removes the soft tissue of the palate at the back of the roof of the mouth. The other is carried out with the aid of a laser that burns two holes in the back of the palate which then contract as scar tissue is formed, leading to greater rigidity and stiffness of the tissues responsible for the problem.

SLEEP PARALYSIS

Sleep paralysis is a condition in which the sufferer wakes up but is totally unable to move. Sometimes hallucinations can occur at the same time which may be frightening, but in most cases the sufferer is otherwise healthy and the sensation lasts no longer than a few moments. Other people may suffer from narcolepsy in association with sleep paralysis and the treatment for this is listed on p. 474.

JET LAG

This occurs as a result of flying across different time zones, which causes the normal body rhythms to be interrupted. It is most frequently experienced when flying from west to east and results in fatigue during the local day, wakefulness at night, poor memory and concentration, and a reduced tolerance for physical and mental activity. Jet lag seems to be worse for people over the age of 30 who are more likely to be in the habit of following a rigid and established daily routine.

Treatment of Jet Lag

It is a good idea to drink plenty of water during the flight and to avoid alcohol and heavy meals. People flying eastwards should attempt to go to bed earlier than usual for a few nights before the journey and people flying in the opposite direction should stay up later. When planning a flight, try to book the tickets so that arrival can be anticipated in the new time zone in the early evening. Going to bed early on arrival will help. On average it can take about 12 to 24 hours to recover for each time time zone that has been crossed and of course making up for the problem can be eased by organising a stop-over with the booking agent en route wherever possible. It is thought that melatonin, a hormone produced by the pineal gland, has an important role to play in body rhythms (or biorhythms). In America this is available as a commercial preparation for the treatment of jet lag, although it is not licensed in Britain as such. There are, however, many aromatherapy products on the market, some of which are even sold in-flight, which can be used either to wake somebody up or make them more sleepy, according to their requirements. However, frequent travellers say that the best thing for jet lag is to adjust your watch to the time at your destination as soon as you get on the plane. Avoid alcohol, drink lots of water, refuse the food served but have fruit instead, and get on with your day when you arrive at your destination, going to bed at local time.

NIGHTMARES AND NIGHT TERRORS

Nightmares are unpleasant and vivid dreams which occur during rapid eye movement sleep and are remembered very clearly when the person suffering the nightmare wakes up. They are especially common in children around the age of 10 and are made worse by nasal congestion and breathing difficulties or by anxiety. In adults nightmares are usually brought on by medications or by emotional trauma.

Night terrors, on the other hand, occur mainly in children and cause a child to wake suddenly in a terrified condition. They are seen at a younger age than nightmares, often starting at about the age of 4 and gradually improving with age.

Terri is 4. She hates going to bed and has to be cajoled to do so by her parents who will often spend a couple of hours reading to her before she drops off. She then wakes screaming, huddled up in a corner. Terri has night terrors, although luckily she rarely remembers the problem in the morning. Hoewever, her parents find it quite distressing to see her begin to scream when not fully aroused from her sleep. When she does wake she doesn't seem to recognise them or her surroundings and furthermore she cannot be easily comforted.

Physical symptoms of anxiety are obvious to see, the child appearing sweaty and agitated with fast pulse and dilated pupils. Within a few minutes, however, the child will go back to sleep and have no recollection whatsoever of the night terror the following morning. Anxiety appears to be the underlying cause although night terrors are not associated with any long-term problems in their own right.

Sleepwalking

Sleepwalking or somnambulism occurs during non-rapid eye movement sleep and does not appear to be associated with dreaming. Certain people seem to be predisposed towards sleepwalking when they get out of bed, wander about for a few minutes and then return to their bed once more. Sometimes anxiety or other psychological problems may be the cause of sleepwalking but often it is something a younger person grows out of and all a parent or partner needs to do is to steer the person gently back to bed and take precautions to keep them out of danger such as blocking off stairs and closing doors. Waking the sleepwalker is not generally helpful.

Narcolepsy

This is a sleep disorder which may or may not be inherited, where there is profound daytime sleepiness and recurring periods of sleep which come on several times every day. These attacks can last from a few seconds to over an hour and can often interfere with daily life. In the majority of cases, there may be cataplexy as well, where there is sudden loss of muscle strength without loss of consciousness. Sleep paralysis (see p. 472) may also occur. The diagnosis can be confirmed by the use of an electroencephalogram (EEG), an electrical recording of brain activity, in which it is shown that the sleep occurs in the rapid eye movement state which paradoxically occurs in these patients while they are still apparently awake.

Treatment of Narcolepsy

It is important to have regular short periods of sleep, which narcoleptics need anyway, but the standard treatment of choice is the use of stimulant drugs to control daytime drowsiness, along with certain anti-depressant drugs to counteract cataplexy.

Good sleep hygiene

* Have a regular bedtime and keep the bedroom for sleep and love-making only.
* No TV or reading newspapers before bedtime since they'll fill your mind with things not conducive to restful sleep.
* Prepare the bedroom by vaporising lavender, clary sage or ylang-ylang oil.
* Have a warm bath before bed preferably with 8 drops of lavender oil in it and perhaps some clary sage.
* Rid yourself of the day's worries by writing them down.
* Have a massage (self-massage if necessary) with relaxing oil, perhaps while listening to some soothing music.
* Have a soothing bedtime drink such as Sleepytime tea or chamomile tea (not drinking chocolate, which contains caffeine).
* Play a meditation tape if you wish.
* Do some final spiritual practice which may include doing your affirmations, some creative visualisation for a wonderful day tomorrow, a quick survey of the good things of today (there must have been some), sending out love and good wishes to as many people as you can, and a final handing over to a higher energy (which you may call God, the universe or your higher self) of whatever you cannot change and simply need to accept.
* Turn over and go to sleep.

Nutritional Healing

Despite the fact that sleep disorders have a variety of causes, it helps as always to go back to basics, to routine, to taking care of ourselves in all ways and to paying attention to what we eat, when we eat and how we eat it. Small nutritious meals spread throughout the day are better than a comparative fast followed by a heavy meal in the evening. Sometimes sleep which is already precarious can be affected by blood sugar becoming low during the long fast of the night. Having a complex-carbohydrate meal at the end of the day will help. Something like pasta with vegetables would be ideal. Also keeping a small snack such as a rice cake by the bed to have if you wake can often help you back to sleep. However, Angie, for instance, has such a severe problem that she will need more help than this. Tryptophan, at one time readily available as a night medication which helped shorten initial insomnia (the time it takes to get off to sleep), is found naturally in warm milk and turkey meat. Alternatively, eating a small high-carbohydrate evening snack such as cereal will help boost natural tryptophan levels. The Vitamin B group, which has long been recognised for its ability to soothe stress and calm jangly nerves, will also help promote sleep. The B vitamins are also important in the synthesis of serotonin and therefore help mood control (serotonin, an important chemical messenger or neurotransmitter, plays a major role in maintaining mood). Vitamin B_{12} has been shown to settle sleep within days and B_6, niacin (Vitamin B_3) and B_1 are also involved in the induction of sleep. REM sleep improves very quickly with niacin, so look for foods containing it (see p. 543). Calcium and magnesium are also important. The caffeine in coffee, tea, chocolate and some soft drinks can leave you unable to sleep, even if taken hours before bedtime, and of course such snacks as Rosalynn has in bed are absolutely counter-productive to sleep. Alcohol may help you get to sleep but will then wake you up a few hours later, leaving you restless and unable to sleep with the temptation to take more to drop off again. Don't do it!

Vitamins and Supplements

Calcium and magnesium supplements can really help if they are taken together (you can buy them as a combined supplement) just before bedtime. They will also help settle restless legs. Vitamin C and the B vitamins mentioned above can be topped up with a supplement. Melatonin, a substance secreted by the pineal gland, can be bought in the USA but isn't licensed in UK. A small dose of say 0.5 mg can encourage sleep although it is important first to put into practice all the other measures mentioned so that a sleep routine can be re-established rather than just depending on medication to make you drop off. Melatonin has the added benefit of being a powerful antioxidant, but avoid it if you are pregnant since researchers in the Netherlands are looking into its possibilities as a birth control device because of its action on the female reproductive system.

Exercise and Lifestyle

Stress is one of the major causes of sleep disturbance and needs to be addressed (see p. 481). Using cigarettes, coffee or alcohol to deal with daytime stress will only upset your sleep at night. Although you may feel an initial calm, nicotine is a stimulant with negative effects on your blood pressure, circulation and brain. Taking extra exercise, outdoors as much as possible, will help and adding breathing exercises will add even more benefit. An evening walk with your dog could round the day off well and put you in the mood for closing the day on a relaxed note. Dashing around in the gym in the evening is more likely to leave you wide awake and stimulated. Try yoga, T'ai chi or Chi gong, or try some gentle movement to music at any time of the day and feel yourself come into a new state of harmony. Opinions vary as to what to do when you wake in the wee small hours of the morning. Some say not to switch on the light since it upsets melatonin production and can lead to further insomnia, although as someone who suffered insomnia for years after a depressive illness, you'll see below that Brenda's way of dealing with it was different.

A PERSONAL NOTE FROM BRENDA

I remember that when I was depressed many years ago, I would awake at about 3 a.m. feeling awful. Initially the idea that I might be the only person awake used to fill me with horror. Worries and pain would flood into my mind and it was the most lonely and lost time of the whole 24 hours. However, as my depression resolved, even though I continued to wake in the night, my attitude to it changed. I would get up and decide what I was going to do with this precious extra time that had been given to me while the house was quiet and there were no demands upon me. It became a special time. Even now I often wake up around that time and write or read and enjoy those creative hours by myself. It ceased to be a problem when I ceased to see it as such.

Complementary Therapies

There are various herbs such as valerian, hops, melissa (lemon balm), chamomile, evening primrose and passion flower which may help to promote sleep without any risk of a hangover. Both passion flower and valerian boost serotonin levels and can therefore also have an effect on mood. St John's Wort, used quite widely for mild to moderate depression (see p. 195), also helps promote natural sleep by improving levels of neurotransmitters. Rosalynn might find either of them useful. Valerian, used for centuries and available either as tablets or drops, unfortunately has a most off-putting smell, although it doesn't cause bad breath. Its beauty is that not only does it promote sleep, but it also reduces tension so that even if you do wake up, you feel less anxious about being awake. Skullcap, used by native Americans, has been researched fairly recently in Russia and found effective. Kava is a herb from the South Pacific where it has been used for centuries for reducing stress and promoting sleep. It appears to have few side effects and is not habit-forming, though there have been some reports of rashes and tummy upsets and it shouldn't be taken by pregnant women or by those taking antidepressant medication. In the homeopathic arena there is Gelsemium, useful where insomnia is due to anxiety.

Vaporising lavender oil in your bedroom for a couple of hours before you go to bed will help prepare an atmosphere conducive to sleep. If you add to that a little clary sage and put both of them in your bath before you settle down into bed, you'll be much more likely to gently float off to sleep. If you could also arrange a gentle massage, perhaps given by a loving partner, then better rest is pretty well assured. Put a beautifully cleansed amethyst in the corner of your pillowcase or have a piece on your bedside table. Some rose quartz would help also. If you like crystals and have some in your bedroom already, take out any clear quartz since their energy may well keep you awake, especially if they're very clear, transparent ones. See if you can get your reflexologist to pay you a house call and do a treatment for you, after which you can retire. If you meditate make sure that you do it early enough to settle down again before bedtime since usually it will stimulate you to feel well and very alert. Acupuncture and Traditional Chinese Medicine can also help.

Emotional and Spiritual Healing

Melatonin levels vary, not only through each day, but also through the course of our lifetime. It's quite natural for us to need less sleep as we get older. The person who may have enjoyed 12 hours' sleep as an adolescent may be satisfied with 7 hours in her thirties and 5 in her seventies. It's important to recognise how much sleep you need. You may be one of those who only needs a little sleep and if so that's fine. Power-napping in the day can be a way of getting the extra you need until your sleep settles down. The basic rule is that the more you worry about not sleeping, the more your sleep will be upset. If you wake, the thing to do is to get up, do something like read or write a letter, then go back to bed and try again. Sometimes after depression, the last thing to settle down is your sleep.

THE ROLE OF MELATONIN IN SLEEP

Melatonin is a hormone secreted by the pineal gland, a tiny but important gland in the brain. Melatonin plays a key role in sleep and wakefulness, and in the control of the internal body clock which also signals the secretion of other hormones. The release of melatonin is stimulated by darkness and promotes sleep. In light, its release is suppressed and wakefulness ensues.

INTEGRATED APPROACH

1. Sleep disorders may be transient, lasting only a few nights, but if they continue for longer than this, talk to your doctor in case there is an underlying problem such as depression.
2. If your partner complains that you snore badly and if you feel as though you've hardly slept, ask your doctor if you might have sleep apnoea, which is a potentially dangerous condition.
3. Eat a small mainly carbohydrate meal in the evenings and have a milky drink.
4. Cut down on stimulants such as coffee and tea at night and try soothing herb teas instead.
5. Try to develop a good routine around bedtime which doesn't involve stimulation by TV, newspapers, etc.
6. Try to use the bedroom only for sleeping and love-making, not as a place to eat, watch TV, etc.
7. Make sure that you have a good vitamin and mineral supplement to augment your diet, and take your Vitamin B and calcium/magnesium supplement at night since they will help reduce tension and promote sleep.
8. Make an effort to rid your mind of the day's worries by writing them down.
9. Do your affirmations and last thing at night create a vision of a good tomorrow, then let go of whatever you cannot change and simply need to accept.
10. There are several complementary therapies which may be very helpful.

Stress

Too much stress turns us into monsters. It makes us act out of character or our personality may appear to change altogether. It makes us lose sight of the very things in life for which we're striving and it makes us forget how and why we're trying to achieve them. Taken to its extreme, excessive stress can ruin our lives and the lives of those around us too. Stress means different things to different people but suffice to say that it is a state we experience when the demands that are made upon us cannot be counterbalanced with our ability to deal with them. It is how we perceive those demands and our ability to cope with them that will ultimately decide whether we feel completely overwhelmed at one extreme or bored stiff at the other. There is a middle road of course when the demands made upon us are stimulating and our coping mechanisms are perfectly adapted to deal with them. This is a satisfying, rewarding and happy situation to be in, but although many of us will have experienced it from time to time, most of us will still go through life in a continual state of flux. Personality largely determines which people are most vulnerable to the effects of stress. Competitive, ambitious overachievers like David (see p. 482) tend to be stressed. They may appear impatient, hurried and highly conscious of the time. They constantly seek to exert control over their environment, and are preoccupied with deadlines, intolerant of delay and generally hostile. In short, they tend to be workaholics. People who are easygoing and calm are less likely to become stressed. They are generally content with their lot in life and are not easily irritated. They appear patient and relaxed.

The Effects of Stress

Like anxiety, most people think that stress is a bad thing, but in fact we would not be as effective as we are without some stress to sharpen our drive and motivate us to do well. In fact the effect of stress on performance is dose-related. When our lives have too little stress we feel bored, uninvolved and understimulated. As demands are made upon us which offer challenge, we become alert and feel more empowered and a level is reached where we can work at peak efficiency with happiness and pride. When stress continues beyond that level, however, we become less efficient in our work and our concentration is marred as we become anxious and overloaded. Eventually exhaustion and burn-out occur. Recognising when we become overstretched and overstressed is important in helping us to achieve our peak performance without the onset of unpleasant symptoms.

When stress becomes excessive or chronic, it affects every system of our bodies as well as our minds. Men and women may respond differently to stress, women often becoming emotional and irritable with headaches, irritable bowel syndrome, anxiety and depression. Men are more inclined to get high blood pressure, their pulse rate rising along with their tempers.

David, a workaholic by nature, developed severe chest pain and felt he couldn't breathe. The doctor was called who found David to be overweight, overworked and stressed out. Investigations to rule out a heart attack proved negative as did blood tests, but David's anxiety was difficult to eradicate even with strenuous reassurance. In-depth scrutiny of his lifestyle, however, showed that as a result of chronic stress, David was suffering from an acute anxiety attack, with all the physical symptoms which that entailed.

In the acute phase of an anxiety attack, the blood flow to the intestines is reduced, impeding the digestive processes. The skin becomes pale and sweaty. The bladder tells us it needs emptying and the sexual organs may be affected so that impotence in men and disturbed periods in women are common. When stress becomes chronic, permanently high blood pressure and chest pain may result. Indigestion, heartburn, ulcers, bloating, wind, diarrhoea and irritable bowel syndrome are seen. The skin may be affected by dryness, rashes, psoriasis and eczema. Headaches, migraines, tremor, confusion, depression and anxiety all present themselves. In terms of emotions, people often feel apprehensive, anxious and lose their sense of humour. There is muscle tension and strain. Overbreathing, feelings of suffocation and asthma can occur and loss of sex drive and abnormal sexual responses are reported. These symptoms of stress affect not only the individual but those who have to live with them as well. Almost every serious illness known to man is contributed to by the manifestations of stress.

The Causes of Stress

Many of life's events can cause unpredictable stress and these include, in the order of greatest importance, bereavement, divorce, separation, a jail sentence, injury or illness, marriage and redundancy. Even life events which are associated with happiness such as pregnancy, change of job and house buying may induce stress. Christmas is another well-known example. Keeping a mental note of how many stressful factors are impinging on you at any one time is useful in planning how to reduce the stresses in your life if symptoms are occurring. Choosing not to move house, change job and have a baby all at the same time, for example, is helpful.

SELF-HELP

There are many ways in which we can ease the pressure on ourselves:

* Limiting the extent to which we agree to take on any more challenges.
* Becoming more assertive, learning to say NO.
* Writing things down often helps to clear anxieties and fears from the mind.
* Becoming better organised and drawing up a life-plan.
* Being optimistic and thinking more about the positive side of things.
* Learning to work more efficiently, managing our time more effectively.
* Being willing to delegate.

* Looking at problems more constructively as challenges.
* Getting our priorities right.
* Taking time for ourselves and for those who are important in our lives.
* Discussing issues with others.
* Learning to work to live, rather than live to work.
* Learning new skills or retraining.
* Taking up a new hobby or pastime.
* Learning to stop rushing about, concentrating on finishing one job at a time.
* Waiting patiently when we have to.
* Avoiding situations which we find particularly irritating.
* Setting ourselves realistic deadlines.
* Stop getting angry about things over which we have no control.
* Learning to relax.
* Becoming less competitive and keeping a sense of humour.
* Taking more exercise.
* Applying moderation in everything.
* Getting enough sleep.

Conventional Treatment

Professional help may be needed when symptoms are chronic and severe. Behavioural symptoms such as overeating, anorexia, increased cigarette smoking and excessive alcohol intake, antisocial behaviour and constant tiredness or depression, require treatment. Physical symptoms such as chest pain, migraine, stomach ulcers, insomnia, back pain, psoriasis and sexual problems are equally deserving of help and details of conventional treatment will be found in the appropriate sections of this book. In some cases short-term medication may be indicated, although in the vast majority of cases, changes in lifestyle are what are needed. When the symptoms have become disabling, the use of sedatives, tranquillisers and antidepressants may well be appropriate in that they allow the sufferer to once again enjoy a better quality of life. However, they should only be used either as a last resort or initially for a very brief period in the lowest dose effective and under close supervision at all times. Sadly, the overprescription of tranquillisers over the last 30 years has led to much chronic abuse with many side effects and high dependence.

Ten tips to reduce stress

1. Slow down your breathing and count your breaths.
2. Try smiling even if you don't feel like it – the very action of moving your facial muscles in that way changes your reaction to the situation.
3. Put up your arms and wave. This also sends chemical signals to your brain which relax you and make you feel better.
4. Laugh more.
5. Always sit down to eat without reading or watching TV.
6. Remember that all things are in balance eventually. If you try to use energy now that you don't really have (e.g. by using coffee or recreational drugs to prop you up) you will have to pay for it later with feelings of exhaustion.
7. Be conscious of your body and regularly make sure that your shoulders are down and your jaw relaxed.
8. Use a routine before bedtime to help you get good-quality sleep (see p. 475).
9. If you have to put out a lot of energy, then you must put a lot in. Make sure you have the best-quality food you can afford and take extra vitamins and minerals.
10. Make a commitment to have some exercise and some relaxation every day.

Nutritional Healing

Reducing caffeine, alcohol and refined sugars, having your meals regularly while sitting down in a calm and pleasant atmosphere, will all go far to helping your body and mind get out of the constant state of rush and overdrive that characterises stress. Protect your immune system (see p. 535) since it needs to be able to protect you from opportunist infections etc. Take extra garlic. As always, be aware of any food allergies which may be stressors, although often the cause is to be found much more simply in the way you live your life. Always try to go back to the basics (see p. 4), even though you may have to renew your pledge to yourself to do so several times before living more healthily becomes a way of life.

Vitamins and Supplements

You do need extra vitamins and supplements. Be sure that you're getting enough of the Vitamin B group which have a naturally calming effect and protect your nervous system, and of course take a multivitamin/multimineral supplement every day. Panax ginseng is perhaps the most powerful anti-stress supplement. For the best results take it on a 3 weeks on and 2 weeks off rotation which will give your adrenal glands time to recover in between. Ashwagandha (winter cherry), mainly a herbal tonic for men, will help to increase energy and vitality, promote natural sleep and generally counteract the effects of stress. Kava tea or valerian will help also. Your levels of Vitamin C, zinc and magnesium are also critical here so make sure that you either eat enough naturally or, if your stress is likely to be ongoing for some time, take a supplement (see p. 543). Please don't simply rely on this to keep you out of trouble, however. Your stress level needs to come down.

Exercise and Lifestyle

The 10 tips to reduce stress (see p. 485) cover this. Do make sure that you have enough exercise since this can be a major factor in reducing stress.

Complementary Therapies

Learning the art of relaxation by using any of the various techniques available can be hugely beneficial. Meditation, aromatherapy, autogenics, biofeedback, homeopathy, acupuncture, acupressure, healing, yoga and counselling can all help.

Take your pick – the list of relieving therapies is enormous. Herbs you may like to try include chamomile, which promotes relaxation and inner peace, and reduces stress, anger and stress headaches; jasmine (also as an oil), which is emotionally soothing, or kava made into a tea. Lavender oil is both soothing and rejuvenating while ylang-ylang soothes nerves, and reduces stress and the insomnia associated with it.

Emotional and Spiritual Healing

There are many voluntary bodies such as the Samaritans and MIND with local groups who can provide a sympathetic ear, advice and information. There will always be a local voluntary branch of Relate nearby to help if the sources of stress are to do with relationships.

> *Chloe found Relate to be useful when the stress in her life had become so great that it had disastrous consequences, not only for her. She had been attempting to juggle the responsibilities of looking after 3 children and a taxing full-time job for some years while her unsupportive husband did little to share the load. One day while attempting to reach an impossible deadline, she drove through a red light and collided with a motorcyclist who lost a leg. Full of guilt, she began to drown her sorrows in alcohol and within a couple of months had developed a moderately severe drinking problem. This in turn put further strain on her marriage. It was only during Relate counselling that the appalling degree of stress in her life was really acknowledged and addressed. Chloe changed her job and her lifestyle and is now content and fulfilled in nearly every emotional department.*

Some people who have spiritual or religious beliefs may find solace and support in their faith and many ministers of religion are highly experienced in dealing with the myriad sources of human stress. Your family doctor may refer you to a clinical psychologist, psychiatrist or psychotherapist. In addition, your local Community Health Council, Citizen's Advice Bureau, Social Services and other community centres are all available. Sometimes just talking to such people is therapeutic.

In your intimate relationships it's important to learn to take time for yourself and for each other. Talking and listening, having time together both within and outside your home, coming home at reasonable hours and both going to bed at similar times, will help you regain the closeness that may have been lost while stress was governing your life. Remember that touch can reduce stress, and just holding hands, having a hug or having a comforting back rub can work wonders, as can love-making of course. In fact giving and receiving love and enjoying a good sense of humour are massively therapeutic.

If you would just stop for a few minutes and look at why you're living your life in such a stressful way and what you're gaining from it, you might be able to see in a blinding flash that it doesn't have to be that way. In fact the risks and potential losses are so great that it just doesn't make sense at all, even though you may feel that you're gaining financially, in kudos, in approval from others, in fame, and many, many other ways. Are you really? And in any case, are those really your goals in life? Is it worth risking your health, relationships, happiness, the happiness of those dear to you, missing the special times with your children that you can never recapture? It's all too easy to work too hard, to try to give everyone the best possible service and then not giving that same courtesy to yourself or your family. The only person who can decide on the priorities, however, is you. If the welfare of your work and your clients and colleagues really *does* come above that of yourself and your family, are you actually listening to your own inner wisdom? By now you may find that you're so addicted to your work, to driving too fast, to mopping up every single bit of work before you leave in the evening, to staying up into the early hours of the morning, that it will take some time and some gentle steps to be able to change things if you're not to fall into an exhausted, withdrawal state.

So why not start by setting yourself realistic goals to begin to downgrade. The goal of finishing half an hour earlier at the office may be easier to achieve than making a commitment that you're always going to be home by 5.30. By now both you and your family are probably sick of your broken promises, so how about discussing it with them and taking only small steps, gradually increasing your goals till you get to the point that your life is more manageable. The same goes for those like Chloe who are constantly dashing about, balancing work and family and for the many women who are also looking after ageing relatives, doing community work, etc. Give yourself a pat on the back whenever you achieve your next goal and keep going. Eventually you'll find yourself in a happier healthier place and will look back and wonder why you did it a different way for so long. Downgrading may be the buzz word but it's amazing how it can revolutionise your life and bring you great joy and peace. Living a comparatively stress-free life, confronting a new way of being, having time to spend on the simpler but ultimately more rewarding aspects of life, can help us find our spirit and become whole.

INTEGRATED APPROACH

1. Remember that stress creeps up on us unawares and can create havoc in our lives.
2. Stop and think and sort out your priorities. Does work really come above partner and family in your book?
3. Set yourself small achievable goals and stick to them.
4. Accept that you may need professional help and if so, ask for it.
5. Try some of the many complementary techniques that can be of enormous benefit.
6. When you have an appointment for yourself, such as having a massage, treat that just as seriously as you would a professional meeting or something you might do for someone else.
7. Symptoms such as chest pain and difficulty in breathing may herald the onset of some complication so don't neglect them.
8. Remember that stress can affect every organ of your body so have regular health checks.
9. If medication turns out to be essential, it should only be used for a brief time at a small dose.

Stroke

A stroke occurs when part of the brain becomes permanently damaged as a result of an interruption of its blood supply. Doctors refer to a stroke as a cerebrovascular accident (CVA). It occurs either because a clot forms in one of the blood vessels supplying the brain or because an existing clot (thrombus) travels to the brain along one of these arteries from a distant site such as the heart. The latter situation is termed an embolus or embolism. Alternatively, a stroke may occur as a result of a haemorrhage or leakage of blood from an artery, either within or near to the brain. The consequences of a stroke are alteration in brain function which, depending upon the site of the brain affected, may lead to numbness, weakness or paralysis. Every year 1 in 500 people in Britain have a stroke, the risk rising with increasing age, men being more vulnerable than women. Although stroke is the condition many of us fear most, as it can render us disabled and dependent on others while our mental functions may be entirely preserved, 30 to 50 per cent of stroke victims make a fairly full recovery from their first stroke. Another third become disabled in some way and up to a third will die within a few days following their stroke. However, even those who are initially paralysed generally learn to walk again. The provision of aids for the home and occupational therapy work is immensely helpful in this regard and only a mere 5 per cent of stroke sufferers ever require full-time institutional care. For thousands, however, the resultant disability from a stroke may become a huge burden to themselves and to their families.

Symptoms

Symptoms of a stroke can develop either very suddenly or much more gradually and will depend on the part of the brain affected, on the underlying cause and the extent of the damage.

Hamish was found slumped in his armchair by the fire by his wife who had popped out for some shopping some half an hour previously. He did not appear to recognise her, was dribbling from the corner of his mouth and was clearly very ill. His blood pressure, when the doctor took it, was alarmingly high. Hamish is one of the 100,000 or so people who experience a stroke every year in Britain.

In severe cases there is an abrupt loss of consciousness which may be followed by coma and death. In milder cases there may be loss of part of the visual field, slurred speech, numbness or weakness in an arm or a leg or difficulty in swallowing. Among the commonest symptoms are headache, dizziness and confusion, visual disturbance, slurred speech and hemiplegia, which is weakness or total paralysis down one side of the body. In women, however, the initial symptoms may be quite vague.

Ruby, 58, felt nauseous with some abdominal pain and had reported feeling very tired over the last few days. She believed that she would just get over what she thought was possibly a tummy bug. Her daughter called her GP in any case and when he questioned her about the presence of chest pain, Ruby said there had been none. Nevertheless he decided to have her investigated at the local hospital but Ruby had a full-blown stroke on the way there.

Since one side of the brain controls the sensation and movement on the opposite side of the body, it is easy to establish on which side of the brain the CVA has occurred. For example, hemiplegia affecting the right-hand side of the body will be the result of a CVA on the left side of the brain. Since the left is also usually the dominant cerebral hemisphere where the centres for language and speech are located, a problem there might also produce slurred speech and an inability to understand other people's spoken words or to express words themselves, known respectively as receptive and expressive aphasia.

The Risk Factors

Generally speaking strokes are relatively uncommon under the age of 60. Thrombosis accounts for up to 50 per cent of strokes, embolism for 30 to 35 per cent and haemorrhage for the remainder.

RISK FACTORS

1. Increasing age: women over 55, men over 60 (haemorrhages due to congenital abnormalities where there is weakness in the walls of the blood vessels in the brain, are more commonly seen in younger age groups).
2. Raised blood pressure (140/90 or higher).
3. Atherosclerosis (hardening of the arteries), which produces narrowing of the arteries and restriction of flow, making thrombosis and embolism more likely.
4. Heart disease or heart attack, which leads to interruption of blood flow and may cause clots.
5. Abnormal heartbeat, which predisposes to clots in the chambers of the heart.
6. Diabetes mellitus, which affects the health of blood vessels especially if there has been poor glucose control over a number of years.
7. Polycythaemia (too many red blood cells).
8. Hyperlipidaemia (too much fat in the blood).
9. Oestrogen in the oral contraceptive or HRT, which makes some women more vulnerable to thrombosis (although risks are lower than in normal pregnancy, when oestrogen levels are naturally raised).
10. Family history of heart attack or stroke (male relative under 55, female relative under 65).
11. Smoking, which increases the risk of clotting and hardening of the arteries.
12. Total cholesterol of 240 mg/dcl or more.
13. HDL (good cholesterol) less than 35.
14. Less than 30 minutes of physical activity at least 3 times a week.
15. More than 20 lbs overweight.

Maggie is 34 and works a tennis coach at her local sports club. When giving a lesson one day she suddenly fell to the ground and was unable to walk or speak. On admission to hospital she was found to have suffered a stroke due to a blood clot which had travelled from a deep vein in her calf. The oral contraceptive pill she had been taking was thought to be a contributory factor. Maggie, despite being fit and athletic, had suffered a stroke.

TRANSIENT ISCHAEMIC ATTACK (TIA)

By definition, a TIA produces identical symptoms to that of a stroke but their duration is less than 24 hours, with all abnormalities recovering within that timescale.

Tom at 84 reported having had a fall which he attributed to having tripped on an uneven footpath. About 3 weeks later he fell in the garden and this time had numbness on the left side of his face with drooping of the corner of his mouth and weakness in his hand. His wife noted that his speech was a little slurred and he seemed rather confused about what had happened to him, although by the following day he appeared fine. A month later, having complained of a headache the day before, he lost the use of his left arm and leg, could not speak and seemed to have difficulty in understanding what was being said to him. Tom has suffered a series of transient ischaemic attacks (TIAs) leading to a major stroke.

As in Tom's case, a TIA may be seen as a warning sign, but the symptoms are just as distressing and alarming to the patient and their relatives. Anybody experiencing a TIA should have the matter urgently investigated since the possibility of a full-blown stroke in the near or distant future is very much more likely. Investigation may often lead to the identification of an underlying abnormality which can be treated.

Diagnosis

A stroke constitutes a medical emergency and even with the milder varieties there can be no way of telling in the initial stages how the stroke will progress or evolve. One of the attending doctor's earliest decisions must be whether to keep the patient at home or whether to admit them to hospital. A lot will depend on their general state of health, their symptoms and their age. There are also a number of other possible diagnoses that need to be considered and these include an infection such as meningitis or encephalitis, a subdural haematoma as a result of a bang on the head some time previously, an abscess or a tumour. The clinical examination will reveal the initial extent of the problem, but tests need to be carried out to identify the underlying cause. Tests would probably include an electrocardiogram (ECG) to test for abnormalities in heart rhythm, a chest X-ray to detect abnormalities in heart size or the presence of abnormalities within the lung, angiography to identify any weaknesses in blood vessel walls or blockages within them, blood tests to look at cholesterol and blood fat levels, and CT or MRI scans to identify abnormalities within the brain and the extent of any damage there.

Conventional Treatment

Initial emergency treatment requires the maintenance of an adequate airway and intravenous or nasogastric tube-feeding in patients who are unconscious or semi-conscious. Dedicated nursing care is needed to prevent the development of bedsores, deep vein thrombosis (DVT) or complicating infections such as pneumonia. Once the cause of the stroke has been established, anticoagulants or thrombolytic treatment to dissolve blood clots can be given for embolisms and thrombosis respectively, and low-dose aspirin is almost universally used to prevent further recurrences of a stroke. Recovery may take at least 9 months to reach its full extent and it is not possible to predict accurately in the early stages how much progress any given patient will make. However, the earlier the treatment the better the healing, and good physiotherapy and speech therapy can aid recovery from paralysis, spasticity or slurred speech.

Nutritional Healing

As you can see from the risk factors box (points 3, 12, 13 and 15), there are some predisposing conditions which can be treated to a great extent with dietary measures, so these play an important role. Alpha lipoic acid is a powerful antioxidant which is useful. The richest natural sources are listed on p. 211. It is part of the synergystic team of antioxidants which help release energy, are necessary for the production of enzymes used in the metabolism of glucose and prevent arteries clogging. Oats will help bring your cholesterol down. Since there is an association between alcohol and high blood pressure, reduce your intake. Foods rich in Vitamin E will protect you, although in this instance, supplements tend not to. Garlic can also reduce cholesterol levels and is much more powerful when taken raw. Foods containing Vitamin C are also essential to control cholesterol levels.

To lower your cholesterol levels:

eat less:	*eat more:*
red meat	fish and poultry
eggs	soya
high fat dairy produce (butter, cream, etc.)	tofu
cakes, pastries, biscuits	fruit and vegetables
salt and salty foods	whole grains
coffee	herb teas
	water
	juices

Vitamins and Supplements

There are some vitamins and supplements that are particularly useful. Melatonin, sadly not yet available in the UK, helps protect stroke victims from further damage when new blood vessels are opened as blockages are removed and a flow of oxygen and free radicals goes through the brain. Lecithin will help to bring your cholesterol down. Vitamin B_6 and folic acid (folate) are protective, as is CoEnzyme Q10. Ginkgo biloba, hawthorn, garlic and cayenne are all useful. Have your magnesium levels checked since a low level may be a risk factor. If you're menopausal, talk to your doctor about the pros and cons of HRT.

Complementary Therapies

Try lavender, lemongrass, peppermint or rose aromatherapy oils or better still get a good aromatherapist to mix a blend for you. Basil will help you regain memory. Hyperbaric oxygen has had some variable results. Have a look at the complementary therapies for depression on p. 195 and institute them. Don't forget music which is healing, soothing and can lift you albeit temporarily into a different place. Do use it – gentle and soothing, emotionally unlocking or vigorous and rousing. All have their place. Massage is essential, both for sufferers who need to have their muscles stimulated and stretched to prevent the formation of contractures, and for those who are in caring roles and who may be straining their muscles by lifting and carrying. See if the massage therapist or reflexologist who comes to give a treatment to the stroke victim can give one to you immediately afterwards while all is settled for a while and you can relax.

Exercise and Lifestyle

TIAs may occur singly, in a series as in Tom's case, or may go on to full stroke within a month or so. See any TIA as an early warning signal and do something about your health now. It is a sad fact that the greatest causes of death in post-menopausal women are heart disease and stroke. Both are a much greater threat than cancer. As we saw in Ruby's case, although women with stroke do have angina and chest pain, they are more likely to have other symptoms such as nausea, abdominal pain or fatigue. So do note such symptoms and talk to your doctor.

Preventative measures include:

* Getting your blood pressure down.
* Exercising for at least 30 minutes 3 times a week which will help reduce your weight, relieving any extra strain upon your heart.
* Having outdoor activities, but even if you're housebound you should still keep as active as possible. Push your doctor or social worker to get you into a day centre.
* Lowering stress, as this will always help.

* Having a pet, which can work wonders, but do be aware of what you and your surroundings can cope with.
* Stopping smoking, although you will then need to do more exercise since sadly it is a fact that smoking does control your weight.

Look at the section on control of diabetes (p. 207) since diabetes can double your risk of stroke. And lastly work to get your cholesterol down. Have it measured regularly and understand what the numbers mean.

Emotional and Spiritual Healing

Much of what has been said in the sections on heart disease, high blood pressure and stress is relevant here. Try to have as much emotional support as possible and, perhaps as important, try to cooperate with the help that's being offered. That is not to say that you have to accept blindly what others are offering if your instinct tells you it's not what you want or need, but do look at the fact that for whatever reason, your ability to do things for yourself may have been temporarily suspended, so there must be a lesson to be learned about being vulnerable and learning to receive from others. Sadly the frustration which accompanies stroke can often make stroke victims difficult to deal with, and if you are a carer, whether male or female, make sure that you have plenty of time for yourself and learn to delegate as much as you can. The first rule for the nurse is to take care of themselves since otherwise there will eventually be no one to look after the situation. There is a lot of professional help available if you manage to mobilise the resources, so check with your doctor, in your local library and with Social Services. For both victims and carers watch out for depression. It is natural that mood will be low at least for some time. However, what is initially a normal reaction to such an awful life event can often slide unnoticed into clinical depression which needs to be vigorously treated. Try to get out as much as you can and keep up with friendships and social life to the best of your ability.

All are healing in themselves, but still try to make space for some formal healing too, which will lift your spirits and allow you to see the greater picture.

INTEGRATED APPROACH

1. Look at the risk factors and deal with as many of them as you can.
2. Should you have a TIA see it as an early warning and do something about your health now.
3. Set up a good eating programme and also take the various supplements you need.
4. Keep positive and cooperate with physiotherapy and other treatments from the beginning to ensure maximum recovery.
5. Accept the help that is available.
6. Take care of the emotional aspects such as frustration and depression.
7. If you are a carer take time out for yourself.
8. Use complementary therapies to heal and keep you at optimum energy levels.

Thyroid Problems

The thyroid gland helps regulate the body's metabolism and energy levels. It is a kind of thermostat which controls the tick-over speed of the body, and symptoms may arise if its function is either increased or reduced. The gland is located in front of the neck, just below the larynx or voice box, and when it becomes visibly enlarged it is known as a goitre. In adults it maintains the speed of metabolism and in children it is important for growth and mental development. A gland may become underactive, overactive or may be affected by tumours.

Underactive Thyroid

If insufficient thyroid hormone is produced, the patient is said to be suffering from hypothyroidism or myxoedema.

Divina, 53, felt lethargic and depressed, was constantly cold all the time and troubled by constipation. Her doctor originally dismissed her symptoms as being part of the menopause. However, as her weight increased and her skin became drier and coarser, a return visit to the doctor led to a blood test for thyroid trouble. The result confirmed an underactive thyroid and after a few days, treatment with thyroid hormone she felt completely invigorated and refreshed. All her old energy came back and within 3 months she was back to her normal weight. Divina had developed an underactive thyroid.

Divina's symptoms are classic. Sometimes there is also puffiness and swelling of the face and hair loss. It is as if the body has slowed down overall and all other functions slow down with it. As well as physical decline there is also slowing down of mental function so that concentration and memory become poor and depression may ensue. In severe cases everything slows down to the point that the person affected may be unable to function at all. The commonest cause is an autoimmune disorder known as Hashimoto's disease, whereby the body's own antibodies for no known reason attack its own thyroid gland. Other causes include the results of surgery for a hyperactive thyroid gland or as a result of radioactive iodine therapy used for the treatment of cancer of the thyroid or hyperthyroidism. Hashimoto's disease appears to affect about 1 per cent of the adult population and older women are especially vulnerable.

Margaret began to find that the collars of her blouses and sweaters were becoming much tighter and when she looked in the mirror she noticed a smooth puffiness at the root of her neck. Her doctor confirmed a thyroid goitre but blood tests showed that her thyroid gland was producing sufficient thyroid hormone. However, her body was manufacturing antibodies which were responsible for the swelling of her gland and she was initially treated with a very small dose of thyroid hormone and some steroids. Margaret had developed Hashimoto's disease.

In children, congenital hypothyroidism may result in cretinism if it remains untreated, resulting in mental retardation, stunted growth and coarse facial features. Treatment of an underactive thyroid involves using replacement thyroxine in tablet form, in a dose sufficient to counteract the symptoms without producing symptoms of hyperthyroidism. The dose is determined by regular blood tests to make sure that serum levels are adequate. Thyroxine hormone is also used to treat some goitres and some forms of thyroid cancer.

Overactive Thyroid

People who have an overactive thyroid are said to be suffering from hyperthyroidism. Symptoms include anxiety, palpitations, weight loss, sweating, diarrhoea and heat intolerance. It is as if the whole body is working too fast and many of the functions of the body work faster accordingly. The commonest cause is Grave's Disease, another autoimmune condition but which in this case results in the production of autoantibodies which stimulate the thyroid gland to secrete increased amounts of thyroid hormone. This affects 1 per cent of the adult population, especially middle-aged women. There may be a number of small nodules which may be felt in the thyroid gland and treatment consists of medication to suppress the activity of the thyroid gland, surgery to remove it (partial or total thyroidectomy) and, in older patients, radioactive iodine to selectively destroy some or all of the thyroid tissue.

TUMOURS

The thyroid gland may be subject to benign or cancerous growths. Benign varieties, adenomas, may be capable of producing too much thyroid hormone, leading to hyperthyroidism. Malignant tumours of the thyroid gland are fairly rare, accounting for only 1 per cent of all cancers. These are seen particularly as a result of radioactive fallout and were commonplace after the nuclear attacks on Hiroshima and Nagasaki and as a consequence of the disaster at the Chernobyl nuclear power plant in Russia. The normal clinical finding is a single firm nodule in the gland. Since it is impossible to tell by examination alone whether this is benign or malignant, scanning is normally carried out to assess the activity of the nodule. Sometimes a biopsy is also taken of a sample of cellular tissue from the nodule for examination under the microscope. Fortunately thyroid cancer has a high cure rate provided it is detected in time and treatment includes total thyroidectomy (removal of the gland), usually with the use of radioactive iodine afterwards to destroy any remaining thyroid tissue. As a result of removal of the gland, thyroid hormone tablets will be prescribed following the operation to prevent symptoms of hypothyroidism.

Tests

Patients suspected of having a thyroid disorder are often given blood tests to determine their hormone levels. Most commonly these measure the hormones produced by the thyroid gland and those that stimulate the thyroid gland to produce them, which come from the pituitary gland. The aim is to ensure that the levels of these hormones stay within normal limits. However, a small percentage of people appear to have clinical symptoms of an underactive or overactive thyroid, even when the blood tests remain within these normal limits. In this case treatment may be adjusted clinically under specialist supervision to render them symptom-free, even though on an assessment of blood tests alone they would not be eligible for treatment.

Sometimes a more sensitive test is to take your core temperature using a thermometer before you get out of bed each morning for a couple of weeks. At this time your temperature will be at its highest. Make a note of it daily. If it is regularly less than 36.5°C, you may well be suffering from mild hypothyroidism even if your blood tests are normal. If it is regularly below 35.5°C, you may have moderate to severe hypothyroidism. Do check with your doctor and ask to see a specialist if necessary. Sometimes what appears to be depression associated with lethargy and lack of interest in doing anything is actually reversible extremely quickly (as it was in Divina's case) when the hormone imbalance is righted.

Nutritional Healing, Vitamins and Supplements

Occasionally there is insufficient iodine in the diet, so adding seafood or sea vegetables such as kelp, dulse, nori and seaweed can help. Kelp taken as a daily supplement can often make the difference between that lethargic state and feeling well without the need for any further treatment. However, since occasionally the problem is caused by having too much iodine in the diet, be careful and have your tests done first. Discuss the results with your doctor and ask their opinion about manipulating your diet or taking supplements. Vitamins A and E are both utilised in the manufacture of thyroid hormone so do take plenty of foods containing these vitamins naturally and add a supplement also. Remember, however, that adding Vitamin A supplements during pregnancy is not a good idea. Your diet alone should contain enough. People with thyroid problems have often been found to have low levels of zinc, so add zinc-containing foods (see p. 545, or possibly a supplement also.

Exercise and Lifestyle

As we have said many times, exercise is good for every organ in your body and the thyroid gland is no exception. Indeed, exercise stimulates thyroid function and helps regulate thyroid hormones. So even if you feel lethargic, exercise will help. Always do breathing exercises. Try walking, T'ai chi, yoga or pilates initially and gradually build up to aerobic exercise.

Complementary Therapies

Although you may well need orthodox treatment, it would be worth having a consultation with a homeopathic physician since homeopathy can be very helpful in prompting your body to right itself and get back in balance. Autogenics may be beneficial, and aromatherapy will help you with lethargy and other symptoms. Vaporising some lemongrass oil or burning lemongrass incense will also help perk you up. Try some voice work (see below) since the whole throat area needs attention.

Emotional and Spiritual Healing

The thyroid is governed by the throat chakra which develops between the ages of 16 and 21, so if you had problems then, you may need to do some work here. Often there will be a history of some difficulty at this time, or even earlier, that will have delayed the development of this chakra which deals with truth, integrity, speech and vocation. Sometimes there will have been difficulty with personal expression of one kind or another and working on throat chakra issues will help. Singing, or at least allowing yourself to speak as you really need to, will clear away a lot of the problems of this area, so do have a consultation with a healer who works with the chakras. Reiki would be good also. If there are definite issues you can remember that still need some working through, then don't hesitate to have some counselling or psychotherapy.

Carly, now in her late thirties, came for healing complaining of lethargy over several years. She had eventually been diagnosed and was on treatment for her hypothyroidism. However, someone had mentioned to her that she might want to look at the possibility of clearing up some of the pain in her past. A healing assessment showed that she had a blocked throat chakra. On direct questioning about her late teens she began to cry about the fact that her mother had died when she was 16 and although she had then taken over caring for her 2 younger siblings, she had never really dealt with her own grief or her anger at the fact that she had not been able to follow her desire to go to university and to study law. Instead she had married early and had children of her own, and although she loved her family very much, she felt that life had somehow passed her by. Over the next few months she became more and more well, her thyroid improving and along with it her energy and her mood. Healing the hurt of the past freed her from its hold and a couple of years later she gained a place to study law as a mature student, fulfilling her ambition at last. She is now happy and healthy, needs no medication and has completely changed her life. Her marriage and her relationships with her children have improved as all have encouraged her and showed their pride in her achievement. Of course in healing the block to her throat chakra, her way was also cleared to open up her spirituality, helping her feel whole for the first time.

INTEGRATED APPROACH

1. Have blood tests and if necessary follow these up with regular core temperature readings.
2. If necessary ask to see a specialist to be treated on clinical grounds even if your tests appear normal.
3. Watch your diet and discuss with your GP whether you may need more or less iodine in your diet.
4. Take regular exercise.
5. Complementary therapies such as homeopathy are helpful.

6. Have a healing assessment especially if you are aware of some trauma between the ages of 16 and 21.
7. Look at whether you have achieved your potential and found your vocation. If not have some work on your throat chakra which may clear the whole throat area including your thyroid.

Tiredness

Tiredness is the most common complaint seen by doctors daily in their surgeries. In fact so many people complain of it that we have a familiar abbreviation for it – TATT or tired all the time syndrome. Often the problem is put down to poor sleep, overwork or dismissed as stress. Sometimes a recent viral infection is blamed and the title post-viral fatigue is used. But the sad truth is that most sufferers are made to feel that they are wasting their doctor's time and should simply pull themselves together. In certain cases they should. If there are underlying causes such as a poor relationship, too much smoking and drinking, a run of late nights and lack of exercise, then that is something that each individual needs to address and a doctor cannot do much about. But when tiredness persists relentlessly and continues despite adequate rest and relaxation, this common and, on the face of it, often trivial complaint may be masking a much more significant problem. A proper diagnosis is therefore vital, so it would be usual for your doctor to inquire not only into your physical health but also into the situation at home, at work, and in your daily life in general. Let's look at some of the most common causes of undue fatigue and then at what you can do to help yourself.

Anaemia

Haemoglobin is the oxygen-carrying component of red blood cells, and when it is reduced in quantity, the supply of oxygen to all the tissues of the body is reduced. This not only produces generalised tiredness, but also pallor, particularly in the face, and breathlessness on exertion. It means that the lungs have to work that much harder to pump the thinner blood around the body to try to make up in quantity what it lacks in quality. For this reason palpitations are common, as is a rapid pulse. Very frequent or heavy periods can be the cause and anaemia in this group of women is not uncommon. Deficiency of iron, Vitamin B_{12} or folic acid (folate) in particular leads to anaemia and often treatment will include replacing these.

INFECTIONS

Any infection, especially one that produces a raised temperature, can lead to tiredness. Some infections such as pneumonia, tuberculosis, glandular fever or a lung abcess will render people absolutely exhausted, although there may well be other symptoms that point to the source of the problem. In ME (myalgic encephalomyelitis) it is notoriously difficult in the early stages to reach a diagnosis and some people may even be accused of making up their tiredness when really they are desperate to carry on a normal life. Many patients with infections as diverse as brucellosis, kidney infections and low-grade gall bladder infections have been told to pull themselves together and snap out of it when their fatigue had a concrete physical basis.

DEPRESSION

Some 15 per cent of the population will suffer depression at some time in their lives and almost all of them will feel chronically tired. Accompanying the fatigue there may be loss of appetite, poor concentration, loss of libido, etc. To add insult to injury, many of the drugs available for the treatment of depression are capable of making the tiredness even more profound especially in the early stages. See p. 195 for other ways of treating depression.

HORMONAL CHANGES

Sometimes fluctuating hormone levels can cause fatigue. The tiredness of pregnancy, menopause, premenstrual syndrome and post-natal depression is well recognised. Even men go through a kind of menopause (sometimes termed andropause) or mid-life crisis when they suffer fatigue and lack of energy, and some authorities believe that this is due to fluctuating levels of the male hormone testosterone.

Boredom and Stress

Not having enough to do can be just as crippling as having too much to do, so those who are bored and unmotivated can feel just as tired as those who are working far too many hours and taking on too much responsibility. The physical and emotional symptoms of stress are listed on p. 482, and the consequences spill over into every area of life as well as the lives of all those around such as partners, family, friends and colleagues, the whole thing becoming an ugly vicious circle. If you are constantly pushing beyond your natural capacity, the results are exhaustion and ill health, either physical, mental or spiritual.

Underactive Thyroid

As you will see from p. 499 the constellation of symptoms here includes tiredness. The problem is much more common in women than in men, particularly in middle age. It is, however, one of the most satisfying conditions in medicine to treat since the response to thyroxine tablets is quick and in no time the patient reverts to their normal healthy state believing that some sort of miracle has happened!

Poor Diet

Sadly we tend to be a nation of overfed but undernourished people. We may eat a lot, but our diet is often over-processed, much of the natural goodness having been lost in the preparation. Food that has sat in a can for a long time or which has been processed and packaged cannot possibly retain the nutrients it once had. If we replace these with more raw and natural ingredients which are ready to release their energy to us, our vitality can be improved immensely. Where our energy is reduced and there is chronic subclinical exhaustion, it is a fact that our pain threshold is lowered and complaints and symptoms increase. If we are overweight and constantly dragging a huge weight around with us, of course we are tired before we start to do anything else. If you doubt this, try the old trick of carrying a few pounds of sugar with you everywhere you go for an hour or so and see how good it feels when you put it down! Have a look at the recommendations on diet on p. 5 and see how far you are from the ideal. Add a few vegetables and fresh fruit juices, herb teas, some magnesium-rich foods such as molasses, nuts, spinach, broccoli, bananas, pumpkin seeds, seafood, dairy produce and baked potatoes to your regime. Reduce your intake of coffee, sugar and alcohol, have regular small snacks, increase your water intake and watch for food allergies. If you can afford organic food, do try it. You'll notice the difference within a few weeks. If not, then try to make sure that all food is washed or peeled very carefully to remove all traces of insecticides and other toxins, and keep a food and symptom diary to see what changes the way you feel.

Supplements and vitamins are simply a must these days since the earth no longer contains enough fulvic acid, an essential for plant metabolism, to allow the food we grow to give us the essentials we need. So a high-potency vitamin and mineral supplement with extra Vitamin C and magnesium would be good. Two teaspoonfuls of flax seed (linseed) oil daily will give you your essential fatty acids. Some Siberian ginseng and royal jelly will help your vitality, and Vitamin E and thymus extract will also help as well as doing great things for your immune system.

MAGNESIUM DEFICIENCY

Some very significant studies on magnesium deficiency have been done over the past 30 years or more. In one double-blind study in the 1960s of over 3000 patients, 75–91 per cent improved and had relief from fatigue. The benefit was noticed within 4–5 days of the start of supplementation and continued even after the supplement stopped 4–6 weeks later. However, few doctors even test for a magnesium level. If you wish to try a supplement, magnesium citrate or aspartate are the best absorbed. You will need 500–1200 mg of magnesium daily taken as 2 or 3 doses.

MEDICATIONS

Many medications are capable of producing tiredness as a side effect. Tranquillisers, antihistamines and antidepressants are notorious for this, but painkillers, blood pressure tablets, muscle relaxants, oral contraceptives, anti-inflammatory preparations, sedatives, corticosteroids and cough medicines can also produce this symptom. Check with your doctor or pharmacist or read the literature that comes with your prescription to see if this could be the case.

HOSPITALISATION

Anyone who has undergone surgery or had a general anaesthetic is likely to develop some tiredness in the immediate aftermath. Some of the tiredness is the result of adjusting to what has happened and your body is telling you that you need rest to heal. Sometimes the problem can seem worse if there has been inadequate preparation for surgery or if there have been unrealistic expectations. Some of your energy will be diverted to the healing process, leaving you feeling lethargic. There may also be side effects from the anaesthetic. Any extended period of time in bed can lead to muscle wasting and a feeling of tiredness and accompanying weakness. Provided the underlying cause has been treated while in hospital, the tiredness should clear in 3–4 weeks.

WEIGHT CHANGE

Many of the functions of the body, including weight control, are governed by various glands. Any of these can develop abnormalities leading to weight changes and fatigue in the sufferer. An underactive adrenal gland will cease to produce steroids, leading to severe weakness and fatigue. In the case of diabetes, the pancreas fails to produce insulin normally, leading to abnormalities in the level of sugar in the blood with resulting weight changes and fatigue. Sometimes inexplicable weight loss is the result of chronic infection or even malignancy. Weight change is a symptom that should never be ignored and the best advice is to see your doctor as soon as possible.

Nutritional Healing, Vitamins and Supplements

The recommendations given in the section on ME are ideal here. Please see p. 349.

Exercise and Lifestyle

If you're isolated, get out of the house very little and exercise even less, one of the symptoms you will undoubtedly have is tiredness. If you add to this smoking and drinking, or partaking in any other activity (such as using illicit drugs) that leaves you full of toxins, then your problems will be compounded. Poor bedtime routine (see p. 468), stress or the inability to relax will add to the problem. Learning to power-nap can be very helpful. Beginning an exercise regime, starting gently perhaps with some yoga, breathing exercises and T'ai chi, will soon help you feel stronger and more capable and much less tired. Your tiredness will start to evaporate as your energy, attitude, mood, sleep, immune function and self-esteem improve. Try Epsom salt baths before you go to bed. You will absorb the magnesium through your skin and get more restful sleep. Too much sleep can make matters worse and you may arise feeling fuzzy-headed and lethargic especially if you have been sleeping in a poorly ventilated room. Practise positive thinking, take holidays, breathe deeply and if necessary change the colour scheme of your home and office since colours can affect our mood and energy levels. Better still have a feng shui expert come in and give you a professional opinion on how to reorganise your space and change colours etc. in order to lift your energy.

Complementary Therapies

Try some of the therapies listed on p. 353. All of them will be good for you.

Emotional and Spiritual Healing

It's amazing how some people continue to do all that they do over long periods despite the fact that they are so tired.

Tara at 32 has 3 small children, one of whom has night terrors, causing the whole family broken nights. Her father had had a stroke and she would visit her parents' home daily to help her mother care for him. To make ends meet she also has a part-time job in the local newsagent's. Her marriage was a little rocky since she was always too tired for sex and if the opportunity came along for an evening out she would opt rather to put up her feet and try to relax. Not surprisingly she was chronically tired, but it would have been easy to look at her lifestyle and leave it at that. Luckily her GP took time to not only listen to her but also to do some routine checks. Since she had been neglecting herself for so long, she had not thought to examine her breasts regularly and was astonished when her GP found a hard lump. The causes for her tiredness were several, including stress, overwork, depression and a developing cancer in her breast.

Deepak on the other hand is grieving for the death of his wife. He has sleepless nights and painful, sorrowful mornings and yet tries to manage to get to work on time and get his children off to school. Added to this he feels socially isolated since he moved from London to the Midlands a few months before his wife died suddenly, and he is far from the support of his family and friends.

Maggie has been crippled by her rheumatoid arthritis, is now wheelchair-bound and has constant pain. Nevertheless she usually manages a smile and a positive cheery comment despite the fact that her life leaves much to be desired. She said that her peace of mind and her faith kept her going when the pain and the chronic tiredness she suffered could have got her down.

People's thresholds for rest and sleep vary greatly. Some people who are exceedingly busy thrive on it and are always full of energy while others need their 8 or 9 hours' sleep and have little stamina. Being isolated like Deepak, depressed and sleeping poorly like Tara, will generally lower your control and make you feel irritable with poor self-esteem, self-confidence and motivation. All of these people need emotional and spiritual support as well as the conventional medical approach. Like Maggie, all would benefit from finding a spiritual connection which could lift both their mood and their energy. Disciplines such as meditation and yoga would be helpful to all of them, although one might wonder where Tara would find the time to fit either into her already busy day. The beauty of meditation, however, is that it improves the quality of your sleep, increases your vitality and perks up your energy to such a degree that the 20 minutes spent doing it are more than recouped by the improved efficiency and effectiveness of the next few hours. For all of them some healing would be good and would help them to relax, refresh, recreate and heal, their tiredness lifting as the rest of their condition and their life improves.

INTEGRATED APPROACH

1. Consult your GP to have a proper diagnosis made and rule out physical causes.
2. Eat well ensuring that you have a good supply of all the nutrients you need.
3. Supplement your diet with vitamins and minerals.
4. Check that prescribed or over-the-counter medications are not the cause of your tiredness.
5. Exercise regularly.
6. Avoid isolation.
7. Get adequate rest and sleep.
8. Reduce stress.
9. Complementary therapies recommended on p. 353.

Urinary Problems

These problems can arise from any part of the urinary tract; that is, those parts of the anatomy responsible for the formation or the excretion of urine: the kidneys, the ureters (the tubes that drain the kidneys), the bladder and the urethra (the tube that empties the bladder to the outside). Disorders may arise in any of these structures and symptoms vary accordingly. Urinary problems are extremely common and many have serious complications such as kidney scarring with kidney failure, or even septicaemia which may be life-threatening. Simple cystitis can lead to severe discomfort and for hundreds of thousands of women it is a recurrent nightmare.

The conventional approach is reasonably good at identifying the underlying causes of such symptoms but all too often antibiotics are prescribed inappropriately where no bacterial infection exists, and not enough advice is given by busy doctors about simple measures the patient can undertake themselves to prevent future problems. A great deal more education needs to be disseminated about urinary incontinence which must be one of the last taboos in British medical circles, as over 3 million sufferers in Britain can readily testify.

Urinary Tract Infections (UTIs)

These include urethritis, cystitis and pyelonephritis, described below. They affect men and women alike. Predisposing factors in men include prostate enlargement and urethral stricture (a narrowing of the tube due to scar tissue). In women, the predisposing factor is pregnancy, which relaxes the smooth muscle around the urethra and ureters allowing infection to ascend upwards. Either sex may have kidney stones, congenital abnormalities, bladder tumours and spinal cord disorders such as spina bifida and spinal cord injury. The latter two conditions prevent complete emptying of the bladder, leading to stagnation of urine and the development of infection. Although frequency (a frequent desire to pass urine) is one of the commonest symptoms of urinary tract infection, it may also be caused by other disorders. Any infections may well make a person want to pass urine frequently, but the volume passed is usually small. Anyone who begins to pass urine in greater quantities than usual without pain should be suspected of having diabetes until proved otherwise. Tests on the urine will rapidly identify the presence of glucose suggestive of this condition.

URETHRITIS

This is inflammation of the urethra, the hollow tube which drains urine from the bladder to the outside. It may be the result of infection or irritation and occasionally it may be due to a stricture. Burning or a scalding sensation when passing urine is the classic symptom and treatment usually consists of dilatation of the stricture using a solid cylindrical metal rod or cutting through the scar tissue using an instrument called a urethrotome. Very occasionally the troublesome part of the urethra is reconstructed surgically, a permanent solution which allows urine to pass through it without discomfort.

URETHRAL SYNDROME

In this condition there is pain or discomfort when passing urine, coupled with the recurrent urge to pass urine very frequently. There may also be lower abdominal pain and even discomfort in the genital area. Middle-aged women at the menopause who have thinning of the vulval tissues are most commonly affected. There is rarely any causative infection to find and the kidneys and bladder appear normal. Psychological factors may contribute to the symptoms. Sometimes oestrogen creams can be helpful. Strong soaps and other detergents should be avoided, as should antiseptic creams of any kind as they can cause an allergic irritation that can exacerbate symptoms. A high fluid intake and scrupulous personal hygiene are recommended.

Cystitis

This is one of the commonest of all the symptoms seen in general practice from which the majority of women will suffer at some stage in their lives. Symptoms include frequency (wanting to pass urine very often) and urgency (cannot wait to go) and there may be low abdominal pain and sometimes the presence of visible blood in the urine. When it is severe, sufferers may even have a slight temperature and feel generally poorly. In more than 50 per cent of cases significant numbers of bacteria can be cultured from the urine while in others there appears to be no bacteriological cause. In some cases, allergy to a condom, to spermicidal cream or to a perfumed bubble bath or other scented soap may be linked with the mechanical irritation of sexual intercourse, a condition often referred to as 'honeymoon cystitis'. The conventional approach to treatment involves appropriate antibiotics once the causative organism has been identified by laboratory tests. You need to drink plenty of fluids and to pass urine at least every 2 hours to dilute the germs in the urine and to flush the system through. Aseptic cystitis, where no germs are responsible, often responds to a high fluid intake and to re-acidification of the urine using cranberry juice, citrate salts or simple lemon barley water. Changes in sexual positions so there is less irritation to the urethra in the front wall of the vagina can help prevent recurrent sexual cystitis.

Pyelonephritis

Here infection ascends to involve the kidneys, and symptoms of high fever, backache, nausea, vomiting and severe malaise can occur. Strong antibiotics are required to eradicate the infection and to prevent it spreading into the bloodstream. Follow-up cultures of the urine should be undertaken to ensure that all micro-organisms have been killed. Without adequate treatment permanent scarring and shrinkage of the kidneys can occur, leading to abnormal kidney function.

INCONTINENCE

The uncontrollable and involuntary passing of urine is referred to as urinary incontinence and it means the bladder is not functioning normally. There are several different types of incontinence. Whilst it is not life threatening, the condition seriously impacts on the quality of life for those affected. However, only 1 in 10 actually get round to seeking medical advice because of the stigma attached to the problem and only 150,000 people are currently receiving advice and treatment. Many of those who do come for help only do so when the problem has begun to have an intolerable effect on their lives. This is despite the fact that most feel unable to travel on long journeys, that their whole life revolves around visits to the toilet and they are afraid to go out shopping or to the gym in case they wet themselves. They need to buy clothes which they find more practical as they are easier to get on and off, rather than those they might feel are more fashionable.

There are three main types of incontinence – stress, urge and overflow.

Stress Incontinence

This means that urine leaks out when the sufferer coughs, sneezes or exercises.

Danielle has 3 children and ever since giving birth to the third has noticed a leakage of urine when she laughs, coughs or even carries heavy shopping bags. She is slightly overweight and when she coughs after her first cigarette of the day she wets herself. Embarrassed by the problem, she has been unable to tell anybody about it and she now avoids going on any journey where she may not be able to find a toilet. She also refuses to go on holiday, much to the puzzlement of her husband. Danielle has stress incontinence due to weak pelvic floor muscles.

This is a classic story. The muscles at the base of Danielle's bladder have become weakened by childbirth, although this can also occur following the menopause, resulting in an inability of the sphincter muscles to fully contract and hold the urine back. Being overweight puts additional strain on these muscles and exacerbates the problem. In Danielle's case she also needs to give up smoking and get rid of her smoker's cough which makes the situation worse.

Urge Incontinence

In urge incontinence, the bladder muscles contract at the wrong time and place, and a person feels a sudden need to pass urine (urgency) which is swiftly followed by incontinence. The cause of this often remains a mystery but sometimes it is the result of a stroke or some other disease of the nervous system such as multiple sclerosis.

This is the case for Gail who is in her early sixties and has diabetes. She experiences a terrific urgency to pass urine but regularly finds she cannot get to the toilet in time and wets herself. The prescription for antibiotics by the family doctor did nothing to remedy the situation and she began to despair that she would ever have a normal life again. However, being taught to empty her bladder fully with a small catheter plus a prescription for some tablets to stabilise the muscles in the wall of the bladder cured her problem.

Overflow Incontinence

This occurs when the bladder does not empty completely and then simply overflows. This may occur as a result of diabetes, spinal damage of some kind or in the presence of an obstruction to the bladder outlet.

Investigative tests for incontinence

There are many diagnostic tests to assess the causes of incontinence. Urinalysis, a simple analysis of a urine sample, is the commonest of these. You will usually be asked for a midstream specimen. This means that the first part of the stream is discarded as it can often be contaminated with germs which frequently inhabit the end of the urethra. Urinalysis includes the physical characteristics of urine (the colour, the concentration and clarity) and the microscopic part of the test detects invisible traces of blood, cellular debris, crystals, pus or bacteria. A drop of urine is then cultured in the laboratory on a special growing jelly called agar to see which micro-organism grows. Chemical testing of the urine can find traces of glucose, blood, protein or bile, a breakdown product of blood. Urine is also occasionally examined for traces of drugs and for human corionic gonadatrophin, a hormone secreted in greater quantities in pregnancy. Additional tests when kidney disease or disorders of other parts of the urinary tract are suspected include ultrasound testing, intravenous urograms (where a radio-opaque dye is injected into a vein followed by X-rays of the kidney) and cystoscopy, whereby a special viewing instrument is passed into the bladder for direct observation. Cystometry measures the pressure within the bladder, and micturating cysto-urothrography forms part of urodynamic studies which look at the flow of urine from the bladder to the outside while the patient is voluntarily voiding.

Conventional Treatment

Bladder retraining reduces the urge to pass urine. You will be asked by your continence advisor to keep a diary of how often you pass water or wet yourself, to see if there is a pattern. This allows for a strategy to be drawn up to retrain your bladder to empty less frequently and under your control if possible.

Medication includes drugs such as propiverine, a bladder antispasmodic that is highly effective in calming an overactive bladder and is very well tolerated. Intermittent catheterisation, a procedure employed to empty the bladder completely 2 or 3 times a day, may be used to treat overflow incontinence. You will be taught to insert a small tube into the urethra which allows the bladder to drain. Sometimes a permanent in-dwelling catheter may be used as an alternative. For stress incontinence which remains troublesome despite the above measures, urogynaecologists who have a special interest in this condition are now using collagen injections to tighten up the muscles in the base of the bladder and this is an increasingly popular and effective method of treatment.

Men with incontinence can use a special penile sheath which is attached to a tube draining into a collection bag. For women, a variety of incontinence pads are available in many shapes and sizes in disposable and non-disposable forms. Plastic sheets or disposable pads for the bed can also help to protect mattresses. All these practical measures and conservative treatments for urinary problems are available on the NHS, either from your GP, from your urologist or urogynaecologist, or from continence advisers and specialists who work as part of the primary health care team in hospitals.

The treatment of urinary incontinence involves self-help measures also. There are measures that you can take to help prevent and clear any of the problems which beset the urinary tract, so first, as always, try to start with the basics of nutrition, exercise and changes of lifestyle.

Nutritional Healing, Vitamins and Supplements

Drinking at least 8 glasses of water each day and preferably a little more (on top of other drinks such as tea and juices, etc.) will generally keep your urinary tract well flushed and will lower the risk of kidney stones. Making the first and the last drink of the day *hot* water will cleanse the system and help detoxify your liver at the same time. Cranberry juice, unsweetened or sweetened with apple juice, makes urine more acidic and less able to support bacteria, so if you're prone to urinary tract infections (UTIs) drink some regularly. During an acute attack of UTI increase the amount of acidic foods (such as grains, seeds, nuts and fish) in your diet while temporarily reducing your intake of fruit and vegetables, flax seed (linseed), fish oils and beans. Try boiling some barley in water for about 20 minutes, then straining and drinking the cooled liquid. It may look unappetising but is very soothing and can stop the symptoms of cystitis in their tracks. Caffeine (found in coffee, chocolate, some canned drinks, etc.) and nicotine both cause bladder irritation and hyperactivity, so they need to be avoided in UTIs and incontinence. If kidney stones are your problem, increase the fibre in your diet and reduce your consumption of refined sugars, animal products, salt, strawberries and purine-containing foods (such as meat, shellfish, herrings, sardines, anchovies and Brewers yeast). Black tea, cocoa, rhubarb and parsley are best avoided. Add garlic to your cooking wherever possible and also eat foods containing potassium (see p. 544). Vitamins A, B_6 and C are essential, although there is probably enough Vitamin C in your diet and taking any extra is not a good idea (see below). Zinc-containing foods will help your body's natural healing process. Check natural sources on p. 545.

All the vitamins and minerals mentioned above (except Vitamin C) can be taken as a supplement if you wish. Some say that Vitamin C in high doses may contribute to the development of kidney stones and although this is debatable, if you already have stones, it would be worth avoiding excess Vitamin C. Aloe vera can help prevent or heal UTIs and folic acid (folate) is helpful too. Some orthodox medications such as Prozac and some muscle relaxants may cause incontinence, so check with your doctor to see if you can find a more natural alternative. If you choose to take a citrate mixture make sure that you dilute it well and drink lots of water.

Execrise and Lifestyle

Good personal hygiene and good sense will improve the situation considerably. Making sure that you bathe or shower regularly is a must, and wearing cotton underwear and allowing good ventilation by wearing stockings rather than tights will help. Make sure that both you and your partner bathe before making love. Urinating after sex will wash the urethra clean and prevent anything from entering the urinary tract. Many women put off going to the toilet for so long that they are incontinent in the last few seconds before finally getting there. Although training your bladder is a good idea, going when you know you must also makes sense. Douching is not necessary and can be harmful by washing infective material up into the pelvic organs. Good toilet hygiene, in which women always wipe backwards away from the urethra, will also minimise any infection from the bowel. Exercise increases blood flow to the pelvic area and also helps tone the muscles there. Kegel exercises are specifically for the pelvic floor muscles and you can do them whenever you remember, whether you're sitting at your office desk or standing at the bus stop. Pelvic floor exercises are designed to tighten the muscles that control the outflow of urine from the bladder and they are similar to the exercises learned in post-natal classes after childbirth. They are taught by NHS physiotherapists in special units in all hospitals. Pelvic tilts, done lying on your back with your knees bent and raising your bottom off the ground, will strengthen the pelvic area.

Complementary Therapies

The classical herbs for problems in the urinary tract are uva ursi and golden seal. Neither should be used during pregnancy, however. Other herb teas you might like to try are buchu, corn-silk, cranberry, nettle and red raspberry leaf. Parsley and golden rod are natural diuretics. Juniper and marshmallow root are both helpful. For cystitis, homeopathy has a variety of remedies including Apis, Belladonna, Cantharis, Dulcamara, Benzoic acid, Lycopodium and Pulsatilla. For incontinence, you could try Causticum. Reflexology and yoga will also help. In the throes of cystitis or a UTI, try laying a towel soaked in some hot water containing a little lavender oil on your lower abdomen while resting and visualising the whole urinary tract being filled with healing light and the pain and inflammation being healed. Make sure that the water isn't too hot, but resoak the towel again fairly regularly to keep the temperature up for as long as you can manage.

Emotional and Spiritual Healing

The urinary tract is the province of the second, the sacral, chakra and some healing to this area will often help. Also look at where you may be being rigid in your life, since the whole essence of this chakra is flexibility and flow, and blocks at the sacral chakra will often result in problems associated with the waterworks. Have a look at issues which were traumatic around the ages of 5 to 8 and see if there's anything you need to clear up there.

Darlene had suffered regular physical abuse as a little girl and had always felt stiff and lacking in grace. She had had problems with her periods all through her adult life, felt stiff in her lower back and sometimes had swollen ankles and fingers. Her personality was rigid too and she had few friends as she was difficult to be with, prickly and unable to give and take. Her short marriage ended because she was unable to relax sexually. Her husband eventually labelled her frigid and had an affair. She has been alone for the last 16 years. It was no surprise when she eventually confided that she has had recurrent urinary tract problems and now is incontinent too.

If any of that sounds familiar to you, why not see a healer who works with the chakras to help you clear any problems of the past which still affect you. Urinary tract problems such as those we have mentioned may respond very well to healing so do try. Incontinence is a problem that most people think will never happen to them and when it does it is usually a great blow to the self-esteem and self-confidence. Not only does it remind us that we're getting older, but it leaves us feeling embarrassed and sometimes unnecessarily ashamed. If we're not careful our quality of life can suffer. So take a little time to be aware of your whole self and have some counselling or psychotherapy if you need to, to get your physical problem into perspective. Sometimes when the emotional is cleared, the physical has a much better chance of healing.

Integrated approach

1. Eat a well-balanced diet including lots of fruit and vegetables with supplements if necessary.
2. Drink at least 8 glasses of water daily as well as other fluids such as herb teas etc.

3. Do pelvic floor exercises regularly to strengthen your muscles.
4. Be vigilant about hygiene and avoid douching.
5. Wear cotton underwear and pads or panty liners, etc. if necessary.
6. Take good care of yourself and that includes having some healing, counselling, etc.
7. Discuss your situation with your doctor and try to be honest about how the problem affects your life.
8. Guilt and shame have no place here. Urinary problems are just like any others and there is help available if you ask for it.

Visual Disorders

Problems occurring in or around the eye are common and include styes, conjunctivitis, puffiness and irritation due to allergy, redness of the white of the eye and floaters, which are harmless shadows that cross the field of vision, especially when you look at a bright background. But none of these actually cause problems with the vision itself. In this chapter we concentrate on problems that do.

A logical and thorough approach is required in the assessment and diagnosis of visual disorders and will often involve your doctor referring you to a specialist.

James, aged 27, woke up one morning unable to focus clearly when he looked straight ahead. He was unable to read his newspaper and began to wonder if he had had some kind of stroke. The doctor, who looked at the back of his eye, observed some swelling of the optic nerve head and diagnosed optic neuritis, a condition suggestive of the onset of multiple sclerosis. James was referred urgently to a neurologist for further investigation.

Flashing lights in the visual field might indicate low blood pressure, impending retinal haemorrhage or temporal arteritis (a condition where the cranial arteries are inflamed, which can cause sudden blindness and migraine). Double vision can arise from something as simple as a squint or as serious as a brain tumour, causing paralysis of one of the extraocular eye muscles. Either or both eyes may be affected. Furthermore, the underlying disorder may lie superficially within the eye or deep within the brain itself, either in the nerve pathways transmitting sensations of sight from the eye, or in that part of the cerebral cortex responsible for interpretation of the signals. The availability of CT scanning, which can show 3-D pictures of the brain in great detail, has greatly advanced the location of deep-seated problems.

Although some people have a genetic predisposition to particular visual problems, by adulthood up to 60 per cent of us may need some kind of vision correction. Degenerative diseases such as macular degeneration are increasing. Yet the most common factors resulting in poor vision – namely poor nutrition, pollution, ultraviolet radiation – are within our control. Optimal nutrition is essential and research from around the world shows that comparatively simple changes in our diet can reap amazing benefits in our visual health. One study found that a diet high in refined sugar, white flour and white rice could raise the risk for developing eye focus distortion (near-sightedness, long-sightedness and astigmatism) by 300 per cent. We shall discuss nutritional measures later.

Visual disturbance can arise from structures in or around the eye itself, in the nervous pathways that transmit the sense of vision to the brain, and within the brain. The doctor's examination is designed to detect which particular part of the anatomy is responsible. Using an ophthalmoscope, every layer of the eye can be examined in turn. If no eye disorder can be identified, the clinical picture may then warrant further investigation using other techniques such as X-rays and CT scanning.

Among the commonest causes of visual disturbance are errors of refraction, sudden loss of vision, glaucoma and cataracts. Each of these is considered separately.

Errors of Refraction

These refer to problems within the eye itself which affect the ability of the eye to focus. They include myopia (short-sightedness), hypermetropia (long-sightedness) and astigmatism (where the curvature of the cornea is not symmetrical and smooth). The vast majority of these problems can be corrected with the use of glasses or contact lenses. Many people now enjoy the quick and safe correction of these refractive errors with the use of laser treatment which in mild to moderate cases can reshape the surface of the eye, avoiding the need for contact lenses or glasses in the future. This technique is still in its infancy, however, for more severe or complex refractive problems.

SUDDEN LOSS OF VISION

Visual loss may be gradual or sudden. It may be complete, it may purely affect the periphery of the visual field, with the central vision being saved, or it may affect the central vision while the peripheral field is spared, the latter producing problems with reading or fine detailed work. Visual loss which comes on gradually may arise from cataract formation, macular degeneration (whereby the central focusing area at the back of the retina becomes less sensitive), chronic glaucoma, blood vessel damage at the back of the eye due to diabetes mellitus and keratopathy (which refers to any disorder of the cornea). Sudden visual loss on the other hand may occur due to injury, inflammation within the eye itself (uveitis), bleeding into the jelly at the back of the eye (vitreous haemorrhage), rupture of a blood vessel in the retina (retinal haemorrhage), disorders of the optic nerve or due to problems within the brain such as a stroke, a tumour or an infection.

GLAUCOMA

Glaucoma is one of the commonest and most serious eye problems affecting the over-sixties and it accounts for up to 15 per cent of all registered blindness in Britain. The pressure of the fluid within the eyeball, which must be maintained in order to retain the shape of the eyeball, rises, causing damage to the sensitive fibres in the optic nerve, leading to loss of vision. There are two main types of glaucoma, chronic simple glaucoma and acute glaucoma.

The chronic form is the most common and generally affects people over the age of 40. Since the early damage to the visual field is peripheral and the central vision is spared, there may be no symptoms for many years until blindness has become advanced. Often there is a family history and for this reason all members of a family affected by glaucoma are entitled to free tests with an optician to help pick up the early signs before there has been too much damage. Chronic glaucoma occurs where the drainage of fluid from the eye is blocked, allowing it to build up.

Acute glaucoma, where the pressure builds up very much more quickly, may occur as a secondary result of an eye injury, an inflammation within the eye (uveitis), or lens dislocation. Symptoms of acute glaucoma include a severe dull pain in or above the affected eye. The vision is cloudy and halos may appear around lights. The patient may also feel nauseated or even be sick, while the white of the eye is often red and the pupil dilated.

The diagnosis of glaucoma is usually made using a technique known as tonometry which involves the puffing of compressed air against the front of the eye, showing a raised pressure level. Ophthalmoscopy (examination using an ophthalmoscope) can also show changes affecting the optic nerve head at the back of the eye, especially cupping, where a small depression is seen at the end of the optic nerve due to the pressure upon it. Finally, the diagnosis can be confirmed and the degree of visual loss assessed by visual field testing, which may reveal blind spots in the periphery of vision.

Conventional Treatment of Glaucoma

Conventional treatment of chronic glaucoma usually involves eye drops such as timolol applied twice a day, although occasionally tablets are prescribed. Treatment is usually necessary for life to prevent further increases in pressure and very occasionally surgery may be required to assist fluid drainage.

The treatment of acute glaucoma is regarded as a medical emergency to prevent permanent and total loss of vision. Initial treatment consists of eye drops, pills, liquids and intravenous fluids to reduce the pressure. Once this is under control, surgery is carried out, the operation being known as a peripheral iridectomy which involves making an incision at the edge of the iris enabling better drainage of fluid away from the eye.

Prevention

Glaucoma can be prevented. Everybody over the age of 40, independent of their family history, should have eye tests at least every 2 years so that they can undergo tonometry which will reveal any previously undetected developing glaucoma. The fairly recent practice of buying off-the-shelf reading glasses, although convenient, tends to allow us to avoid the essential eye exams that are part of an assessment with an optician, so think carefully before continuing to self-prescribe your spectacles. Chromium has often been found to be low in patients with glaucoma and therefore a supplement would be useful. Cod liver oil seems to help reduce intraocular pressure, as do ginkgo biloba and Vitamin C.

Cataracts

A cataract develops when the lens of the eye becomes opaque and cloudy. Once it has reached an extent where visual loss is considerable, surgical extraction of the lens can be carried out, replacing the faulty lens with a clear artificial one, a tiny implant that is splinted on the iris and usually obviates the need for any other form of corrective refraction such as glasses or lenses. Sometimes, however, glasses or contact lenses are still required for reading. The operation is dramatically effective, as Dorothy found.

> *Remarkably fit for her age, 72, Dorothy had enjoyed her fairly isolated existence in her country cottage in deep Gloucestershire where she was in telephone contact with friends and relatives and thoroughly enjoyed reading. However, as her vision gradually faded and she found that she could no longer read even larger print, she began to feel depressed and lonely. She had first one cataract removed, then 6 months later the other, which restored her sight almost miraculously, giving back her quality of life and lifting her clinical depression.*

Most people have the operation under general anaesthesia, although elderly patients who could not tolerate general anaesthesia well can have it done under a local anaesthetic. Almost all patients are discharged within 48 hours and, if they are to have glasses prescribed, will have an assessment some 2 months later by which time healing of the incision at the front of the eye will have taken place and the cornea will have gone back to its normal shape.

Nutritional Healing

People who consume less than 3½ servings of fruit per day have an increased risk of cataract. Bilberries are particularly good for preventing or slowing the formation of cataracts. The amino acids glutathione, L-cysteine and L-glycine all help prevent cataracts and it has been reported that melatonin (not yet licensed in the UK) may inhibit cataract formation.

The *Journal of the American Medical Association* reported that those consuming large amounts of carotenoids from green leafy vegetables have a 43 per cent reduced chance of developing macular degeneration. Carrots are a rich source of Vitamin A which is important for the function of the cells of the retina. Dark green leafy vegetables, broccoli, cabbage, cauliflower, sprouts and fennel are full of antioxidants which help prevent or reverse damage due to free radicals. However, you may like to also take a supplement, since there is such overwhelming evidence that antioxidants help, and yet the amounts necessary to treat and sometimes reverse changes are too large to get from diet alone. Cold-water fish, flax seed (linseed) oil and bilberries are good sources of the essential fatty acids. Sulphur-rich foods such as eggs, garlic and asparagus, and herbs and spices such as marjoram, ginger and cayenne, added to your cooking, will support and protect your vision. Food should be fresh and as simple as possible. Avoid frying or eating leftover food.

Vitamins and Supplements

Other supplements you would be wise to add are Vitamins A and D which are essential for healthy eyes. Vitamin A has a particularly beneficial action on the cells of the retina.

Other essentials are Vitamins B and C, carotenoids, selenium, magnesium, calcium, zinc and the omega-3 fatty acids. Bioflavinoids can improve the health of the tiny blood vessels of the eye, help prevent the breakdown of collagen and fight free radicals. Lutein (found naturally in spinach and broccoli) protects from macular degeneration. Ginkgo biloba, gotu kola or hawthorn berry will improve circulation.

Exercise and Lifestyle

Aerobic exercise helps the eyes as it does every other part of the body. Breathing exercises also help improve the circulation. Eye exercises are helpful in some conditions. Smoking again comes under criticism here and is a particular risk factor for macular degeneration (together with being a Caucasian woman over the age of 75 with high blood pressure). Steer clear of smokey atmospheres and other kinds of pollution. Try to always work in a good light and take regular breaks if you work at a computer. Also protect yourself with a computer screen that reduces flicker. Writing on an angled surface is said to be less of a strain on your eyes. If you have a lot of old amalgam fillings think seriously about talking to your dentist about having these replaced. As always prevention is better than cure, so always protect your eyes from the sun (especially between the hours of 10 a.m. and 3 p.m.) with a good pair of sunglasses which block 100 per cent of UVA and UVB light. Also remember to wear protective goggles if you are doing anything which may be dangerous such as cutting wood or working with metal or if you work in extremely bright light such as when welding. Should you be involved in any incident where you may have suffered a splinter of glass, metal or wood to your eye, seek immediate attention at your local accident and emergency room or eye hospital. Sometimes fragments are impossible to detect by simple examination and need a professional assessment.

Complementary Therapies

Herbs to try include bilberry, pine bark and grape seed, either in tablet form or made into a tea. Other therapies that have something to offer include relaxation, meditation, acupuncture, acupressure, reflexology, biofeedback, yoga and Traditional Chinese Medicine.

Emotional and Spiritual Healing

Many of us fail to truly value our eyes and our sense of sight until they are threatened. If you're in the position of reading this before you have any problem, then please look carefully at the preventive measures you can use. Depression, anxiety and fear are only some of the negative emotional accompaniments of visual problems. Psychotherapy or counselling can help here, and sometimes a group situation is very beneficial. If your vision is becoming worse do try to look for the positive and be willing to accept all the help and support you are offered. The fear of blindness needs to be acknowledged and dealt with, while a great deal of support may be necessary to help reduce stress as much as possible and encourage the development of new skills. You will find that the Royal National Institute for the Blind (RNIB) has a lot to offer and you don't need to be completely without sight to ask for their help. Do ask your doctor about having a counsellor and also about someone to give you any financial assistance you may require and to help assess your needs for various aids in the home. Although you may resist such things as learning Braille, it could enhance your life enormously and give you back the independence you appear to have lost, thereby improving your self-confidence and self-esteem. While the pain of losing something as precious as your sight cannot be underestimated, with a positive outlook you will find that life still has much to offer. Bitterness, resentment and anger, although understandable, are in the end not only a waste of energy but actively counter-productive. Talk to your counsellor about these feelings and if necessary have some formal psychotherapy. Spiritual healing can help and your healer may focus on the brow chakra which is associated with vision. You may also be asked to look at what in your life you are unwilling to see, and while this may sound rather strange, sometimes it can help to reflect on this and come to terms with whatever you need to acknowledge in your life. Try to live a life that is as full as possible and enjoy the fact that your other senses will compensate a great deal if you allow them to develop. Whatever the physical situation, your inner sight and wisdom can continue to grow and your spirituality can give you a sense of peace that is greater than anything you have previously experienced.

INTEGRATED APPROACH

1. Have regular eye examinations from age 30 onwards, if your eyesight has started to deteriorate or if you have a relative who has glaucoma.
2. Seek urgent medical advice for any sudden change including pain in the eye or loss of vision.
3. Take care to protect your eyes from sunlight by wearing good sunglasses.
4. Wear protective goggles when necessary to prevent injury.
5. Eat a good diet with plenty of antioxidants and vitamins. Supplement where necessary.
6. Avoid pollution which will affect your eyes.
7. Ask for help with practical aids etc. and also for help in dealing with the feelings that accompany any deterioration of your vision.
8. Complementary therapies and healing can be very helpful, especially in the early stages.
9. The RNIB will be a source of support both practically and emotionally.

Appendix 1

The Immune System

The immune system consists of the lymph nodes, spleen, thymus and tonsils, together with specialised white blood cells such as macrophages and mast cells, and chemicals in the bloodstream, especially complement factors, interferon and interleukin.

Lymph nodes filter foreign particles, bacteria and cell debris out of the fluid which flows between cells and which, when collected in lymphatic vessels, is known as lymph. Lymph nodes contain B lymphocytes, white blood cells, which can initiate the production of antibodies.

The spleen produces white blood cells, destroys bacteria, old red blood cells and platelets, while also acting as a reservoir of blood for emergencies. The thymus produces T-cells which are of three kinds: helper cells, which help other white cells to function; suppressor cells, which inhibit white cells from functioning, and cytotoxic cells, which attack and destroy foreign tissue, cancer cells and cells infected with viruses. If there are too many helper cells and not enough suppressor cells, the body will start to attack itself and autoimmune disorders such as rheumatoid arthritis and lupus may result, as well as allergic reactions. If there are too many suppressor cells and not enough helper cells, there is a deficiency of the immune system. The tonsils provide a defence system for the throat and act like a sponge, mopping up infective material.

White blood cells produce antibodies to illness or infection. Natural killer cells, whose function it is to destroy diseased or infected cells, are reduced in cancer and chronic infections and also in chronic fatigue syndrome. Macrophages gobble up foreign particles, bacteria and cell debris, while mast cells release histamine in allergic reactions. We can enhance natural killer activity by giving up smoking, having regular exercise, adequate rest, a mainly vegetarian diet and maintaining a sensible weight. Nutritional deficiencies (especially in children and the elderly), too much sugar and high cholesterol will suppress their activity. A high-complex carbohydrate, low-protein diet together with a high-potency multimineral and multivitamin supplement, exercise (including breathing exercises), a positive mental attitude, relaxation and sleep, all support the immune system. The ability of white cells to destroy micro-organisms is markedly affected by the ingestion of refined sugar. For up to 5 hours after eating a high-sugar snack, immune function is depressed possibly due to the fact that sugar competes with Vitamin C for transportation sites across membranes. It is therefore better to fast from sugar for a few days when you have an infection. Obesity and alcohol consumption also reduce immune activity. Breastfeeding babies for 4 months or more gives infants immunity from many diseases and also helps them have a healthy immune system for life.

Echinacea and astragalus are the two classical botanicals which enhance immune system function. Echinacea needs to be taken every few hours at the start of illness (especially viral) and then tailed off. There is nothing to be gained by taking it constantly. It is better during the winter months if you feel you need protection to take it for perhaps 10 days, then stop for 10 days and start again, repeating the pattern for 3 months or so. Astragalus works rather differently and should be available in most health-food shops. Vitamin A is an anti-infective agent which acts by maintaining the health of the skin and the mucous membranes which line the body, making it particularly useful in respiratory disorders. It has an overall effect of increasing the action of white blood cells, improving antibody response to infection, having a direct antiviral action and promoting the function of the thymus. It needs to be used with caution, however, and should never be taken as a supplement by women who are pregnant or at risk of becoming pregnant because of its association with birth defects when taken in high doses. It has a remarkable effect upon children's recovery from measles and the reduction in possible complications, often even after a single dose. Vitamin

C is a powerful antioxidant, even more so when taken alongside Vitamin E. Add the B vitamins, especially B_6, B_{12} and folic acid (folate), and you already have a good supporting system. Zinc supports thymus activity and helps in the production of T-cells, while carotenes also protect the thymus and help in the fight against viruses. Iron and selenium are protective of the immune system and although taking what is available in a multimineral supplement should generally be enough, take extra if you're under particular stress (but see p. 481 on anaemia and iron before doing so).

Don't forget that your body, mind and spirit are connected and that the health of one will intimately affect the health of the others. There is little point in having a good diet with supplements if you then spend your time being negative, gossiping about people or sending out hateful, vengeful vibes. Thoughts and feelings have biochemical reactions associated with them, and you will only be healthy if you detoxify your mind and spirit as well as your body. Perhaps one of the best-researched methods of doing just that is meditation, although healing in any form will help and will have an effect upon your immune system. As always, however, the responsibility is yours to then carry on the good work. You will eventually get to the point that you will not allow your body to take in toxic substances, and hopefully you will see that your mind will not be healthy unless you have the same rules there also. Bad news, malicions conversation, acts which offend your integrity, will all affect you just as dramatically and you will learn to avoid them in a bid to remain in harmony and balance throughout.

Appendix 2

The Energy System

The whole universe consists of energy in one form or another and human beings, as parts of the macrocosm, are no exception to the rule. We also consist of molecules held together by constant vibration. However, our physical body, that part of us which is visible, has sensation and which we can touch, is not where our true reality ends. In fact around our physical body there are layers of energy which are still very much part of us and which are collectively known as the aura or human energy field. Some people are able to see this, many more are able to sense it or feel it and be aware on a subtle level of when it is invaded by others – when our personal space is encroached upon. But whether you can or cannot feel, touch or see it, it is certainly there and has a great bearing on how you feel, how you interact with others and how they interact with you, and the state of your physical health.

Within the aura there are many areas where the flow of energy is much more organised and flowing at a different speed. These whirlpools of energy are called chakras. Some of them are quite large and are called the major chakras, some are smaller, the minor chakras, and then there are many tiny ones over joints and acupuncture points. Ideally there should be a free flow of energy throughout our aura, our chakras and our physical body, which keeps us well and balanced. However, depending upon what happens to us throughout our lives, our aura can become the repository for pain and discomfort and leave us unable to be our best, and our chakras either fail to develop fully, become distorted or damaged and result in our natural energy being blocked.

The chakras also allow for a free flow of energy between us and others, but much more than that, their health governs our health and emotional state. Each of the 7 main chakras governs a particular area of our physical body, part of our emotional development, our hormonal state and much more. Since each of them should develop in sequence from the time of our birth, trauma at various times of our lives can distort or arrest our development leaving us with problems which may at first be difficult to understand.

For instance, should you have suffered trauma in your very early days, say up to the age of about 4 or 5 years old when your root chakra is developing, then you are likely to have difficulty with your sense of belonging, feeling secure and having good self-esteem, and you may find yourself compensating for such insecurity by drinking, taking drugs, being depressed or having an eating disorder. Physically you may have difficulty with your sexual organs.

Problems a little later, between the ages of about 5 and 8 at the time of development of the sacral chakra, may result in having difficulties with relationships, being rigid in both mind and body and in having problems with simply going with the flow. In a physical sense you may also have difficulty with flow, so that the systems of the body that are filled with fluid – your circulation, lymphatics, urinary system and menstrual flow in women – may be problematic. Sexual difficulties are common here.

Your solar plexus chakra develops between the ages of about 8 and 12 and problems at this time will usually result in difficulties with your own power, being either aggressive or feeling powerless and helpless. The will is affected and you may feel either headstrong or weak-willed. Your ability to be prosperous will also be affected and you may forever be struggling to make ends meet no matter how hard you try. In a physical sense you may have digestive problems among other things. Some healing of this chakra can remedy the problem.

Your heart chakra develops between the ages of 12 and 16. Trauma during this time will usually render it difficult for you to truly love and feel loved, to empathise with others and be compassionate. You may feel cold and unmoved by things or conversely so easily moved that you can hardly function because you get involved in everyone else's problems. Your heart chakra also governs your heart and lungs, so a blocked heart chakra can often result in problems in these organs with high blood pressure, chest problems and heart disease.

Between the ages of 16 and 21 your throat chakra develops and allows you to come to understand what is right for you, to communicate this well to the world and to define your own integrity. Problems here can make it difficult to stand up for who you are, to say it as it is, be self-assertive and find your vocation in life. In a physical sense your throat, tonsils and thyroid as well as your hearing can be affected by blocks in this area.

The brow chakra develops in some people between ages of 21 and 26 although in some it never develops at all. This chakra allows us to see things in a different way and to develop a sense of inner vision, a capacity to see things from all points of view and to visualise a greater picture. It lifts us to a more spiritual way of life where there is much more richness as our inner life becomes part of our everyday experience. Problems here can cause difficulties with our actual vision but also with memory and other brain functions.

The seventh chakra is the crown which, located directly above your head, develops after the age of 26 and sometimes not at all. It allows us to experience universal love which frees us from the ties of the world and gives us a completely new experience of transcending the mundane and entering into a calm and peaceful place where we are free and intensely happy, albeit sometimes for only seconds at a time initially. Meditation can help us achieve this quite remarkable state which can profoundly affect our total wellbeing.

If there are problems at one chakra, then, because all are interconnected, problems in other areas develop also, rather like a domino effect.

The chakras are spinning at different speeds and are different in size and colour. The root chakra in good health is red, the sacral orange, the solar plexus yellow and the heart green. The throat is a beautiful sky or turquoise blue whereas the brow is deep blue or even purple. The crown when developed is either deep purple or white. They are usually brought back to their full capacity by clearing whatever hurt us at the time of their development, healing the pain, forgiving those who harmed us and learning to see our lives as a series of challenges and lessons which help us grow to be who we really are capable of being.

Although this brief description of the energy system is intended to help you understand references to the chakras in the text, you may find yourself called to read in much more detail how to lift yourself beyond a state of feeling well and into a place of positive happiness and health. If so, then we recommend that you read Brenda's book, *The Rainbow Journey* (Hodder & Stoughton, 1998).

APPENDIX 3

Vitamins, Minerals and their Sources and Functions

VITAMIN	NATURAL SOURCES	MAIN FUNCTIONS
Vitamin A	Coloured fruits and vegetables, dairy produce, eggs, fish oils, liver	Promotes healthy skin, hair and inner membranes, night vision, resistance to infections especially respiratory; lowers risk of heart disease; helps immune system; shortens duration of illness and may protect against some cancers; helps improve vitality and growth
Vitamin B_1 (thiamine)	Yeast, brown rice, whole wheat, oats, peanuts, pork, vegetables, milk	Promotes growth; aids carbohydrate digestion; essential for normal function of nerves, muscle, heart and brain; improves mental attitude
Vitamin B_2 (riboflavin)	Liver, kidney, milk, yeast, cheese and most of those as for B_1	Promotes healthy hair, skin and nails; helps in growth and reproduction; helps in digestion
Vitamin B_3 (nicotinic acid or niacin)	Lean meat, whole wheat, green vegetables, beans, yeast	Helps lower cholesterol; helps control blood pressure; promotes good circulation; takes part in carbohydrate metabolism; increases energy; good for healthy skin
Vitamin B_6 (pyridoxine)	Meat, fish, egg yolks, cantaloupe melon, cabbage, milk, brown rice, peanuts, soya, wheatgerm	Helps in fat and protein metabolism; a natural diuretic; helps minimise premenstrual symptoms

Vitamin B_{12} (cyanocobalamine)	Liver, kidney, beef, pork, eggs, milk, cheese, fish	Essential for red blood cell production; promotes growth; promotes a healthy nervous system; improves circulation and balance; helps memory; enhances immunity, especially in the elderly
Choline (lecithin)	Egg yolks, brain, liver, heart, green leafy vegetables, peas, beans, wheatgerm	Lowers cholesterol; aids memory; helps detoxify the liver; is necessary for fat metabolism and nervous system function
Folic acid (folate)	Dark green leafy vegetables, liver, kidney, yeast	Promotes healthy skin; prevents neural tube defects in the fetus; improves lactation; helps prevent anaemia; essential for protein metabolism; essential for red blood cell formation
Inositol	Fruits, nuts, grains, milk, yeast, cantaloupe melons	Lowers cholesterol; helps keep hair healthy; helps prevent eczema; helps relieve diabetic neuropathy
Vitamin B_5 (pantothenic acid)	Liver, kidney, yeast, eggs, wheat, peas, molasses, whole grains, cereal	Helps promote healthy skin, hair, nails and central nervous system; promotes antibody production and wound healing; reduces stress and fatigue; aids digestion
Vitamin C (ascorbic acid)	Citrus fruits, berries, kiwi fruit, peppers, cabbage and other green vegetables, broccoli, many other fresh foods	An antioxidant; helps wound healing, maintenance of mood; antibody production; reduces fatigue; is anti-cancer agent; helps with viral infections such as common cold; is necessary for absorption of iron; essential in digestion and absorption of many foods; lowers cholesterol; helps reduce risk of heart attack; protects against allergy; strengthens collagen and other connective tissue, and many other such functions

Vitamin D (calciferol)	Oily fish, fat, dairy produce, or manufactured internally from cholesterol and sunshine	Necessary for calcium absorption and therefore for healthy teeth and bones
Vitamin E (tocopherol)	Wheatgerm oil, whole grains, avocados, meat, eggs, green leafy vegetables	An antioxidant; slows ageing process; protects from heart disease; an anti-cancer agent; improves stamina; helps prevent cataracts; enhances immune system; promotes healthy skin
Vitamin K	Dairy produce, yogurt, egg yolks, alfalfa sprouts, broccoli, cabbage, cauliflower and many other fresh fruits and vegetables	Essential to blood clotting mechanism, liver function and menstruation; may inhibit cancer formation
Vitamin P (bioflavinoids)	Fruits (especially the pulp under the rind of lemons and oranges), vegetables, seeds, nuts	Strengthens capillary walls; augments the effectiveness of Vitamin C by preventing its breakdown in the body; helps immune system cope with colds and other respiratory infections

MINERAL	NATURAL SOURCES	FUNCTIONS
Calcium	Milk and other dairy produce, sesame seeds, broccoli, spinach, almonds, figs	Builds and maintains bones and teeth; necessary in blood clotting mechanism; promotes stamina and vitality
Boron	Negligible	Works with calcium, magnesium and Vitamin D to help maintain bone health and prevent osteoporosis
Chromium	Negligible	Works with insulin in sugar metabolism; also utilised in protein metabolism

Cobalt	Negligible	Necessary for production of Vitamin B_{12} and therefore for red blood cell production
Copper		Used in iron metabolism and building red blood cells
Fluorine	Now in drinking water	Essential for dental health and prevention of caries
Iodine	Kelp and other sea vegetables, seafood, often added to table salt	Growth and energy as part of thyroid function
Iron	Meat	Part of haemoglobin and essential for the oxygen-carrying capacity of red blood cells
Magnesium	Whole grains, wheat bran, green leafy vegetables, almonds, bananas, apricots, beans, some fruit	Normal function of heart, muscle and nerve tissue; used in Vitamin C and calcium metabolism; reduces stress; can help reverse osteoporosis
Manganese		Essential for production of enzymes and for effective use of Vitamins B_1 and E
Phosphorus		Essential for bones and teeth and connected with the action of Vitamin D and calcium
Potassium	Green leafy vegetables, bananas, spinach	An electrolyte whose serum level is essential to the function of many tissues, especially the heart, and to fluid balance
Selenium		Stimulates the immune system; an anti-cancer agent; works with Vitamin E
Sodium		Works with potassium to maintain fluid balance

Sulphur		Promotes healthy nails, skin and hair
Vanadium		May function like insulin
Zinc	Pumpkin and sunflower seeds, beans, ginger, parsley, carrots, oysters, lamb, liver, brewer's yeast, fish, wheatgerm	Promotes wound healing; necessary for carbohydrate and protein metabolism; maintains various enzyme activities; essential for male hormone production and prostate function

Useful Addresses

Although your GP, local library or community centre may be able to give you information on the various therapies, associations, etc. mentioned in the text, you may find the following list useful. In most cases the name of the society or association will be self-explanatory, but where we feel this not to be the case we have added information in parentheses. While we have made every effort to ensure that the information is correct at the time of going to press, we realise that phone numbers change, so please check where necessary.

Useful Addresses for Complementary Therapies

Institute for Complementary Medicine
PO Box 194
London SE16 1QZ
Tel. 0171 237 5165

The British Holistic Medicine Association
179 Gloucester Place
London NW1 6DX
Tel. 0171 262 5299

Research Council for Complementary Medicine
60 Great Ormond Street
London WC1N 3JF

British Complementary Medicine Association
St Charles Hospital
Exmoor Street
London W10 6DZ
Tel. 0181 964 1205

Community Health Foundation
188–196 Old Street
London
EC1V 9FR
Tel. 0171 251 4176

The Council for Acupuncture
179 Gloucester Place
London NW1 6DX
Tel. 0171 724 5756

Society for the Teachers of the Alexander Technique
20 London House
266 Fulham Road
London SW10 9EL
Tel. 0171 351 0828

Aromatherapy Organisations Council
3 Latymer Close
Braybrooke
Market Harborough
Leicester LE16 8LN
Tel. 01858 434242

British Association of Art Therapists
11a Brighton Road
Brighton BN2 3RL

British Association for Autogenic Training and Therapy
18 Holtsmere Close
Garston, Watford
Herts WD2 6NG
Tel. 01932 675501

International Association for Ayurveda
PO Box 3043
Barnet
Herts EN4 0QZ

The Bach Centre (for Bach Flower Remedies)
Mount Vernon
Sotwell, Wallingford
Oxon OX10 0PZ
Tel. 01491 834678

British Chiropractic Association
29 Whitley Street
Reading
Berks RG2 0EG
Tel. 0734 757557

Action Against Allergy
24–26 High Stret
Hampton Hill
Middlesex TW12 1PD

Hygeia College of Colour Therapy
Brook House
Avening, Tetbury
Glos GL8 8NS
Tel. 01453 832 150

Osteopathic Information Service
PO Box 2047
Reading
Berks RG1 4YR

The Affiliation of Crystal Healing Organisations
46 Lower Green
Esher KT10 8HD
Tel. 0181 398 7252

The Flower and Gem Remedy Association
Laurel Farm Clinic
17 Carlingcott
Peasetown St John
Bath BA2 8AN
Tel. 01761 434098

The Confederation of Healing Organisations
Suite Judy, 2nd Floor
The Red and White House
113 High street
Berkhamstead
Herts HP4 2DJ
Tel. 01442 870 660

General Council for Consultant Herbalists
Grosvenor House
40 Sea Way
Middleton-on-Sea
West Sussex PO22 7SA

The Homeopathic Association
27a Devonshire Street
London W1N 1R J
Tel. 0171 9935 2163

Royal Homeopathic Hospital (for homeopathy and yoga therapy)
56–57 Great Ormond Street
London WC1N 3HR
Tel. 0171 833 7267

British Naturopathic and Osteopathic Association
Frazer House
6 Netherall Gardens
London NW3 5RR

British Society for Medical and Dental Hypnosis,
National Office
17 Keppelview Road
Kimberworth
Rotherham SG1 2AR
Tel. 01709 554 558

SAD Association
PO Box 989
London SW7 2PZ

The British Society for Music Therapy
25 Rosslyn Avenue
East Barnet
Herts EN4 8DH
Tel. 0181 368 8879

British Society of Nutritional Medicine
Acorns
Romsey Road
Cadnam, Southampton
Hants SO4 2NN

Royal College of Psychiatrists
17 Belgrave Square
London SW1
Tel. 0171 235 2351

British Association for Counselling
1 Regent Place
Rugby
Warwickshire CV21 2PJ
Tel. 0178 8578 328

For information about Magnetic Therapy, please contact Dr Tim Ridge on 0181 363 7575.

Healing Tao Foundation (for information on Chi gong)
PO Box 195
85 Marylebone High Street
London W1M 3DE
Tel. 0171 224 1817

The British Reflexology Association
Monks Orchard
Whitbourne
Worcester WR6 5RB
Tel. 0188 6821 207

The Shiatsu Society
5 Foxcote
Wokingham
Berks RG11 3PG
Tel. 0173 4730 836

International Association of Spiritual Psychiatrists
The Ravenscroft Centre
6 Ravenscroft Avenue
London NW11 0RY
Tel. 0181 455 3743

International Association for Voice Movement Therapy
7c Ballards Lane
Finchley
London N3 1UX
Tel. 0181 693 9202

Yoga for Health Foundation
Ickwell Bury
Biggleswade
Bedfordshire SG18 9EF
Tel. 0176 762 7271

Transcendental Meditation
Tel. 0990 143733

Useful Addresses for Conventional Treatments

Abortion

National Abortion Campaign
The Print House
18 Ashwin Street
London E8 3DL
Tel. 0171 923 4976

British Pregnancy Advisory Service
Austy Manor
Wootton Wawen
Solihull
West Midlands B95 6BX
Tel. 0345 304030

Brook Advisory Centre
165 Grays Inn Road
London WC1X 8VD
Tel. 0171 713 9000/8000

The Miscarriage Association
c/o Clayton Hospital
Northgate
Wakefield
West Yorks WF1 3JS
Tel. 01924 200799

Addictions

Alcoholics Anonymous
PO Box 1
Stonebow House
Stonebow, York
North Yorks Y01 2NJ
Tel. 01904 644026

Narcotics Anonymous
PO Box 1980
London N19 3LS
Tel. 0171 730 0009

Gamblers Anonymous
PO Box 88
London SW10
Tel. 0171 384 3040

AIDS

Body Positive
51b Philbeach Gardens
London SW5 9EB

National AIDS helpline
PO Box 5000
Glasgow G12 9BL

Terence Higgins Trust
52–4 Grays Inn Road
London WC1X 8JU

Allergies

British Society for Allergy and Environmental Medicine
PO Box 28
Totton
Southampton SO40 2ZA
Tel. 01703 812124

Action Against Allergy
PO Box 278
Twickenham
Middlesex TW1 4QQ

International Society for Orthomolecular Medicine
16 Florence Avenue
Toronto
Ontaria
Canada M2N 1E9
Tel. 416 733 2117

Medic Alert Foundation
12 Bridge Wharf
156 Caledonian Road
London N1 9UU

Anxiety, Panic, Phobias and Obsessions

Be Not Anxious
Chichester
West Sussex
Tel. 01243 572500

Arthritis

Arthritis Care
18 Stephenson Way
London NW1 2HD
Tel. 0800 289170

Asthma

National Asthma Campaign
Providence House
Providence Place
London N1 0NT
Tel. 0345 010203

Attention Deficit Hyperactivity Disorder (ADHD)

Hyperactive Children's Support Group
71 Whyke Lane
Chichester
West Sussex PO19 2LD
Tel. 01903 725182

Backache

National Back Pain Association
16 Elmtree Road
Teddington
Middlesex TW11 8ST
Tel. 0181 977 5474

Bereavement

CRUSE Bereavement Care
Cruse House
126 Sheen Road
Richmond
Surrey TW9 1UR
Tel. 0181 332 7227

Blood Disorders

Childhood Cancer and Leukaemia
c/o The Kerith Centre
Church Road
Bracknell
RG12 1EH
Tel. 01344 304080

Cancer

Bristol Cancer Help Centre
Grove House
Cornwallis Grove
Clifton
Bristol B58 4PG

British Association of Cancer United Patients (BACUP)
3 Bath Place
Rivington Place
London EC2A 3JR
Tel. 0800 181199

Women's Nationwide Cancer Control Campaign (WNCCC)
Suna House
128–130 Curtain Road
London
Tel. 0171 729 2229

Chest problems

British Lung Foundation
78 Hatton Garden
London EC1N 8JR
Tel. 0171 831 5831

Depression

Depression Alliance
35 Westminster Bridge Road
London SE1 7QB

Diabetes

British Diabetic Association
10 Queen Anne Street
London W1M 0BD
Tel. 0171 323 1531

Digestive Disorders

British Digestive Foundation
3 St Andrews Place
London NW1 4LB

Eating Disorders

Eating Disorders Association
Sackville Place
44 Magdalen Place
Norwich NR3 1JU
Tel. 01603 621414

Overeaters Anonymous
PO Box 19
Stretford
Manchester
Tel. 01426 984674

Eczema

National Eczema Society
163 Eversholt Street
London NW1 1BU
Tel. 0171 388 4800

Epilepsy

National Society for Epilepsy
Chalfont St Peter
Gerrards Cross
Bucks SL9 ORJ
Tel. 01494 601300

Headaches

British Migraine Association
178a High Road
Byfleet
West Byfleet
Surrey KT14 7ED

Heart Disease

British Heart Foundation
14 Fitzharding Street
London W1H 4DH
Tel. 0990 200656

Family Heart Association
PO Box 33
Maidenhead
SL6 9UX
Tel. 01628 522177

Cardiomyopathy Association
40 The Metro Centre
Tolpits Lane
Watford
Herts WD1 8SB
Tel. 01923 249977

HYSTERECTOMY

Women's Health
52 Featherstone Street
London EC1Y 8RT
Tel. 0171 251 6580

INFERTILITY

British Agencies for Adoption and Fostering
Skyline House
200 Union Street
London SE1 0LX

Child
Charter House
43 St Leonards Road
Bexhill-on-Sea
East Sussex TN40 1JA
Tel. 01424 732361

Human Fertilisation and Embryology Authority
Paxton House
30 Artillery Lane
London E1 7LS

Issue (The National Fertility Assocation)
509 Aldridge Road
Great Barr
Birmingham B44 8NA
Tel. 0121 344 4414

ME

ME Association
Stanhope House
High Street
Standford-le-Hope
Essex SS17 0HA
Tel. 01375 361013

Action for ME
PO Box 1302
Wells
Somerset BA5 2WE
Tel. 08991 122976

Persistent Disease Research Foundation
4 One Tree Lane
Beaconsfield
Bucks HP9 2BU

MEMORY PROBLEMS AND DEMENTIA

Age Concern
Astral House
1268 London Road
London SW16 4ER

Alzheimer's Disease Society
Gordon House
10 Greencoat Place
London SW1P 9PH

MENOPAUSE

The Amarant Trust
St Andrews House
26 Brighton Road
Crawley
West Sussex RH10 6AA

Women's Nutritional Advisory Service
PO Box 268
Lewes
East Sussex BN7 2QN

MENSTRUAL PROBLEMS

Women's Health
52 Featherstone Street
London EC1Y 8RT

MULTIPLE SCLEROSIS

The MS Society
25 Effie Road
London SW6 1EE
Tel. 0171 371 8000

OSTEOPOROSIS

National Osteoporosis Society
PO Box 10
Radstock
Bath BA3 3YB

PREGNANCY/POST-NATAL DEPRESSION

Family Planning Association UK
2–12 Pentonville Road
London N1 9FP

National Childbirth Trust
Alexandra House
Oldham Terrace
Acton
London W3 6NH
Tel. 0181 992 8632

Pre-eclampsia Society
12 Monksford Drive
Hullbridge
Hockley
Essex SS5 6DQ

PROSTATE PROBLEMS

The Prostate Association
Stanley House
22 Paradise Street
Rugby
Warwickshire CV21 3SZ

SCHIZOPHRENIA

The Mental Health Foundation
37 Mortimer Street
London W1N 8JU
Tel. 0171 580 0145

MIND (The Mental Health Charity)
15–19 Broadway
London EC5 4BQ
Tel. 0181 522 1728 or
0345 660163

SEXUAL PROBLEMS

Brook Advisory Centres
Tel. 0171 713 9000

Relate
Herbert Gray College
Little Church Street
Rugby CV21 3AP
Tel 01372 464100

Sexwise
Freephone 0800 282 930

SLEEP DISTURBANCES

The British Snoring and Sleep Apnoea Association
How Lane
Chipstead
Surrey CR5 3LT
Tel. 017375 557997

SKIN DISORDERS

Acne Support Group
PO Box 230
Hayes
Middlesex UB4 OUT
Tel. 0181 561 6868

Psoriasis Association
Milton House
7 Milton Street
Northampton NN2 7JG
Tel 01604 711129

STROKE

The Stroke Association
CHSA House
123–127 Whitecross Street
London EC1Y 8JJ
Tel. 0171 490 7999

Thyroid Problems

British Thyroid Foundation
PO Box 97
Clifford
Wetherby
West Yorks LS23 6XD

Urinary Problems

The Continence Foundation
The Dene Centre
Castle Farm Road
Newcastle upon Tyne NE3 1PH
Tel. 0191 213 0050

Visual Disorders

Royal National Institute for the Blind
224 Great Portland Street
London W1N 6AA
Tel. 0171 388 1266

Bibliography

Age-Proof Your Body: Your Complete Guide to Lifelong Vitality, Elizabeth Somer (Morrow, 1998).

Alternatives to Over the Counter and Prescription Drugs, Michael Murray (William Morrow & Co).

Anatomy of the Spirit, Carolyn Myss, Ph.D. (Bantam, 1997).

Aromatherapy: A Lifetime Guide to Healing with Essential Oils, Valerie Gennari Cooksley (Prentice Hall, 1996).

The Arthritis Cure, Jason Theodosakis, MD (St Martin's Press, 1997).

Autogenic Training, Dr Kai Kermani (Thorson, 1990).

Brain Longevity, Dharma Singh Khalsa, MD (Warner, 1997).

Breast Cancer? Breast Health, Susan S. Weed (Ash Tree Publishing, 1996).

The Carnitine Miracle, Robert Crayhon (M. Evans & Co, 1998).

The Complete Encyclopedia of Natural Healing, Gary Null, Ph.D. (Kensington, 1998).

The Complete Guide to Natural Sleep, Dian Dincin Buchman (Keats Publishing, 1997).

The Consumer's Guide to Homeopathy, Dana Ullman, MPH (Tarcher, 1996).

Deadly Drug Interactions: The People's Pharmacy Guide, Teresa and Joe Graedon (St Martin's Press, 1997).

Death by Deception, Shannon Quinn (R.F. Quinn, 1996).

Detox Yourself, Jane Scrivner (Piatkus, 1998).

Dr Braly's Food Allergy and Nutrition Revolution, James Braly, MD (Keats Publishing, 1992).

Doctor, What's the Alternative?, Hilary Jones (Hodder & Stoughton, 1998).

Earl Mindell's Supplement Bible, Earl Mindell (Simon & Schuster, 1998).

Eat Right for Your Type, Peter J. D'Adamo (G.P. Putnam & Sons, 1997).

Encyclopedia of Natural Medicine, Michael Murray, MD, and Joseph Pizzorno, MD (Prima, 1990).

Everybody's Guide to Homeopathic Medicines, Stephen Cummings MD, (Tarcher, 1984).

Everyone's Guide to Cancer Therapy, Mallin Dollinger, MD, Ernest H. Rosenbaum, MD, and Greg Cable (Andrews McMell Publishing, 1997).

Feet First: A Guide to Reflexology, Laura Norman (Fireside, 1988).

The Five Elements of Self Healing, Katherine Ketcham (Harmony Books).

Food for Life, Oliver Gillie (Hodder & Stoughton, 1998).

Foods that Fight Pain, Neal Barnard (Harmony Books).
Garlic: The Miracle Nutrient, Earl Mindell (Keats Publishing, 1994).
A Grief Remembered, C.S. Lewis (Faber, 1966).
HEA Guide to Complementary Medicine and Therapies, Anne Woodham (Health Education Authority, 1994).
Healing Visualisations, Gerald Epstein, MD (Bantam, 1997).
Healing Yourself with Light, LaUna Huffines (H.J. Kramer, 1994).
The Heart's Code: Tapping the Wisdom and Power of our Heart Energy, Paul Pearsall (Broadway Books, 1998).
Herbal Defense: Positioning Yourself to Triumph over Illness and Aging, Robyn Landis and Karta Purkh Singh Khalsa (Warner, 1997).
Herbal Medicine, Dr Rudolph Weiss (Beaconsfield, 1988).
The Homocysteine Revolution, Kilmer McCulley (Keats Publishing).
I'm Too Busy to be Stressed, Dr Hilary Jones (Hodder & Stoughton, 1997).
In Search of Woman's Passionate Soul, Caitlin Matthews (Element, 1997).
Kava: The Pacific Drug, Vincent Lebot, Mark Merlin and Lamont Lindstrom (Yale University Press, 1992).
The Little Book of Hugs, Cathleen Keating (Running Press, 1998).
The Little Prince, Antoine de Saint-Exupéry (Wordsworth Editions, 1995).
Love and Survival: The Scientific Basis for the Healing Power of Intimacy, Dean Ornish (HarperCollins, 1998).
Meditating to Achieve a Healthy Body Weight, Laurence LeShan, Ph.D. (Doubleday, 1994).
The Menopause Manager, Mary Ann Mayo and Joseph L Mayo, MD (Fleming H. Revell, 1998).
The Modern Book of Stretching: Strength and Flexibility at Any Age, Anne Kent Rush (Dell Publishing, 1997).
Nature's Cures, Michael Castleman (Bantam, 1997).
Nutritional Influences on Illness, Melvyn R. Werbach, MD (Keats Publishing, 1991).
Perfect Health, Deepak Chopra (Bantam, 1990).
The Pocket Guide to Naturopathic Medicine, Judith Boyce, ND, LAc (The Crossing Press, 1996).
Power Eating: Build Muscle, Gain Energy, Lose Fat, Susan M. Kleiner and Maggie Greenwood-Robinson (Human Kinetics, 1998).
The Power of Positive Thinking, Norman Vincent Peale, (Mandarin, 1990).
Prayer is Good Medicine, Larry Dossey (Harper San Francisco, 1997).
The Rainbow Journey, Dr Brenda Davies (Hodder & Stoughton, 1998).
Rituals of Healing: Using Imagery for Health and Wellness, Dossey Achterberg (Bantam, 1994).
Savoring the Day, Judith Bean Hurley (Morrow, 1997).

The Scientific Validation of Herbal Medicine, Daniel Mowry (Keats Publishing, 1991).

Seven Pillars of Health, Jay Solomon (Prima, 1997).

Skin Deep: A Mind/Body Program for Healthy Skin, Ted Grossbart and Carl Sherman (Heath Press, 1992).

Spirit Child, Isabel Kirton (Findhorn, 1998).

The Spirited Walker, Carolyn Scott Kortge (Harper San Francisco, 1998).

Subtle Aromatherapy, Patricia Davis (Daniel, 1991).

Successful Aging, John W. Rowe MD and Robert L Kahn, Ph.D. (Pantheon, 1998).

Thin for Life Daybook, Anne M. Fletcher, RD (Houghton Mifflin, 1998).

The Tibetan Book of Living and Dying, Sogyal Rinpoche (Rider, 1998).

Total Recall: How to Boost Your Memory Power, Joan Menninger, Ph.D. (University of North Carolina, 1998).

Use Your Head, Tony Buzan (BBC Books, 1995).

A Woman's Book of Life, Joan Borysenko, Ph.D. (Riverhead Books, 1996).

Women's Bodies, Women's Wisdom, Dr Christiane Northrup (Piatkus, 1995).

Younger at Last, Steven Lamm (Simon & Schuster, 1998).

Index